AQUATICS ACTIVITIES HANDBOOK

The Jones and Bartlett Series in Health Sciences

Aquatics: The Complete Reference Guide for Aquatic Fitness Professionals
Sova

Aquatics Activities Handbook
Sova

Basic Law for the Allied Health Professions
Cowdrey

Basic Nutrition: Self-Instructional Modules, Second Edition
Stanfield

Biological Bases of Human Aging and Disease
Kart/Metress/Metress

The Biology of Aids, Third Edition
Fan/Conner/Villarreal

The Birth Control Book
Belcastro

Children's Nutrition
Lifshitz

Complete Guide to Step Aerobics
Brown

Contemporary Health Issues
Banister/Allen/Fadl/Bhakthan/Howard

Drugs and Society, Third Edition
Witters/Venturelli/Hanson

Essential Medical Terminology
Stanfield

First Aid and CPR
National Safety Council

First Aid and Emergency Care Workbook
Thygerson

Fitness and Health: Life-Style Strategies
Thygerson

Golf: Your Turn for Success
Fisher/Geertsen

Health and Wellness, Fourth Edition
Edin/Golanty

Healthy People 2000
U.S. Department of Health and Human Services

Health People 2000—Summary Report
U.S. Department of Health and Human Services

Human Anatomy and Physiology Coloring Workbook and Study Guide
Anderson

Interviewing and Helping Skills for Health Professionals
Cormier/Cormier/Weisser

Introduction to Human Disease, Second Edition
Crowley

Introduction to Human Immunology
Huffer/Kanapa/Stevenson

Introduction to the Health Professions
Stanfield

Medical Terminology (with Self-Instructional Modules)
Stanfield/Hui

The Nation's Health, Third Edition
Lee/Estes

Personal Health Choices
Smith/Smith

Principles and Issues in Nutrition
Hui

Sexuality Today
Nass/Fisher

Teaching Elementary Health Science, Third Edition
Bender/Sorochan

Weight Management the Fitness Way
Dusek

Weight Training for Strength and Fitness
Silvester

Writing a Successful Grant Application
Reif-Lehrer

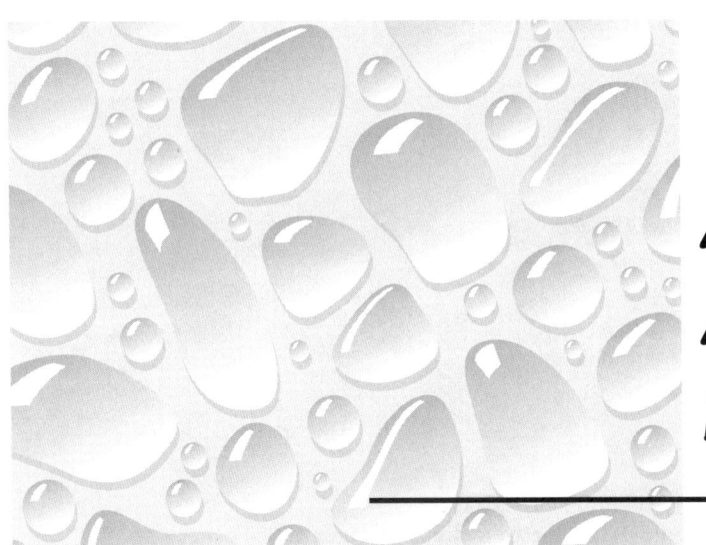

AQUATICS ACTIVITIES HANDBOOK

Ruth Sova, M.S.
Aquatic Exercise Association

Jones and Bartlett Publishers
Boston   London

Editorial, Sales, and Customer Service Offices
Jones and Bartlett Publishers
One Exeter Plaza
Boston, MA 02116

Jones and Bartlett Publishers International
P.O. Box 1498
London W6 7RS
England

Copyright © 1993 by Jones and Bartlett Publishers, Inc.
All rights reserved. No part of the material protected by this copyright notice may be reproduced or utilized in any form, electronic or mechanical, including photocopying, recording, or by any information storage and retrieval system, without written permission from the copyright owner.

Library of Congress Cataloging-in-Publication Data
Sova, Ruth.
    Aquatics activities handbook / Ruth Sova.
      p.   cm.
    Includes bibliographical reference and index.
    ISBN 0-86720-280-7
    1. Aquatic exercises.   I. Title.
GV838.53.E94S67   1992
613.7'16--dc20   91–16578
                                                                                                                                           CIP

Copyeditor: Alyce Dubec
Design and Production: Karen Mason
Cover Design: Melinda Grosser for *Silk*
Prepress: The Courier Connection
Printing and Binding: Courier Westford

Photo credits:

Kurt J. Sova, photographer

Companies: Aquatic Fitness Products, Aquatoner, Danmar Products, D. K. Douglas Co., HydroFit, Hydro-Tone, J & B Foam Fabricators, Omega Corporation, Speedo Activewear, Sprint Rothhammer, and SuitMate

The author does not necessarily endorse any of the products or associations discussed in this book.

Printed in the United States of America
97 96 95 94 93   10 9 8 7 6 5 4 3 2 1

CONTENTS

Forewords ix
Preface xi

CHAPTER ONE / Aquatic Exercise 1

Overview 1
Overall Fitness 2
    Hypokinetic Disease 2
    Mind and Body 2
Physical Fitness 3
    Major Components of Physical Fitness 3
    Minor Components of Physical Fitness 5
    Principles of Exercise 5
KEY WORDS 7
SUMMARY 7

CHAPTER TWO / Types of Aquatic Exercise 8

Format for Cardiorespiratory-Conditioning Classes 8
    Warm-Up 8
    The Cardiorespiratory Workout 10
    Cooldown 11
    Toning 11
    Flexibility 12
Types of Aquatic Exercise Programs 12
    Water Walking 12
    Shallow-Water Jogging 14
    Water Aerobics 17
    Water Toning 18
    Strength Training 20
    Flexibility Training 22
    Aqua-Power Aerobics 24
    Sport-Specific and Sports-Conditioning Workouts 26
    Bench or Step Aerobics 28
    Interval Training 30
    Deep-Water Exercise 31
    Circuit Training 33
    Plyometric Training 35
    Relaxation Techniques 36
Choosing an Aquatic Fitness Program 37
KEY WORDS 38
SUMMARY 38

CHAPTER THREE / Nutrition and Weight Control 40

Nutrition 40
    Water 40
    Guidelines for Good Nutrition 41
Weight Control 42
    Fads and Fallacies 42
    Approaches to Weight Loss 43
Set-Point Theory 45
KEY WORDS 45
SUMMARY 45

CHAPTER FOUR / Aqua Physics 46

General Information 46
    Water Resistance 46
    Water Buoyancy and Cushioning 48
KEY WORDS 48
SUMMARY 49

CHAPTER FIVE / Workout Intensity 50

Using Heartrate to Measure Intensity 50
    Terms and Definitions 50
    Using Heartrates 52
    Heartrate, Oxygen, and Caloric Consumption 53
    Aquatic Heartrate 54

Comparison of Land and Water Exercise Intensities 57
Alternate Intensity Evaluation Methods 58
    Rate of Perceived Exertion 58
    Respiration Rate 59
    "Talk Test" 59
KEY WORDS 60
SUMMARY 61

CHAPTER SIX/ Pool Environment 62

Pool Conditions 62
    Pool Bottom 62
    Water Temperature 63
    Water Depth 63
    Sun Exposure 64
KEY WORDS 64
SUMMARY 64

CHAPTER SEVEN/ Special Populations 65

Basic Precautions 65
    Health History and Physician's Approval 65
    Overexertion 66
Special Populations 66
    Older Adults 66
    Obese Individuals 68
    Prenatal 69
    Arthritic Individuals 69
    Individuals with Low-Back Pain 70
    Individuals with Knee Problems and Chondromalacia Patella 71
    Children 71
KEY WORDS 72
SUMMARY 72

CHAPTER EIGHT/ Equipment 73

Equipment Information 73
    Equipment Principles 73
    Precautions and Contraindications 75
    Population Contraindications 76

Equipment Types 76
    Weights 76
    Jugs 76
    Towels 77
    Pull Buoys 77
    Water Wings 77
    Kickboards 78
    Margarine Lids and Frozen Dinner Plates 78
    Balloons, Balls, and Beach Balls 78
    Deep-Water Vests and Belts 78
    SpaBells 79
    Hydro-Fit 79
    Aerobic Workbench 79
    SPRI Tubing, Bands, and Belts 80
    Hand Paddles 80
    Dynabands 80
    Styrofoam Barbells 81
    Styrofoam Discs 81
    Aqua Gloves 81
    B-Wise Swim Fitness Bar 82
    Hydro-Tone 82
    Aquatoner 82
Aquatic Aids 83
    Aquarius Water Workout Station 83
    Aquarius Rehabilitation Tank 83
    Relaxation Tanks 83
    Shoes 83
    Exercise Clothing 84
Music 85
    Sources 85
    Mediums 85
    Tempo 85
    Styles 86
    Copyright 86
KEY WORDS 86
SUMMARY 86

CHAPTER NINE/ Choreography 87

Muscle Balance 87
A Catalog of Movements 88
    Starting Positions 88
    Arm Movements 88
    Individual Moves 89
    Successful Combinations 132

KEY WORDS 135
SUMMARY 135

CHAPTER TEN/ Muscle Groups 136

Alignment and Muscle Balance 136
Movements for Major Muscle Groups 137
KEY WORDS 141
SUMMARY 141

CHAPTER ELEVEN/ Workouts 142

Sample Class Programs 142
    Strength Training 142
    Water Walking 143
    Aerobics 145
    Toning 146
    Flexibility 147
    Aqua Circuit Training 148
    Sport Specific 149
    Bench Aerobics 150
    Deep Water: Using Flotation Vests or Belts 151

CHAPTER TWELVE/ General Program Safety 154

Programming Information 154
    Certification Standards 154
    Contraindicated Exercises 154
    Preventive Measures 156
    General Problems 157
KEY WORDS 161
SUMMARY 162

CHAPTER THIRTEEN/ Resources 163

Aqua Wear 164
Choreography 164
Consultants 165
Equipment 165
Filters, Chemicals, and Air Products 175
Health Products 177
Music Sources 177
Organizations 178
Pool Products 180
Publications 181
    Books 181
    Catalogs 184
    Magazines and Newsletters 185
Shoes 186
Signs and Charts 187
Skin and Hair Care Products 187
Training and Workshops 188
Video- and Audiocassettes 189

Glossary 191

References 199

Index 203

FOREWORDS

By Kathie Davis

— Executive Director, IDEA: The Association for Fitness Professionals

Aqua exercise has become a very popular form of exercise over the past decade. What was once a seasonal response to summertime heat has become the year-round answer to consumer needs. Since it is possible to reap the rewards of a stimulating workout while remaining cool, many diverse populations have taken to the pool. Aqua classes are not only good for the pregnant, overweight, injured, and senior; they are great for anyone seeking variety in his or her exercise program.

A 1989 survey of aqua professionals across the nation by IDEA: The Association for Fitness Professionals showed that 92% of aqua leaders reported "unparalleled growth" in their classes and a shift toward younger people jumping into pool classes. Classes are now being offered for all age levels and abilities—from slow muscle movements for the arthritic to fast-paced, high-energy water circuits.

Aqua exercise, as a part of the fitness movement is here to stay. By reading this book, you are sure to gain a lot of valuable and useful information.

By Dr. Joanna Midtlying

— Professor Emerita, Ball State University

Ruth Sova's *Aquatics Activities Handbook* is a superb, comprehensive, and up-to-date presentation about aquatic exercise. It is the essential reference for the aquatic fitness student.

The author treats the reader to an overview of similarities and differences between land and water exercise and general fitness concepts. Sova masterfully states and restates basic aquatic and fitness facts, and systematically expands and applies relevant facts to each style of in-water exercise. Findings from research investigations of aquatic exercise are interwoven, in nontechnical terms, into the body of the text to further stimulate the intellectual pursuit of fitness-related information.

The clarity of Sova's presentation in lay terms of all major muscle groups and their functions, makes for easy reading and a more knowledgeable fitness consumer. Examples of water exercises for each muscle group are complemented by essential information about body alignment and muscle balance, and concepts of nutrition and weight control.

The subject matter is extensive. Each style of water exercise, ranging from water walking and jogging to aquatic power aerobics and deep water exercise, receives in-depth treatment by the author. College and community water exercise students are introduced to strength and flexibility training, body toning, and conditioning for sport-specific activities, and other styles that comprise the full spectrum of aquatic exercise.

Sample water workouts and guidelines for water workout intensities provide significant help to the fledgling and advanced aquatic fitness student or instructor. Guidelines for sources, selection, and use of aqua equipment and music, and identification of pool conditions and water depths for safe, productive water exercise, further aid in program planning for water exercise.

Special populations will discover that one or more styles of water exercise may effectively accommodate individual fitness needs. All populations are encouraged to alternate water exercise styles or to combine styles to meet and sustain specific fitness goals.

Each chapter of this book contains essential information. Key concepts are summarized at the end of each chapter. The text is functional and the reading is compelling. This handbook is a treasure for all aquatic consumers who wish to make informed choices about personal fitness through aquatic exercise.

By Dr. Alison Osinski

—Aquatic Consulting Services

Ruth has been involved in the development of structured water fitness programs from the early days of the industry. Her pioneering role in making the public aware of the benefits of water exercise is recognized by leaders in the field and by aquatic fitness devotees throughout the world. By developing this text, Ruth has provided a needed resource for students wanting to know more about the benefits of aquatic exercise.

In this book, Ruth provides general fitness information, then goes on to explain how exercising in the water differs from land-based exercise programs. For the student, she discusses class organizational and safety guidelines, and provides sample class outlines. A variety of both shallow- and deep-water fitness activities are introduced. Modifications for special populations, contraindicated exercises, information on eliminating hazards associated with participation in water fitness programs, and equipment available to modify exercises or add variety to exercise routines is discussed. Specific benefits of the various exercises including their affect on muscle groups are included. The physical, social, and psychological benefits of participating in water exercise are cited.

After reading this informative handbook, the reader is bound to join the ever-expanding ranks of water fitness enthusiasts working out and getting healthy in pools all across the country.

PREFACE

Aquatic exercise is the most exciting, effective, and exhilarating way to work out. I am thrilled that you are involved in my favorite way to fitness.

The aquatics industry is growing and changing quickly, and the rapid growth challenges us to remain informed. A knowledge base like the one presented in this book will help us to move safely and effectively toward positive results.

Aquatic exercisers must have a wide spectrum of knowledge to work out safely in the pool. This book has been written to be a thorough resource to answer this need.

We can learn from problems encountered by other fitness industries. Overuse injuries have occurred in both joggers and aerobic dancers. What can we do to protect ourselves? Enthusiasts in any segment of the fitness industry have always faced particular problems. What can we do to protect ourselves from chronic exposure to heat and humidity? What about our unique environment? What is the safest program for someone with a bad back? What exercises can obese children perform?

Since it is difficult to be an authority on every topic, I found specialists to review each section. I want to thank this diverse group. Dani Riposo assisted with the fitness concepts and is widely quoted in the nutrition section.

Alison Osinski reviewed the safety issues, and Bud Sova and Jack Wasserman assisted with the biomechanics of aqua physics. Vicki Chossek, Peg Windhorst, and Joanna Midtlying, reviewed material content, and Karl Knopf, June Lindle, Julie See, and Angie Nelson gave editorial advice. Mr. Jun Konno also reviewed content with an international perspective. Varied aquatic equipment manufacturers provided us with photographs. The Aquatic Exercise Association, Vicki Chossek, Dani Riposo, and Nicole Sova provided technical assistance.

In addition to the technical support, I would like to thank the following for their valuable assistance: Karen Mason, Graphic Design and Production Services, for assistance with the book's production; Nicole Sova for transcribing the manuscript; Kurt Sova for the photography; Bud Sova for financial support; the Aquatic Exercise Association staff, Vicki Chossek, and the Jalkanen family for their support; Alyce Dubec for help editing the manuscript; and Joe Burns, editor and vice president of Jones and Bartlett Publishers, for assistance with this book.

Because of all their help, this book is a comprehensive reference tool for each of us to use as we exercise, buy new equipment, or have any specific questions about aquatics.

AQUATICS ACTIVITIES HANDBOOK

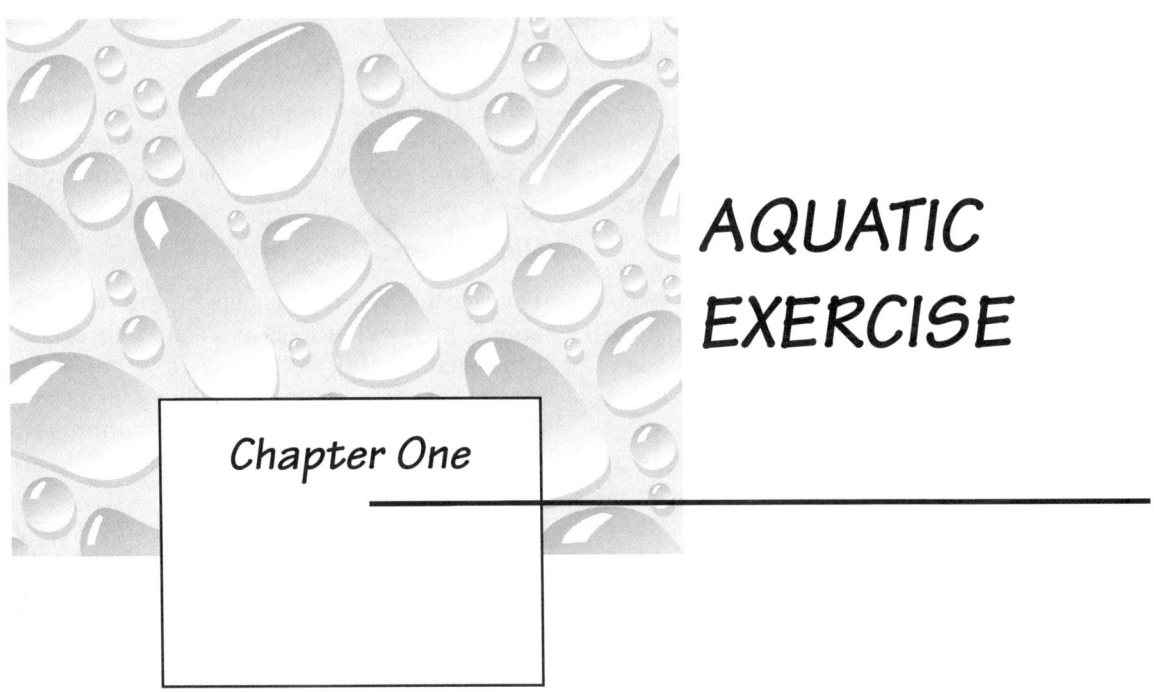

AQUATIC EXERCISE

Chapter One

OVERVIEW

The concept of aquatic exercise is an idea whose time has certainly come. The jogging craze of the late sixties and seventies, the aerobic dance frenzy of the seventies and early eighties, and the pursuit of total fitness through cross training that brings us into the nineties have matured into an intelligent pursuit of health and fitness. Exercise is the fountain of youth, and everyone wants to drink from it.

Like almost everything in life, jogging, aerobic dance, and cross training have proven to be less than perfect. As more people have joined in the bouncing, jumping, jogging, and pumping, reports of minor injuries have become more frequent. The impact experienced during these sports has created countless exercise dropouts. As Baby Boomers move into middle age, they are demanding a fitness program that will enable them to continue exercising for the rest of their lives, despite joint problems and reduced flexibility they may eventually experience.

Thus, aquatic exercise has become a major exercise alternative in our fitness-conscious society. It is a perfect mix of water and workout. Since the movements are performed in chest-deep water, these programs appeal to the swimmer and nonswimmer alike.

The buoyant support of the water effectively cancels approximately 90% of the weight of a person submerged to the neck. This dramatically decreases compression stress on weight-bearing joints, bones, and muscles. Since it is thought that most movements done in the water involve only concentric muscular contractions, muscle soreness is minimal. The possibility of muscle, bone, and joint injuries is almost completely eliminated. Individuals concerned with excess pressure on their ankles, knees, hips, and back can now increase their strength, flexibility, and cardiovascular endurance with safe aerobics: aquatic exercise.

Buoyancy makes the program ideal for many people who have painful joints or weak leg muscles and cannot participate in alternative exercise programs. Special populations—such as those with arthritis or other joint problems, obesity, and back problems, as well as pre- and postnatal women, sedentary individuals, and those recovering from injury or surgery—are prime candidates for aquatic exercise.

With the body submerged in water, blood circulation automatically increases to some extent. Water pressure on the body also helps to promote deeper ventilation (breathing) of the lungs. With a well-planned activity, both circulation and ventilation increase even more.

Flexibility work is increased and performed more easily in water because of the lessened gravitational pull. It is much easier to do leg straddles or side stretches in water. Many individuals can do leg bobbing or jogging in water who could never do so on land. The resistant properties of water also make it a perfect exercise medium for the well-conditioned individual who is looking to accomplish more in less time. The resistance of the water makes taking a simple walk a challenging workout, testing muscular endurance and strength and cardiorespiratory fitness. Vigorous water exercise can make a major contribution to individual flexibility, muscular strength and endurance, body composition, and cardiorespiratory fitness.

There are many kinds of aquatic exercise programs to choose from. This book describes many and offers sample programs. Variations can be made by combining or alternating programs to suit an individual's specific needs.

In this book, the term **aquatic aerobics** or water exercise will refer to vertical exercise in the water with the participant submerged to chest or shoulder depth. Most aquatic exercisers stand in chest-deep water or work out vertically in the deep end (diving well) of the pool while using buoyant devices.

OVERALL FITNESS

Overall **fitness** may be defined as a combination of physical, mental, and emotional well-being. It implies a positive outlook on life with enough strength and stamina to perform daily tasks with energy to spare for leisure pursuits.

Hypokinetic Disease

For reasons we are just beginning to understand, physical fitness is related to overall fitness and total well-being in a variety of ways. Unfortunately, our society is largely sedentary, which conflicts with the inherent purpose of our bodies, namely, that they are designed for movement.

Movement helps to keep us healthy. Without movement, our bodies begin to deteriorate. Sometimes that deterioration is mistakenly chalked up to age instead of disuse. The deterioration that results from inactivity has caused a whole new syndrome of disease in our society, diseases that are hypokinetic. **Hypokinetic disease** is a condition caused by or aggravated by inactivity. (*Hypo* means "not enough." *Kinetic* means "movement.")

Common examples of hypokinetic disease are heart disease, back pain, obesity, ulcers, and blood vessel diseases, such as atherosclerosis. Hypokinetic mental disorders include insomnia, lethargy, depression, and anxiety. Hypokinetic diseases also include metabolic disorders, such as adult-onset diabetes and hypoglycemia; bone and joint disorders, such as osteoporosis and osteoarthritis; and the stress disorders of constipation and mood swings.

The physically fit person, besides having a reduced risk of hypokinetic disease, is more likely than his or her unfit neighbor to feel good, look good, and enjoy life. He or she can work and play more effectively; is more creative; and is less likely to suffer from anxiety, depression, and psychosomatic illness.

Mind and Body

The mind-body connection in overall fitness works in reverse also. That is, the emotionally stable person with a positive attitude will be less likely to suffer from physical diseases. Dr. Thomas McKeown, a prominent English physician, said, "It is now evident that the health of man is determined predominantly, not by medical intervention, but, by his behavior, his food, and the nature of the world in which he finds himself" (Conrad, 1979, pp. 30–31). Practicing muscular and mental relaxation techniques, visualization, self-responsibility, cognitive concepts, imagery, and positive affirmations will all help in gaining overall fitness.

Mental Attitude

The mental attitude of the regular exerciser is improved not only by a psychological phenomenon but also by a physical one. While the exact effects of powerful hormones called *endorphins* are not clear yet, they seem to be related to pain, emotions, the immune system, exercise, and the reproduction system. The feelings of well-being that come with vigorous exercise have been traced to endorphins. They also may have an effect on mental problems. For instance, patients experiencing depression often have low levels of endorphins.

Mental Sharpness

The mind-body connection also correlates with mental sharpness, alertness, and sometimes intelligence. A study at Purdue University found that after working out three times a week for six months, one group was not only 20% fitter but scored 70% higher in a test of complex decision making (Welch, 1989).

Overall fitness should be a goal for all people. This book will cover aspects of the physical portion of fitness. It is a guide to achieving physical fitness through water exercise.

PHYSICAL FITNESS

Major Components of Physical Fitness

There are five major aspects or components of physical fitness:

1. Cardiorespiratory endurance
2. Muscular strength
3. Muscular endurance
4. Flexibility
5. Body composition

When working toward physical fitness, many people include only one or two of these five aspects in their workout plan. All five components are interrelated yet separate enough that a person can be fit in one aspect but not in the others. A truly fit person will include all aspects of physical fitness in his or her workout and will be fit in each one.

Cardiorespiratory Endurance

Cardiorespiratory endurance, or fitness, involves the ability of the heart and blood to supply oxygen from the respiratory system to the cells of the body during sustained exercise. To increase this component of physical fitness, aerobic exercise must take place.

In order to be aerobic, the exercise must be continuous, involve the body's large muscles (the quadriceps, hamstrings, and gluteals in the legs and buttocks), and last for at least 20 minutes. An individual should work at a perceived exertion level of "somewhat hard" to "hard" and/or elevate the heartrate into the working zone. (See Chapter 5 for more information on heartrates and perceived exertion.) To improve cardiorespiratory endurance, an aerobic workout should be repeated at least three times a week. Leaping, kicking, jogging, and walking in the water will increase the workload on the cardiorespiratory system so that endurance benefits can be obtained.

Exercise is usually associated with its cardiac benefits. A recent study has shown that lack of exercise may be the single risk factor most clearly associated with future coronary disease (Riposo, 1985). Regular cardiorespiratory exercise has been shown to improve, to varying degrees, almost all of the commonly accepted risk factors that can be changed: lack of exercise, elevated cholesterol, elevated triglycerides, lowered high-density lipoproteins

DIAGRAM 1-1 Primary Risk Factors for Coronary Heart Disease

1. Hypertension (high blood pressure)
2. High blood lipids and cholesterol levels
3. Cigarette smoking
4. Obesity (overweight)
5. Family history of heart disease (close blood relative died suddenly before age of 55 or family history of high cholesterol, Marfan's syndrome, or enlarged heart)
6. Atherosclerosis (hardening of the arteries)
7. Diabetes
8. Sedentary lifestyle (lack of physical activity)
9. Stress
10. Age (women, risk greater after menopause; men, risk increases proportionately with age)
11. Sex (men more at risk than women until age of 50–60, then both are equal)

(HDL), hypertension, smoking, obesity, stress, and diabetes (glucose metabolism). Myocardial efficiency is also markedly improved, as evidenced by decreased resting pulse and decreased heartrate at the same workload during exercise. This means that after doing a specific workout program for about eight weeks, the body adapts, making it easier for an individual to do that same program. The effect of

DIAGRAM 1-2 Secondary Risk Factors for Coronary Heart Disease

1. Asthma or other allergies
2. Arthritis or other joint problems
3. Anxiety
4. Use of medications, alcohol, drugs
5. Current activity
6. Recent surgery
7. Previous difficulty with exercise (chest discomfort, dizziness, extreme breathlessness)
8. Pregnancy status

exercise on the heart alone makes it a valuable prescription for both physicians and patients (see Diagrams 1–1 and 1–2).

Muscular Strength

Muscular strength is the ability of a muscle to exert great force in a single effort. It is usually attained by lifting weights. To achieve muscular strength, each muscle group works submaximally (about 60% of the maximum ability) for about eight repetitions. After all muscle groups have been worked, the entire workout is repeated once or twice.

Water offers a natural resistance or weight. Paddles, water-tight weights, webbed gloves, and special weight-training equipment can all be used to intensify the force of the workload in the water.

Muscular Endurance

Muscular endurance is the ability of a muscle to repeat a contraction with a moderate workload over a long period of time. Ten to thirty repetitions of any movement build up endurance rather than strength. A workout involving 10 repetitions working each muscle group can be done three times.

Muscular endurance and toning can be achieved sooner with the water's resistance than with endurance workouts on land. Moreover, there is minimal risk of injury due to the cushioning effect of the water.

Flexibility

Flexibility is the ability of limbs to move the joints through a normal range of motion. Flexibility workouts include static stretching of each major muscle group for 30 to 60 seconds. Only muscles should be stretched, not tendons or ligaments.

Due to the lessened effect of gravity in the water, the joints can be moved through a wider range of motion without excess pressure, and long-term flexibility can be achieved.

Body Composition

Body composition is the proportion of fat body mass to lean body mass. It should not be confused with being overweight or underweight, since it does not deal with weight. In fact, eliminating fat body mass and increasing lean body mass may increase the total body weight. A desirable amount of body fat for women is 18% to 20%. The well-conditioned female athlete normally has 16% to 18% body fat. Men should have 10% to 12% body fat. Male athletes usually achieve 7% to 8% body fat.

The average person burns 450 to 700 calories while performing one hour of aerobic exercise. In the water, 77% of the calories burned come from fat stores, thus reducing the fat mass in a body. Muscle tissue (lean body mass) growth is stimulated while moving through the water resistance.

Minor Components of Physical Fitness

Other components of fitness listed by sports physiologists are called minor components or skill-related components. Skill-related fitness is related to performing motor skills, such as playing soccer or walking a tightrope. The skill-related components of physical fitness are:

- **Speed**—the ability to perform a movement in a short period of time
- **Power**—the ability to transfer energy into force at a fast rate (a combination of strength and speed in one explosive action)
- **Agility**—the ability to rapidly and accurately change the position of the entire body
- **Reaction time**—the amount of time elapsed between stimulation and reaction to that stimulation
- **Coordination**—the integration of separate motor activities in the smooth, efficient execution of a task
- **Balance**—the maintenance of equilibrium while stationary or moving (static and dynamic balance).

All of the fitness components, both health-related and skill-related aspects, are trainable; that is, they will show improvement when subjected to appropriate activity.

Principles of Exercise

Six basic principles of exercise must be understood in order to create a sound exercise program:

1. Overload
2. Progressive overload
3. Adaptation
4. Specificity
5. Reversibility
6. Variability

Overload

The **overload** principle states that if an increase in demands is made on a muscle or system, that body part will respond by *adapting* to the increase. If adequate rest and good nutrition accompany the overload, there will be an increase in strength or efficiency. Improvement cannot occur unless overload is present. Training occurs by means of the overload principle.

Progressive Overload

Progressive overload is also sometimes called progressive resistance. It is the principle of gradually increasing overload. If the overload or stress is increased too quickly, injury, pain, or exhaustion may result instead of proper training. "No pain, no gain" is a fallacy. Only in competitive athletics, where participants are willing to take enormous risks for the possibility of superior performance, does this slogan have any merit, and even then, it is questionable.

All training of exercise programs should follow the principle of progressive overload. Trying to do too much, too soon paves the way for exhaustion, pain, and possible injury. Programs should begin at low intensity, for a short duration, with minimum frequency, and gradually increase the overload in each category. Training occurs by means of the overload principle.

Adaptation

Adaptation is also called *training*. It is an improvement in the fitness level that results when the body adapts to overload. Place greater work demands on a muscle (including the heart) than it is used to performing, and it will respond by getting stronger. Stretch a muscle longer than it is accustomed to being stretched, and it will become more flexible. Expose muscles to sustained activity for longer than they are accustomed to, and muscular endurance will increase.

The body will adapt to the stresses or overload placed on it so that an increase in overload can be made. By the same token, if the overload is less than normal for a specific component of fitness, there will be a decrease in that particular component. Keeping the overload at a constant level will maintain the current level of fitness.

Specificity

The principle of **specificity** states that only the muscle, body part, or system that is being overloaded will adapt and improve. Thus, a stretching program will not improve cardiorespiratory fitness. Just as overload is specific to each component of fitness, it is also specific to each body part. Those muscle groups being overloaded are the only ones that develop. Weight training for the hamstrings will do nothing for the biceps.

In order to see improvements in all the major components of fitness, the program has to be designed specifically to overload each component. In order to have muscle balance in a workout, the workout must be designed to involve all the muscles equally.

Reversibility

Reversibility means that fitness benefits cannot be stored by the body. Several days without a workout means the training level will start to decline. It is generally thought that it takes 12 weeks to improve the fitness level and only 2 weeks to see it decline.

Variability

Variability is a principle that most people ignore. It states that adaptation or fitness improvements are enhanced by varying the intensity, length, or type of workout. Variability adds to the training effect.

The popular fitness concept of **cross training** uses variability as its foundation. Athletes who have hit fitness plateaus have been able to move to higher levels of fitness through cross training. Rather than do the same fitness activity for every workout, athletes do different types of workouts on different days. Runners can use deep-water running, biking, and water strength training to increase their fitness levels. Swimmers can use cross-country skiing, water walking, and weight lifting. Any change in the type, intensity, or length of the workout will enhance fitness improvements.

Reasons for cross training include:

— an optimal development of all components of physical fitness
— an enhanced motivation toward exercise adherence
— injury prevention due to avoidance of overtraining
— development of balance with opposing muscle groups
— effectiveness in weight-loss programs
— an overall increase in general physical fitness

All training or adaptation works on the principle of stressing the body and letting it recover in a stronger form. Too often, exercisers make the mistake of repeating the same workout, day after day. That can stress the same muscles and joints until an injury occurs.

In designing an exercise program to provide maximum physical and mental health benefits, activities to promote all the major components of fitness should be included. Cardiovascular work should be integral to the program, since cardiovascular fitness is most important for total well-being. Strength and flexibility work enable people to perform their daily tasks with ease, as well as help protect them from back pain. Body composition can be favorably altered by endurance and strength training.

Many of the skill-related fitness components can also be included in a basic exercise program. We know that if a person's goal is to improve in a particular sport, training in the specific fitness components and movement coordinations of that sport are necessary for optimum improvement. Nevertheless, it is easy to incorporate into a series of exercise routines movements to improve speed, agility, reaction time, balance, and coordination with a resultant improvement in overall fitness.

Taking time at the end of each exercise session for conscious voluntary relaxation is important. Slow stretches and guided relaxation add a feeling of mental and physical release that has also been shown to have important health benefits.

KEY WORDS

Aquatic aerobics
Buoyancy
Fitness
Hypokinetic disease
Cardiorespiratory endurance
Muscular strength
Muscular endurance
Flexibility

Body composition
Speed
Power
Agility
Reaction time
Coordination
Balance

Overload
Progressive overload
Adaptation
Specificity
Reversibility
Variability
Cross training

SUMMARY

— The concept of aquatic exercise is an idea whose time has come.
— Exercise is the fountain of youth, and everyone wants to drink from it.
— The buoyant support of the water effectively cancels approximately 90% of the weight of a person submerged to the neck.
— Flexibility work is increased and performed more easily in water because of the lessened gravitational pull.
— There are five major components of physical fitness: cardiorespiratory endurance, muscular strength, muscular endurance, flexibility, and body composition.
— Minor components of physical fitness are: speed, power, agility, reaction time, coordination, and balance.
— Six basic principles of exercise are: overload, progressive overload, adaptation, specificity, reversibility, and variability.
— Minor components of physical fitness are: speed, power, agility, reaction time, coordination, and balance.
— Taking time at the end of each exercise session for conscious voluntary relaxation is important.

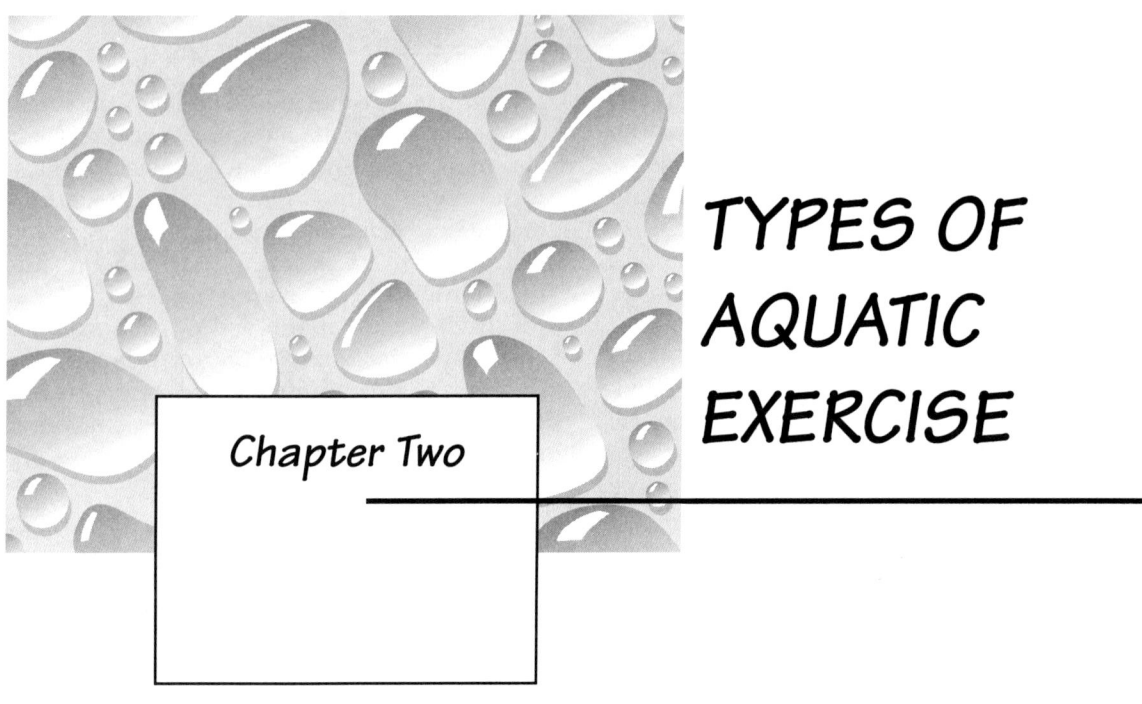

TYPES OF AQUATIC EXERCISE

Chapter Two

The format of aquatic exercise programs varies, depending on their goals. Almost any program or program variation follows either the aerobic or nonaerobic class format. Programs focusing on cardiorespiratory conditioning, such as water aerobics, water walking, deep-water programs, and circuit training, follow the *aerobic* class format. Programs that focus on muscular endurance, strength, or flexibility follow a *nonaerobic* class format.

FORMAT FOR CARDIORESPIRATORY-CONDITIONING CLASSES

Warm-Up

The **warm-up** is a combination of three different class segments that increase body temperature. The warm-up allows the exerciser to safely exercise at a high intesity. Water cardiorespiratory (aerobic) classes usually begin with a warm-up lasting 5 to 10 minutes. Three types of warm-ups needed for program safety include the musculoskeletal warm-up (called the thermal warm-up), the prestretch, and the cardiorespiratory warm-up.

Thermal Warm-Up

The warm-up portion begins with a **thermal warm-up.** The thermal warm-up is aimed at the skeletal muscles on the surface of the body responsible for movement, as well as the bones that support them. It involves gentle movements, done with control, using a small range of motion that is gradually increased. This part of the warm-up is designed to bring increased bloodflow to muscles and soft tissues surrounding joints, to increase internal body temperature, and to release synovial fluid.

During the thermal warm-up, internal body temperature should increase one to two degrees. This is achieved when more oxygen is released to the muscles as the body prepares for a vigorous workout. To understand the importance of raised muscle temperature, think of chemistry lab experiments. Some chemical reactions occur only when heat is applied; others are more effective when a specific temperature is used.

Similarly, the human body's chemical reactions occur best at certain temperatures. The raised muscle temperature is ideal for chemical reactions that occur when exercising vigorously. Raised temperature also makes muscle fibers more pliable, which reduces the likelihood of injury when kicking, jogging, pushing, and pulling during a vigorous workout.

Joints also benefit from the thermal warm-up. A joint is any place where two bones come together. Bones are held to each other by *ligaments.* The entire joint is encased in a thin, silklike film called *synovial membrane.* When movement occurs, the membrane secretes a lubricant called *synovial fluid,* which helps the joint glide rather than grind. The release of synovial fluid is one reason students move better after class than before. Exercise lubricates joints.

The thermal warm-up should last approximately three to five minutes. Major muscle groups should be used the same way they are used during the aerobic portion of the workout. All major muscle groups and joints should be used in isolation exercises and in low- to moderate-intensity exercises. Beginning slowly, using short levers and a reduced range of motion, stimulates the release of synovial fluid that lubricates joints and allows the body to gradually warm up. The later portion of the thermal warm-up can incorporate movements with a fuller range of motion, long levers, and more powerful contractions of each muscle group.

Prestretch

The **prestretch** is the next part of the warm-up. It is designed to prevent injury during a high-intensity workout. Stretching muscles that are tight from everyday living is important. Although any major muscle groups can be stretched at this point, it is important to stretch the gastrocnemius and soleus (calf), iliopsoas (hip flexors), hamstrings (back of the thigh), low back, and pectoral (chest) muscles during this portion of the workout. Stretches are usually held for 5 to 10 seconds during the prestretch. (Specific explanations of stretches are found in Chapter 9.)

The prestretch is designed to lessen the likelihood of injury during an upcoming workout. It is important to keep the body temperature at a comfortable level during stretches. If participants become chilled, muscles will contract, and injury may result if stretching continues. Keeping the upper-body limbs moving during lower-body stretches and vice versa helps to keep the muscles warm and pliable.

Cardiorespiratory Warm-Up

The **cardiorespiratory warm-up** is the last portion of the warm-up. It includes exercises with an increased range of motion and more moderate intensity. The purpose of the cardiorespiratory warm-up is to gradually overload the heart, lungs, and vascular system. It is safest and most efficient to allow those parts to adjust gradually to the increased demands. This is true for all systems in the body.

Vigorous exercise makes the body demand more oxygen. At the same time, skeletal muscles cause a milking action on veins, making blood return to the heart more rapidly. This creates an overload on the heart. The heart responds by beating more beats per minute, more forcefully. A gradual overload of this type is easier on the heart than a sudden, dramatic one.

The lungs operate automatically but are not self-powered. Muscles are responsible for changing the size of the rib cage. The change in the amount of lung space affects the atmospheric pressure inside the lungs. The change in pressure causes the lungs to inflate and deflate. **Respiration,** or breathing, increases.

As the body's need for oxygen increases, the respiration muscles contract and relax more frequently, so that additional breaths are taken per minute. They also contract more forcefully, causing deeper ventilation in the lungs. The result is that the body can process more oxygen and eliminate more waste gases.

Just like the heart, the respiration muscles adapt efficiently to a gradually increased demand for oxygen.

This part of the warm-up further increases oxygen demands on the heart and elevates the core temperature of the body. For example, muscle temperature may increase as much as four degrees Fahrenheit during the entire warm-up portion. The cardiorespiratory warm-up usually lasts three to five minutes.

In order to keep body temperature up during the prestretch segment, some exercisers intersperse moves that warm and stretch a muscle group. (An example of this technique is found in Chapter 11 in the water aerobics, water-walking, and circuit-training sample workouts.)

Some aquatic exercisers feel a warm-up is unnecessary or too time consuming for their workouts. Research has shown that beginning a workout with high-intensity, vigorous exercise abnormally increases arterial blood pressure, which in turn causes heart stress. Other research has shown that warming up before a workout significantly reduces abnormal electrocardiograph readings during the vigorous phase (Cisar and Kravitz, 1989). These findings indicate that a warm-up is important to the safety of participants.

In conclusion, an effective warm-up produces many benefits; namely, it will:

— increase muscle fluidity, which improves contraction efficiency
— increase the force and rate of muscle contraction
— improve muscle elasticity and the sensitivity of the stretch reflex
— increase the flexibility of tendons, which reduces the risk of injury
— improve metabolic reactions in the muscle which promotes more efficient use of carbohydrates and fats
— increase maximal oxygen intake rate and worktime to exhaustion

The Cardiorespiratory Workout

The aerobic portion of the workout is considered the "calorie-burning" portion. The goal of this portion is to improve the cardiorespiratory system. The American College of Sports Medicine (ACSM) has made recommendations for the quantity and quality of training for developing and maintaining cardiorespiratory fitness, body composition and muscular strength, and endurance in the healthy adult (ACSM, 1990a). These guidelines address the following aspects of an aerobic exercise or **cardiorespiratory workout**:

1. *Mode*—the type of exercise necessary
2. *Duration*—the length of each workout
3. *Intensity*—how challenging the workout is for the cardiorespiratory system
4. *Frequency*—how many times a week the workout should be repeated

If a workout does not follow the guidelines for each of these four aspects, it is not considered a cardiorespiratory or aerobic workout.

Mode

The ACSM guidelines (1990a) state that in order to create the overload necessary to achieve cardiorespiratory fitness, the **mode** must be a large-muscle activity that is maintained continuously and is rhythmic in nature. This means that the large muscles in the body, such as gluteals, hamstrings, and quadriceps, must be used continuously during the aerobic portion of the workout. According to these guidelines, a workout using only upper-body movements would not qualify as aerobic. The legs also must be moving continuously for conditioning to occur.

Duration

The ACSM guidelines (1990a) regarding **duration** say that each workout should have a continuous aerobic portion, lasting between

20 and 60 minutes. Most exercise leaders consider 20 to 30 minutes the average for the aerobic portion of their classes. Classes with a longer aerobic portion usually are of lower intensity and best for students with poor fitness levels who need to improve their body composition. Long-duration, low-intensity classes are shown to be excellent "fat burners." Longer duration, however, can also lead to overuse injuries. Students should gradually build up to longer aerobic sessions. The principle of progressive overload (discussed in Chapter 1) should be followed.

Intensity

The ACSM guidelines (1990a) regarding **intensity** state that the exercise intensity of the aerobic portion should be in a range of 50% to 85% of maximum oxygen uptake or maximum heartrate reserve, or 60% to 90% of maximum heartrate. (More in-depth information regarding heartrate and workout intensity can be found in Chapter 5.) Beginning students should work at low intensity for a short duration until adaptation begins. Only people in excellent physical condition should work at an intensity in the upper portion of the range.

Frequency

The ACSM guidelines (1990a) regarding **frequency** state that a workout should occur three to five times a week in order to achieve results. Working out fewer than three times a week does not improve cardiorespiratory fitness levels. Working out more frequently than five times a week prevents the body from rebuilding and causes overuse injuries.

Cooldown

The cooldown usually lasts about five minutes and uses large, lower-intensity, rhythmic movements. The purpose of the cooldown is to aid the return of blood to the heart at a low enough intensity to allow the heart to move toward a resting level. The cooldown prevents the pooling of blood in the extremities, reduces muscle soreness, and assists in the elimination of metabolic wastes.

The cooldown in a pool is especially important because of water pressure. If a participant leaves the pool while still in the aerobic portion of the workout, dizziness can occur. When exercising at a challenging intensity, blood vessels dilate to allow for increased bloodflow during the workout. In water exercise classes, it is thought that blood vessels are pressurized by the water and do not dilate to the extent they would during land-based exercise. When exiting the pool, the lessened effect of air pressure compared to water pressure allows the blood vessels to dilate further, causing a drop in blood pressure. This can cause the participant to feel light-headed or dizzy or to actually pass out.

Toning

If **toning** or calisthenics is included in the workout it usually follows the cooldown. Trunk, upper-body, and lower-body exercises are done at pool edge or with buoyant devices that hold the participant off the bottom of the pool. (Review Chapters 9 and 11 for toning exercise ideas.)

Muscular Endurance

Some exercisers work on muscular *endurance* with many repetitions, and others work on muscular *strength* with fewer than 15 repetitions. If muscular strength is desired, students should be able to fatigue the muscle in fewer than 15 repetitions. The same exercises can be used for endurance and strength, but the level of overload and, therefore, difficulty has to increase. Exercise difficulty can be increased by using a larger range of motion, slower repetitions, more difficult exercise modifications, or aquatic exercise equipment. Students should use force in each move to challenge the muscles and keep the body at a comfortable temperature.

Muscular Strength

If strength training is used during the toning portion, it should follow the ACSM guidelines (1990a) for resistance training. Strength training of moderate intensity, sufficient to develop and maintain fat-free weight, should be an integral part of an adult fitness program. The recommended minimum is one set of 8 to 12 repetitions of 8 to 10 exercises that condition the major muscle groups at least 2 days per week.

The toning portion of the workout can last 5 to 15 minutes. Upper-body toning often is incorporated into the cooldown to conserve time. Because of the buoyancy of water, participants must be strongly encouraged to put forth the necessary effort to make water exercise effective. It is easy to cheat during water exercise because of the buoyancy and the relaxing effects of the water.

Occasionally, an instructor or student will decide to do the toning portion of a class following the thermal warm-up. There is some controversy among leaders in the field regarding the sequence of exercise classes in terms of whether the cardiorespiratory segment should precede or follow the toning work. Since no definitive research has been completed on this issue, each instructor must make a professional judgment based on the type of class he or she has and what is preferred.

Flexibility

The water aerobics class should always end with a poststretch or **flexibility** section that lasts about five minutes. If the water is warm (over 86 degrees), this section can be extended. All the major muscles used or toned during the workout should be stretched during this time. (Sample flexibility exercises are included in Chapters 9 and 11.)

The purpose of the poststretch is to provide long-term flexibility, help prevent muscle soreness, further lower the oxygen demands on the heart, and reestablish the body's equilibrium. Each muscle should be stretched beyond its normal resting length to the point of tension but not pain. If participants become chilled during the poststretch, they can get out of the pool and stretch on the deck.

Flexibility is important. Exercise leaders have a responsibility to make sure students leave class in better shape than when they arrive. Stretching at every class is one way to make sure of that.

Some aquatic exercise programs combine the toning and flexibility portions of the class to keep the student's body temperature comfortable and to be sure that the muscles being stretched are warm and pliable. For example, after doing toning exercises for the hamstrings, participants would stretch the hamstrings. Following toning of the abductors, students would stretch the abductors. (The sample deep-water workout in Chapter 11 has an example of mixing toning and flexibility.)

TYPES OF AQUATIC EXERCISE PROGRAMS

Water Walking

Definition

Water walking is simply striding in waist- to chest-deep water at a pace fast enough to create the overload necessary for cardiorespiratory benefits. The type of stride used should vary to ensure use of all the major muscle groups in the lower body. Most frequently, the foot action involves a heel strike, followed by rolling onto the ball of the foot and finishing with a strong push off the toes. Stride length will vary according to the participant's height, leg length, strength, and stride, as well as the water depth. The type of walking—for instance

DIAGRAM 2-1 Water Walking

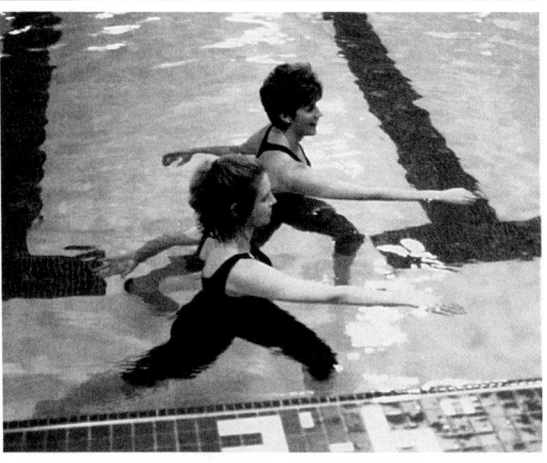

forward, sideways, or backward, with toes pointed in or out, with legs straight or bent, or on toes or heels—determines the muscles being used. Upper-body muscles also should be varied by using stroke, backstroke, figure eights, punching, and jogging arms. Walking sideways usually offers less resistance and can be less exertive. Arm and directional variations also can vary the intensity.

Format

The program should follow the format for an aerobic-conditioning class. It should begin with a thermal warm-up, prestretch and cardiorespiratory warm-up, followed by the aerobic portion, the cooldown, toning, and poststretch.

Equipment

Most water walkers use no equipment, but wearing webbed gloves, like those made by Sprint/Rothhammer or Hydro-Fit, and resistant leg equipment, such as the Hydro-Tone boots, makes the walk more challenging. Walkers also can add variety by using buoyant leg equipment and different resistant, weighted, or buoyant pieces of upper-body equipment on different strides or laps.

Water Depth

Walkers usually begin in hip- to waist-depth water and walk to armpit depth before returning to shallower water. Some lucky walkers have the same depth during the entire route. Shallow water (hip to waist depth) is easier to walk in, and the pace will be faster. Deep water (midriff to shoulder depth) is more difficult to walk in and the pace will be slower. Using the same tempo for shallow and deep walkers generally does not work. Along the same lines, using the same music for shallow and deep walkers is not effective. Deep water (midriff to shoulder depth) is better suited to water jogging (see the following section).

Comparison to Land Workout

A study done at the Nicholas Institute of Sports Medicine, Lenox Hill Hospital, New York, shows that the number of calories burned during water walking increases with the depth of the water (Koszuta, 1988). The study compared dry-land walking and water walking at ankle, knee, and thigh depths and found the optimum depth to be at the thigh. Walking three miles in one hour at thigh depth was shown to burn 460 calories. Unfortunately, this study did not include a test at waist- to chest-depth water with the increased water resistance.

Purpose/Benefits

The major purpose of water walking is to improve cardiorespiratory endurance. Additional benefits include improved muscular endurance, flexibility (if some long strides are incorporated), and an improved body composition. Water walkers also enjoy the social benefits of group participation.

Common Errors

The two most frequent mistakes made in water walking are: (1) leaning forward while walking, and (2) using the same stride for the majority of the walk.

Proper **body alignment** is essential, and an individual should think about it during the entire walk. The head should be held in a neutral position with the chin centered, the eyes should look straight ahead (not up or down), the shoulders should be back and relaxed, the rib cage should be lifted, and the abdominals should be pulled in with the buttocks tucked under (pelvic tilt). If viewed from the side, the walker's ear, shoulder, and hip should be aligned. Walkers who lean forward probably are trying to go too fast and can compromise the low back. Maintaining good body alignment also improves abdominal and back muscle strength. Walking strides should be slow and controlled. The exception to the upright alignment is race walking in water. Race walkers lean forward slightly. Race walking is not recommended for the general population.

The second error—using the same stride for most of the workout—encourages muscle imbalance. Many walkers use their usual walking stride in the water. However, the normal walking stride contributes to overly tight hip flexors. Varying the stride allows participants to offset the natural muscle imbalance everyone has. By simply backing up, participants can ensure the use of the gluteals, hip flexors opposing muscle group. Changing to other strides allows equal use of the adductors, abductors, hamstrings, and quadriceps. Walkers should use stride variations that involve different major muscle groups to ensure **muscle balance.** Each stride should be used for an equal amount of time, unless a specific alternative plan has been set up.

Arm variations also are important. The pectoral muscles are usually tight, so using the trapezius and rhomboids against water resistance is important. Triceps should be used to offset their imbalance with the biceps. (Arm and stride variations with the muscle groups they involve are listed in Chapter 9.)

A study done at the Human Performance Laboratory at the University of Georgia in Athens, Georgia, comparing water and land walking, found that water walkers got the same benefits walking 1.5 to 2 miles an hour (2.5 to 3.3 km/hr) as land walkers got at 3.5 to 8 miles an hour (5.8 to 12.4 km/hr) (Vickery, Cureton, and Langstaff, 1983). Moreover, studies done by Dr. Robert Beasley (1989) at Southern Florida State University found that oxygen uptake while walking 7 miles per hour (11.7 km/hr) on land correlated to the oxygen uptake while walking 1.8 miles per hour (2.9 km/hr) in water.

(A sample water-walking workout is in Chapter 11.)

Shallow-Water Jogging

Definition

Shallow-water jogging is much like water walking, but it is done with bounding or leaping steps. Participants who jog in the water are pushing up and partially out of the water and bouncing as they move through the water, as opposed to walkers who stride with no bounce. Like water walkers, joggers also vary their stride by moving backward, forward, and sideways with heels kicking up behind, knees high in front, knees out to the sides, legs straight, or jogging on toes or heels. Long, slow strides should be varied with short,

DIAGRAM 2-2   Water Jogging

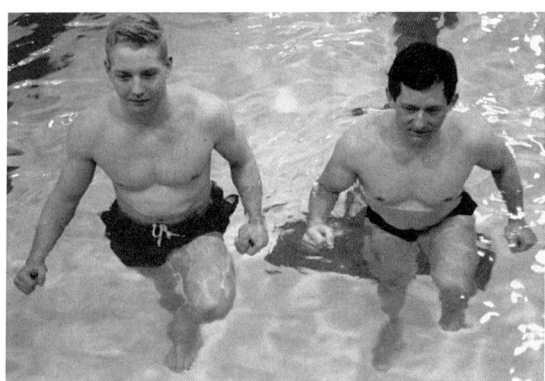

fast strides. Arm movements also should be varied, using backstroke, stroke, side push, punching, and jogging arms to provide upper-body muscle balance. (Stride and arm variations are listed in Chapter 9.)

Format

The water-jogging program should follow the format for an aerobic-conditioning class, beginning with a thermal warm-up, prestretch, and cardiorespiratory warm-up, followed by the aerobic portion, the cooldown, toning, and poststretch.

Equipment

Water joggers need no equipment but can vary the intensity of the workout by adding lightly resistant or weighted upper-body equipment, such as webbed gloves (Sprint/Rothhammer's Water Gloves or Hydro-Fit's Wave Webs) or one-half to one-pound wrist weights. Well-conditioned participants can jog with buoyant bells (by J & B Foam, B-Wise, Nuvo Sport, or Sprint/Rothhammer), heavier weights, or highly resistant equipment. Light ankle weights can be used and will not interfere with the stride but may offset some of the buoyant benefits of water jogging. If the purpose for water jogging is prevention or recuperation from injury, adding ankle weights is not recommended. Adding resistant or buoyant equipment may interfere with the stride for most participants. Well-coordinated, highly conditioned athletes may be able to use buoyant or resistant equipment on their legs. (Precautions regarding equipment in Chapter 8 should be noted.)

Water walkers need to be sure the pool bottom is comfortable for their feet. Some water joggers need to wear special aquatic shoes to protect their feet. Shoes increase drag, which increases the intensity of the workout, but they also prevent blisters, cushion the feet, prevent slipping, and help absorb the shock of impact. Joggers may want to wear aquatic shoes or running shoes. Shoes with black soles may leave marks on the pool bottom, so joggers should wear white-soled shoes or shoes with nonmarking soles.

A *tether* is another piece of equipment that water joggers may need. If the pool is small, joggers will become bored with frequently changing direction. Using a tether system keeps the jogger in place while he or she still expends energy to meet the cardiorespiratory requirements. The tether system involves tubing that attaches to the edge of the pool or the stair or ladder rail. The participant wears a belt around his or her waist that attaches to the tubing. The runner tries to move forward but the tether keeps him or her stationary. Students using a tether system should wear shoes to protect the bottoms of their feet.

Water Depth

Water jogging can be stressful to joints if done in water shallower than waist level. The apparent weight loss of 90% in shoulder-depth water is reduced to about 50% at waist depth. The impact of bare feet on a concrete or tile pool bottom at this depth can cause stress fractures and other overuse injuries. Midriff to shoulder depth seems to work best for shallow-water joggers. Some joggers wear buoyant belts and jog into the deeper end of the pool (5 to 12 feet) before returning to the shallow end. (For more information on deep-water jogging, see the Deep-Water Exercise section, later in this chapter.)

Most shallow-water joggers prefer to keep their arms in the water to increase the resistance for upper-body toning, endurance, and workout intensity. Using arms out of the water and overhead can destabilize the body as it moves through the water, causing alignment concerns.

Comparison to Land Workout

A study was done comparing land-running times to water-running times in an attempt to find equivalents in distance for energy expended (Osinski, 1989). This study found that an individual can run one-quarter mile in the water in the same amount of time it takes to run one mile on land. If participants are looking for a water-jogging pace guideline, this study may be beneficial.

Purpose/Benefits

The purpose of water jogging is to improve cardiorespiratory endurance and achieve all the benefits associated with it—muscular endurance, flexibility (if long strides are used), and improved body composition.

Common Errors

Water joggers make three common mistakes: (1) jogging on the toes, (2) using the same stride for the bulk of the workout, and (3) leaning forward. On land, jogging is a heel-strike sport with the heel usually landing first. In the water, jogging often is done with the forefoot landing first. Too often, the participant never follows through to bring the rest of the foot down. Jogging on the toes can lead to general muscle soreness (torn tissue), tightness and shortness in the calf muscle, shin splints (a pain in the front of the shin), and if done in water that is too shallow, stress fractures (broken bones in the foot) or other overuse injuries. The jogger should always press the heel down to the pool bottom before pushing off again.

The second mistake—using the same stride for the major part of the workout—leads to severe muscle imbalance and injury. Many joggers use their usual jogging stride in the water. However, the normal jogging stride contributes to overly tight hip flexors. Varying the stride allows participants to offset the natural muscle imbalance everyone has. By simply backing up, participants ensure use of the gluteals, the hip flexors' opposing muscle group. Changing to other strides allows equal use of the adductors, abductors, hamstrings, and quadriceps. Joggers should use stride variations that involve different major muscle groups to ensure muscle balance. Each stride should be used for an equal amount of time, unless a specific alternative plan has been set up.

Arm variations also are important. The pectoral muscles are usually tight, so using the trapezius and rhomboids against the water resistance is important. Triceps should be used to offset their imbalance with the biceps. (Arm and stride variations with the muscle groups they involve are listed in Chapter 9.)

The third problem—leaning forward while jogging forward through the water—is often a sign of trying to move too fast, which compromises the low back. Maintaining good body alignment also improves abdominal and back-muscle strength.

Proper body alignment is essential and should be thought of during the entire workout. The head should be held in a neutral position with the chin centered, the eyes should look straight ahead (not up or down), the shoulders should be back and relaxed, the rib cage should be lifted, and the abdominals pulled in with the buttocks tucked under slightly (a partial pelvic tilt). If viewed from the side, the jogger's ear, shoulder, and hip should be aligned. Joggers who lean forward probably are trying to go too fast and can compromise the low back. Most jogging strides should be slow and controlled.

The exception to the upright alignment is race jogging in the water. Race joggers lean forward slightly. Race jogging is not recommended for the general population.

Studies have concluded that the effects of water resistance and buoyancy make high levels of energy expenditure possible with relatively little movement and strain on lower-extremity joints (Evans, et al., 1978). This suggests that water jogging may be a valuable alternate mode of conditioning for developing and maintaining work capacity and cardiovascular fitness.

A study was done comparing land-running times to water-running times in an attempt to find equivalents in distance for energy ex-

Frequency refers to the number of times an activity is repeated in a week.

A three- to five-minute cooldown with low-intensity, fluid, walking-level movements, followed by a poststretch of at least five minutes finishes the workout. Stretches during the prestretch only need to be held 10 seconds. Poststretches should be held 30 seconds.

Equipment

Most water-toning classes encourage students to use upper- and lower-body equipment after adapting to water exercises without equipment. Webbed gloves (by Sprint/Rothhammer or Hydro-Fit), paddles (by Sprint/Rothhammer), frisbees, buoyant bells (Nuvo Sport, Inc. Spa Bells, B-Wise fitness bars, J & B Foam), Dynabands, SPRI tubing and bands, the Aquarius Water Workout Station, small buoyant balls, and wrist weights all can be used to work the upper body. Balls, kickboards, buoyant bells, Aquarius, and resistant devices, like Spa Bells and Hydro-Tone, all can be used for middle-body work. Buoyant, weighted, and resistant ankle cuffs or boots can be worn to work the lower body. Stretchy exercise bands also can be used for lower-body toning. (More information regarding equipment is provided in Chapter 8.)

Water Depth

Because students usually stand at the pool edge for water toning, midriff depth seems best. Participants can stand flat on the supporting leg and keep the body stabilized while doing lower-body exercises with the other leg. At this depth, participants also are able to bend the knees slightly to immerse the entire muscle group being used during upper-body toning. During portions of the workout some classes use buoyant devices, such as Sprint/Rothhammer kickboards, body buoys, and deep-water vests or belts. Because of the amount of buoyancy the devices afford, many students can stay in midriff-depth water during the buoyant portion of the class. Others may have to move to deeper water to keep their feet from touching the pool bottom during the exercises.

Comparison to Land Workout

Toning in water produces quicker results than toning on land because of the water's resistance. Many of the same exercises used in land-based toning classes are used in a vertical position in the water. Unlike land-based programs, water toning participants may become chilled in the water. Using more muscular force during each exercise helps keep the body temperature in a comfortable range. Increased muscular force keeps the students from cheating or doing the move without power, and, therefore, ensures better results.

Purpose/Benefits

The benefits of water toning are increased muscular endurance and muscle mass. Increased muscle mass has a direct effect on improving body composition. If full range of motion is used, flexibility also is enhanced.

Common Errors

All the exercises must be controlled and done correctly. A general rule to test the safety of a move's speed is control—if the move is controlled and the rest of the body is stable and aligned, the speed usually is safe.

It is not a good idea to "go for the burn" during this type of exercise. Many water toners experience the burn when they begin a program. After a few weeks, as the body adapts, the burn occurs less frequently. The burn is a sign of built up **lactic acid.** The exerciser should stop a move that is causing the burn and jog in the water for 20 to 40 seconds until the muscle gets the oxygen it needs and the sensation dissipates.

DIAGRAM 2–5 Strength Training

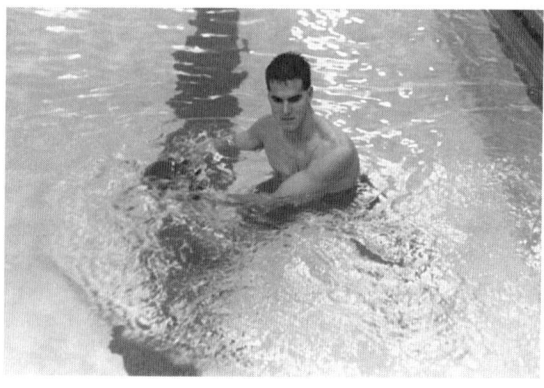

Strength Training

Definition

Strength training in the water is a program aimed specifically at body building. Actual weight-lifting moves, such as squats, bicep curls, knee extensions, and elbow presses, are done in the pool during this workout. In order to attain muscular balance and reduce the risk of injuries, all major muscle groups should be strengthened during a workout, including quadriceps, hamstrings, low back, abdominals, chest, upper back, shoulders, biceps, and triceps. Working all major muscle groups is important for a comprehensive and safe workout. Training just some of the muscles produces less significant results, encourages muscle imbalance, and may cause muscle injuries.

Format

A strength-training program begins with a thermal warm-up and prestretch. Since this is not a cardiorespiratory workout, no cardiorespiratory warm-up is necessary. The strength-training moves immediately follow the prestretch. Each muscle group that is strengthened during the workout must be stretched again later. This final flexibility stage can be done either at the end of the workout or after the last set in which the muscle group is used.

Use Slow and Controlled Moves with a Minimum of Momentum. It is important to perform the strength-training moves in a slow and controlled manner. Fast movements place too much stress on the muscles, connective tissues, and joints. Fast-strength training is less effective and more dangerous than slow-strength training. Participants can work with more resistance if they move quickly through the movements, but it is momentum, not muscles, doing the work. Slow training uses more muscle tension, more muscle force, and more muscle recruitment and is safer and more effective.

Full Muscle Extension to Complete Muscle Contraction. Full-range-of-motion movements should be used in strength training. This not only ensures a full **muscle contraction** but also allows the opposing muscle to stretch. Using a short range of motion has limited value on the muscle being strengthened and may lead to reduced joint mobility. To test for full range of motion in a joint, contract the muscle and move the joint without resistive equipment. When equipment is added, the joint should be able to move to full flexion and stop just short of full extension.

Systematic, Gradual Progression. The principle of progressive overload is extremely important in strength training. Resistance and reps should be gradually increased. The training stimulus must gradually overload in order to allow muscles, bones, connective tissues, and joints to adapt without injury. More demanding workouts require more recovery time.

Equipment

Some unconditioned people can do strength training in water without equipment. Highly conditioned athletes require some type of resistance equipment.

Hydro-Tone is a type of resistant equipment used for upper-, middle-, and lower-body exercises. Aquarius Water Workout Station also is used with success. Participants should never hold their breath while using resistance equipment. Exhale during the exertive lift or press, and inhale during the return or rest portion. The equipment should be gripped easily, because a clenched grip can increase blood pressure.

Almost all strength training in the water is done with equipment, based on the principle of resistance. (See Chapter 8 for more information on types of aquatic equipment.) Buoyant equipment does not work well because only one muscle of each muscle pair strengthens from the buoyancy offered. Weighted equipment approved for use in the water is not heavy enough to create the overload needed to achieve strength benefits.

Water Depth

Strength trainers usually stand in water of midriff to armpit depth. Lower-body exercises usually are done standing at pool edge. Participants stand flat on the supporting leg and keep the body stabilized while doing exercises with the other leg. At this depth, they also are able to bend the knees slightly to immerse the entire muscle group being used during upper-body exercises.

Comparison to Land Workout

Unlike land-based strength training, water strength training seems to use little or no eccentric contractions if exercises are done with resistance equipment. Because of the resistance of water, all strength-training exercises will involve only concentric muscle contractions. If extremely buoyant equipment is used, eccentric muscle contractions occur as the equipment and limb move up toward the surface of the water. If heavy weights are used, eccentric contractions will occur as they do on land.

Purpose/Benefits

The main benefit of strength training is increased muscular strength and muscle mass. Increased muscle mass, which occurs when muscle protein increases and muscle fat decreases, has a direct effect on improving body composition. Muscular endurance also improves. Strength training also improves muscular balance and neuromuscular action and increases the structural integrity of muscles, connective tissues, and bones as it builds strength and density. Moderate levels of strength training also reduce the likelihood of injury. Sports enthusiasts find a strong relationship between gain in strength and gain in speed for sports involving running, cycling, and swimming.

After age 20, without strength training a body loses approximately one pound of muscle every two years. That means at age 40 someone who weighed 150 pounds at age 20 and who did no strength training will have replaced 10 pounds of muscle with 10 pounds of fat. Moreover, for every pound of muscle lost, the metabolic rate goes down about 50 calories a day. For every pound of muscle gained, the metabolic rate goes up about 50 calories a day. Strength training is necessary to keep a youthful fat-to-lean ratio in body composition.

Many exercisers believe they will build big muscles if they strength train. That is not true. Few men and fewer women have the genetic background to build big muscles. Those who have the genes to build large muscles must work long and hard to achieve them.

Strength training is particularly important for women because it staves off osteoporosis, a potentially crippling condition caused by loss of bone mineral.

Common Errors

Injuries common to weight lifters can occur in water if students begin with too much resistance, or too large a range of motion, or if they move too fast. All exercises must be controlled and done correctly. A general rule to check the safety of the move's speed is control—if the move is controlled and the rest of the body is stable and aligned, the speed usually is safe. Correct form is vital. When muscles are too fatigued to maintain correct form, the exercise should be stopped.

Without actual weight in the water, strength trainers may slow down as they tire and, in effect, reduce the weight with which they are training. The participant must be continually conscious of supplying maximum effort. Some students enjoy working with a metronome or music at a specified number of beats per minute to keep them from slowing down.

Participants should maintain the natural curve of the spine and keep feet parallel, knees soft, abdominals contracted, chest open, shoulders down and slightly back, and the back of the neck open. Instructors and students alike will be able to watch for postural imbalances by using these hints for good form. Hyperextension of the lumbar area of the spine, hip flexors, knees, and elbows should be avoided.

Strength-training program participants must remember to include the thermal warm-up, prestretch, and poststretch portions of the program. Muscles and joints must be warmed, lubricated, and prepared for the work they will do. The intensity in strength training is determined by the amount of resistance used in the water. Duration refers to the number of reps performed of each move within a specific time period, and the number of times each group of reps is performed (sets). In general, strength training requires an overload in the amount of resistance.

According to the rule of specificity, when designing a program for strength development, high resistance and low reps should provide maximum effectiveness. Frequency refers to the number of times per week an activity is performed. All muscle groups that are strengthened should be stretched at the end of the workout or at the end of the use of that muscle group.

Guidelines

In early 1990, the ACSM set specific guidelines for resistance training programs (ACSM, 1990a). The ACSM **resistance guidelines** state that the frequency should be at least two times a week. This is considered a minimum standard and should be increased as conditioning occurs. It generally takes 48 hours for the body to repair and rebuild itself to a greater level of strength after a strength-training workout. Workouts, therefore, should be equally spaced throughout the week. Taking too little time between workouts can result in counterproductive workouts.

The ACSM duration guidelines recommend a minimum of 8 to 10 different exercises during the workout. Each exercise should be performed at least 8 to 12 times (reps). This would make up one set. While one set is the minimum considered for training to occur, more conditioned students should do multiple sets. Most muscles should be adequately stressed with 60 to 90 seconds of continuous contraction against a heavy resistance. That usually converts to 8 to 12 reps.

The guidelines also state, "Resistance strength training of a moderate intensity, sufficient to develop and maintain muscle mass, should be an integral part of an adult fitness program" (ACSM, 1990a). This strong recommendation by the ACSM points to the benefits of strength training for all adults. The latest studies also show that moderate-intensity strength training is excellent for the older adult (Strovas, 1990).

The intensity for most programs is 70% to 80% of the maximum resistance a participant can move. A general rule is that the resistance is too great if a student cannot repeat the exercise at least 8 times in a row. There is not enough resistance if the student can repeat the exercise more than 12 times.

Flexibility Training

Definition

Flexibility-training participants stretch different muscle groups to improve their long-term flexibility. Flexibility often is an ignored component of fitness.

DIAGRAM 2-6 Flexibility Training

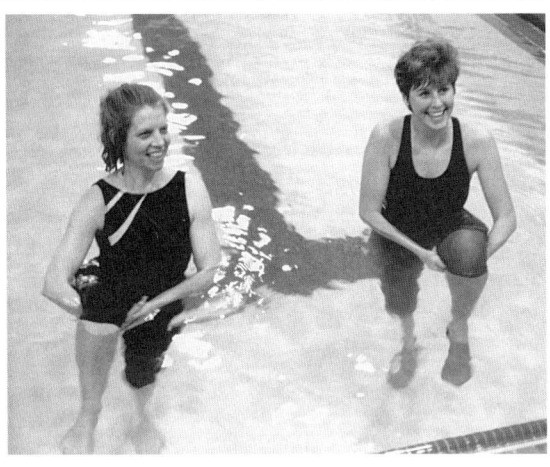

If a muscle is only trained to contract, it loses its ability to stretch as far as it should, resulting in permanently shortened muscles. Most aquatic-fitness programs, such as toning, aerobics, and weight training, concentrate only on training the muscles to contract. Each aquatics program should include a flexibility segment.

Participants often are confused between the terms *muscle* and *joint* when attempting to understand how a flexibility class works. Muscles are *elastic*, which means they can stretch and have the ability to return to their normal position. Tight muscles, either from daily activities or from overuse in an exercise class, shorten the range of motion in the joints they move. Increased range of motion in all joints is the goal of a flexibility class. The goal is achieved by stretching the muscles that move the joints. The joint is not stretched, the muscle is. The stretched muscle, in turn, increases flexibility and, therefore, range of motion in the joint.

Muscles that are tight from daily activities need special attention during a flexibility program. Most people are round shouldered and need to stretch the pectorals. Tight hip flexors and gastrocnemius also need special attention during the program.

Format

During a flexibility-training class, students warm up a muscle group and then move to a 30- to 60-second stretch of that muscle group. For example, students may do knee extensions for 30 to 60 seconds followed by a 30- to 60-second stretch of the quadriceps. Hamstrings with knee flexion can be worked next and then stretched. Intensity is determined by overload or the amount of lengthening of the muscle beyond its resting length. The duration is determined by the type of stretching being done, how long each stretch is done, and how often each stretch is used. A frequency of three times per week is recommended for flexibility training. Care must be taken in flexibility training not to overload in ways that are harmful to the body. Muscles, like taffy, are more pliable when they are warm. Muscle temperature is greatly affected by water temperature. If muscles are warmed before stretching, safer stretching will occur.

Only static, never ballistic, stretches should be used. Fast, jerky, bouncing (**ballistic**) stretches can cause injury to tendons and microscopic tears to muscle tissue. Muscles are protected by a stretch-reflex mechanism. When a stretch is begun, a nerve reflex sends a message to contract through the brain to the muscle fibers. If a ballistic stretch is used, muscles will contract when the next bounce occurs. Attempting to stretch a contracted muscle can cause injury.

Static stretches also trigger the **stretch-reflex** mechanism to respond, but the static stretch overcomes the mechanism and allows flexibility to occur. The muscle fibers contract at the beginning of a stretch, but if the stretch is held at that point (and not pushed further), the nerve sends a signal through the brain to relax the muscle fibers again. When that occurs, the stretch can be taken a little further before the stretch-reflex responds again. Using the stretch-reflex concept in the program helps increase flexibility. Participants should move to the point of mild tension and then relax while holding the stretch in that position. After about 10 to 15 seconds, they can increase the stretch by a fraction of an inch until they feel mild tension again and then relax as they hold the stretch in that position. If the tension does not decrease, the participant should ease off the stretch and hold it at that point.

Equipment

Most flexibility students require no equipment. The edge of the pool and sometimes a bar just below the water surface can be used during this kind of class. The Aquarius Water Workout Station allows good flexibility positioning and flexibility work. Some participants use buoyant devices, such as Sprint/Rothhammer kickboards, pull buoys, buoyant ankle cuffs or boots (such as Hydro-Fit), and bells (such as J & B Foam, B-Wise, and Nuvo Sport Spa Bells), to assist in holding the joint in a full-range-of-motion stretch. This is not recommended for the unconditioned or beginning student.

Water Depth

Average pool depth for the flexibility class is midriff level. Students should immerse problem joints (stiff joints, areas recovering from injury or surgery, and hot joints) during the warming and stretching segments. Flexibility classes also can be done in the deep end of the pool if students wear buoyant belts. Flexibility programs usually are offered in water over 86 degrees.

Comparison to Land Workout

Flexibility programs in the water work well because of the lessened effect of gravity on the joints. Exercisers are able to stretch further without undue tension. Unlike land-based flexibility exercises, almost all water-stretching exercises are done in a vertical position. Although fewer stretch positions can be used for each muscle group, those used are extremely effective.

Purpose/Benefits

The purpose of flexibility training is to increase the range of motion in each joint by elongating the muscles that move the joint. Depending on the intensity of the warm-up before stretching, the program also could increase muscular endurance and body composition.

Tight muscles can hamper joints from moving in a full range of motion. They also can pull the body out of proper alignment. A well-rounded stretching plan helps prevent muscle imbalance, and increased flexibility promotes a full range of motion.

Common Errors

The two most frequent mistakes in water-flexibility classes are (1) stretching cold muscles, and (2) stretching too far. When concentrating on flexibility, many students ignore or minimize warming a muscle before stretching it. If that happens, injury may occur. Cold muscles should not be stretched. Warming the muscle brings blood and oxygen to it, making it pliable. Warming also allows synovial fluid to lubricate the joint that moves the muscles. This allows a more comfortable, larger range of motion stretch.

Too often, students feel they should stretch until it hurts. The phrase most frequently used to describe a proper stretch is *move to the point of tension, never pain*. If performed correctly, a stretch elongates a muscle to a greater length than its resting length. Students should feel the stretch but never feel uncomfortable. Overall flexibility improves with proper stretching.

Aqua-Power Aerobics

Definition

Aqua-power aerobics is a program that combines cardiorespiratory conditioning

DIAGRAM 2–7   Aqua Power

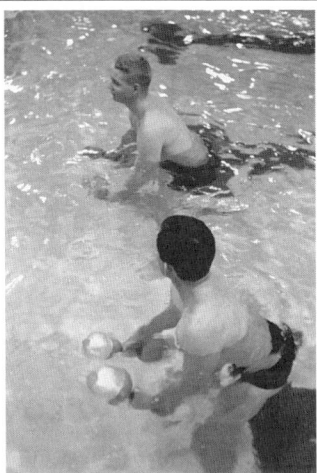

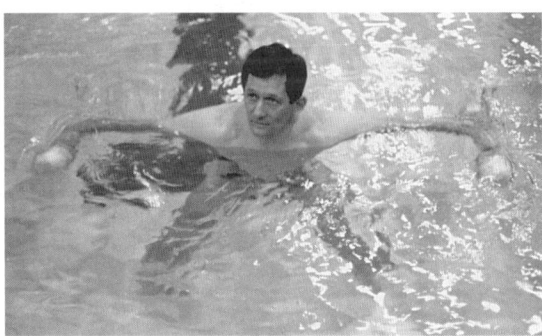

(aerobics), strength training, and muscle toning in the aerobic portion of the workout.

Format

The class follows the usual aerobic format of thermal warm-up, prestretch, cardiovascular warm-up, aerobics, and cooldown, but it eliminates the toning portion before the final flexibility segment. Exercises are used that strengthen muscles against the water's resistance while elevating the demand for oxygen. Many low-impact-type moves—such as lunges, squats, and sidekicks—can be used. Moves are done slowly and with control and power. Explosive muscle force is used in each move. More reps are used if muscle toning is desired with the aerobics. Fewer reps and more resistance are used for aerobics with strength training.

Equipment

Equipment often is used after students have mastered the moves and have adapted to the exercise level without equipment. Webbed gloves (by Hydro-Fit or Sprint/Rothhammer), wrist and ankle weights, Dynabands (through Fitness Wholesale catalog), SPRI exercise bands and tubing, buoyant ankle and wrist cuffs (by Hydro-Fit or Sprint/Rothhammer), and any lightly resistant product can be used. Advanced aqua-power aerobics students may want to experiment with more highly resistant and buoyant equipment, such as Nuvo Sport Spa Bells, B-Wise Fitness Bars, or Hydro-Tone. (See Chapter 8 for more about equipment information.)

Water Depth

Beginning classes use waist-depth water to make students feel more comfortable and successful in performing power moves. In shallow water, exercisers concentrate better on leg movement and proper technique. More advanced classes usually use deeper water (chest depth) for added effectiveness.

Comparison to Land Workout

Land-based power-aerobic workouts are based on the concept of first using an exerciser's body weight and then adding additional weight with wrist and ankle weights. Because of the lessened effect of gravity in water, aqua-based power-aerobic workouts first use the water's resistance and then increase the intensity with the kinds of equipment mentioned above.

Purpose/Benefits

The purpose of aqua-power aerobics is to increase cardiorespiratory fitness, muscular endurance and muscular strength, and to improve body composition.

Flexibility also can be enhanced through the flexibility segment at the end of the class.

Common Errors

The most difficult tasks in an aqua-power class are teaching correct technique to students and helping them understand that slow moves can be aerobic. Some instructors have students review power moves on the deck to demonstrate technique. In water, students need to maintain a proper alignment and learn to use explosive muscle force in the correct portion of the move.

Exercisers who are accustomed to faster, bouncing moves may need a class handout explaining heart rates, oxygen consumption, and aqua-power exercises. Those with little muscle mass may at first have trouble working at an aerobic-conditioning intensity level.

Sport-Specific and Sports-Conditioning Workouts

Definition

Sport-specific workouts are aerobic workouts that are designed to assist sports enthusiasts in developing the muscle strength and flexibility, skills, agility, balance, and coordination needed in their sport.

Format

The format of the workout begins with the traditional thermal warm-up, stretch, and cardiorespiratory warm-up. Power, balance, coordination, and sports skills and patterns are worked on during the aerobic portion. The concept of interval training can be used during the aerobic portion of the workout. Strength conditioning or muscle endurance can be worked on following the cooldown. Flexibility for specific needs follows the strength-conditioning or muscular endurance portion.

Sport-specific conditioning can be done for enthusiasts in most sports, including baseball,

DIAGRAM 2–8 Sport Specific and Sports Conditioning

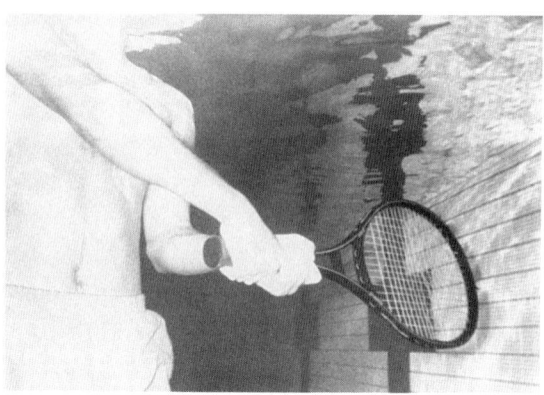

Sport Specific

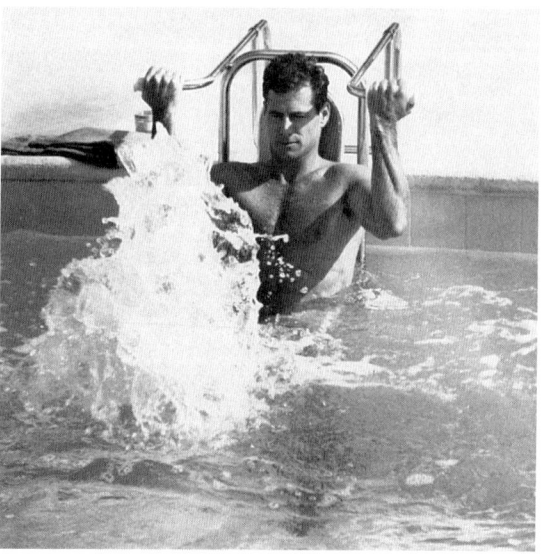

Sports Conditioning

javelin, biking, running, downhill skiing, tennis, weight lifting, football, soccer, cross-country skiing, and track and field. Enthusiasts from different sports can take part in the same aqua aerobics class if different stations are used and time is spent interviewing participants before they enroll. The entire class would stay together during the warm-up and for some of the agility, coordination, and speed drills in the aerobic portion of the class. That ensures muscle balance in the workout. Participants then would move around the pool from station to station, each of which is designed to assist athletes in developing the skills and strength needed in their particular sports. If equipment is needed, it would be at pool edge at the station.

Following the specific exercises, the class would come together again for the cooldown, upper- and lower-body strength exercises (once again for muscle balance), and the flexibility segment. If sport-specific flexibility is necessary, it would follow the group flexibility segment and be done at stations.

If the goal is to improve in a particular sport, the instructor and student need to look at the requirements of that sport:

— What muscles need to be especially strong? Which need to be particularly flexible?
— Is speed important? If it is, is it speed moving forward, backward, or laterally? Is it speed of limb movement?
— What kinds of agility and coordination are required?
— What specific skills are needed?

Note where the student feels aches, pains, and stiffness after the sport so those areas can be conditioned against injury.

Equipment

The actual equipment that is used in the sport can be used in the pool. Baseball bats, golf clubs, and tennis racquets are seen in pools during sport-specific workouts. It is important to note that the equipment, like any aquatic equipment, should always be used with control and safety in mind. Aquatic equipment like Hydro-Fit, Hydro-Tone, Aquarius, B-Wise Fitness Bars, Nuvo Sport Spa Bells and SPRI tubing and Dynabands are used in sport-specific training to help stretch, strengthen, and tone specific muscles. It is also used to simulate moves in the sport. (See Chapter 8 for additional information on equipment.)

Water Depth

Water depth often is dictated by the sport. Runners and soccer players may want to improve conditioning in deep water. Baseball players, tennis players, and golfers need to be in water deep enough to accomplish an underwater swing or stroke. Speed drills usually begin in shallow water (hip to waist depth) and move deeper (midriff to armpit) as the workout progresses. Agility and coordination drills work well in midriff to armpit depth if they are designed for the upper body. Baseball drills for coordination, balance, and agility in fielding a ground ball, and turning and throwing obviously work best in shallower water.

Comparison to Land Workout

Sports-conditioning and -training workouts in water closely compare to those on land. Exercisers can challenge the muscles they use in their sport more easily with water resistance. They can increase muscular strength, agility, balance, and aerobic conditioning without the stress of land-based sports drills.

Purpose/Benefits

The purpose of sport-specific training can be as varied as the participant's needs. Most programs have aerobic or cardiorespiratory and body composition improvements as their main goals. Improved muscular endurance, flexibility, and muscular strength usually are secondary goals.

Common Errors

The most common mistake made in sport-specific training is working only on strengthening those muscles needed during the sport. A goal in this type of program should be creating muscle balance in the athlete. All major muscle groups should be used. Determine the major muscle groups used in the sport and develop agonists and antagonists equally.

Flexibility too often is ignored, even though its importance in injury prevention is well documented. All major muscles should be stretched, with special attention given to those muscles that need to stretch during the sport.

Sport-specific classes usually are designed for fit or conditioned participants who want to increase their abilities in their chosen sports. They generally are not classes for beginners or unconditioned individuals.

Bench or Step Aerobics

Definition

Bench aerobics or step workouts are aerobic workouts that mimic the Harvard Step Test for cardiorespiratory fitness. (During the test, participants step up and down on a bench for three minutes and then check working and recovery heartrates.) Rather than have participants step up and down on a bench for just three minutes, the step workout makes up the entire aerobic portion of the class. Participants use stairs in the pool or weighted benches taken into the pool to step up and down in a rhythmic fashion. Moving the body vertically against gravity creates an intense aerobic workout that focuses on the lower body. Such a workout may be called step training, step or bench aerobics, power-bench workouts, or Step Reebok. It is a high-intensity, low-impact workout.

Format

The class begins with the traditional thermal warm-up, stretch, and cardiorespiratory warm-up. The aerobic segment usually lasts 20 to 40 minutes and is made up exclusively of stepping up and down in a variety of patterns. Traditional cooldown and flexibility segments follow the aerobic portion. The flexibility segment should give special attention to the quadriceps, gluteals, and hamstrings, because they do the bulk of the stepping work. A strength or toning portion can be included between the cooldown and flexibility portions, but it normally is excluded because of the toning achieved during the aerobics portion. Depending on water depth, an upper-body strength or toning portion can be included during the cooldown. If the pool is shallow, additional upper-body toning against the water's resistance is needed.

Equipment

A bench or step such as the Aerobic Workbench is the only equipment needed for the program. Benches used in the pool usually are weighted with diving weights to hold them in position. Benches should be stable to ensure safety. The bench can vary from two to twelve inches in height. Four- to eight-inch benches usually are recommended, because they will

DIAGRAM 2–9   Bench Aerobics

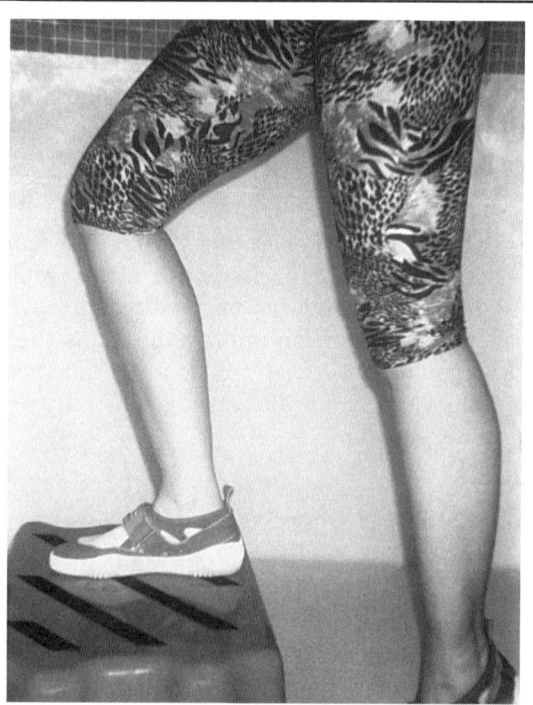

accommodate most fitness levels. The step should not flex the knee beyond 90 degrees.

Other aquatic equipment can be used to make the workout more challenging. Holding resistant devices, like Hydro-Tone, make a more intense leg workout. Using wrist weights will give good upper-body toning if normal press and fly moves are used. Using Hydro-Fit or Sprint/Rothhammer's buoyant ankle cuffs can increase the intensity of the workout for the gluteals and hamstrings as the student steps down. Using SPRI's waistband with tubing adds the upper-body work necessary to balance the workout.

Water Depth

Average water depth for step training should be midriff level. Step training offers a higher level of intensity because the body pushes more water out of the way when stepping out. If a student feels too buoyant or does not have control of the steps, the water level should be lowered.

Comparison to Land Workout

Studies done by Drs. Lorna and Peter Francis at San Diego State University show that land-based step training offers the energy expenditure of running at a seven-minute-per-mile pace with the amount of impact shock to the lower limbs produced by walking (Aldridge, 1990). The impact in water is lessened even more. Bench aerobics on land offers the resistance of gravity and body weight when stepping up. In water, the body works against the resistance of body weight, some gravity, and some water resistance. When stepping down in the water, the body needs to work against water resistance and buoyancy.

Music

Music used during the workout helps keep students on a cadence that challenges them. The tempo used for step classes is usually 100 to 110 beats per minute. Strom-Berg Productions is the only music service that has created a tape specific for aquatic step-training. For more information see the Resources chapter (Chapter 13) of this book in the music section.

Purpose/Benefits

Step-training benefits include cardiorespiratory improvement, increased muscular endurance, and improved body composition. Flexibility gains can be made if a flexibility portion is included at the end of the workout. Muscular strength can improve if additional equipment is used. Balance and coordination also will improve.

Step training is popular among conditioned men and women. Women often appreciate the additional work for the thighs and buttocks, and both women and men enjoy the challenge of this athletic workout.

Common Errors

Students need constant encouragement and advice to help them maintain proper alignment and correct technique. They should step to the center of the platform, keep shoulders back, chest up, buttocks tucked under hips, and knees soft. The entire sole of the foot should make contact with the bench when stepping up. When stepping down, the ball of the foot touches first and then the heel. The knees should not lock on the step up or on the step down. The body always should be carried tall with shoulders centered over the hips. Leaning backward or forward during any portion of the step training is unnecessary and could cause muscle imbalance or injury. The feet should usually start and finish next to each other.

The most common mistake made in step training is using the same step pattern for the entire workout. Add variety to the workout by stepping or walking around, in front, or to the sides of the bench. This provides a better opportunity for muscle balance. Overuse of the quadriceps and hip flexors can cause knee and back injury.

Interval Training

Definition

Interval training is an exertive exercise program usually reserved for well-conditioned athletes. The program can, however, be modified for less-conditioned people. Interval training simply means a workout that combines high-intensity portions with moderate- or low-intensity segments.

During continuous aerobic training, the exercise program is organized so the workout intensity remains in the target heartrate zone during the entire workout. The intensity begins at the low end of the target zone and gradually increases to moderate and high intensity before tapering back to the low end. Interval training is unique in that it is based on short bouts of intense exercise, during which the workout intensity is at the top end of the target zone. These high-intensity bouts are separated by recovery periods, during which the workout intensity is at the low to moderate portions of the target zone. This technique trains the athlete to maintain near-maximum heartrate for a longer total time than would be possible with continuous training. This type of training uses the anaerobic metabolic pathway. The primary fuel is intramuscular glycogen.

DIAGRAM 2–10   Interval Trailing

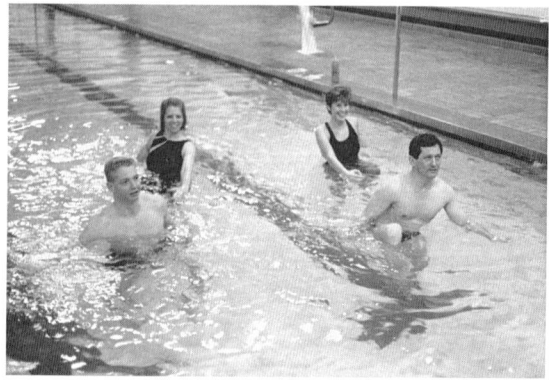

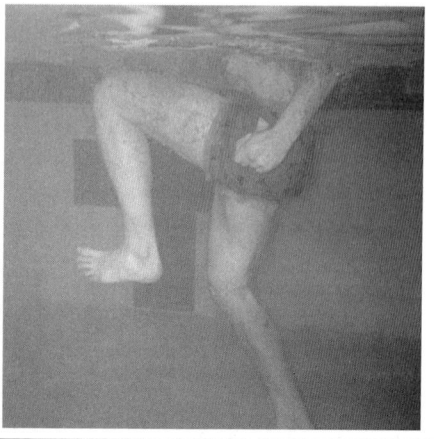

Format

Intervals usually are done as part of the aerobics portion of a workout. The format for a cardiorespiratory workout includes a thermal warm-up, prestretch, and cardiorespiratory warm-up. The aerobics portion usually begins with three minutes of aerobics at low or moderate intensity. Approximately 75 seconds are allotted for the high-intensity interval before returning to moderate or low intensity for three more minutes. Five to seven cycles are done during the aerobics part of the program before cooling down, toning, and stretching.

A **cycle** is the combination of one low- (or moderate-) and one high-intensity set. The low- to moderate-intensity portion is usually at 60% to 75% of the target heartrate. The high-intensity part of the cycle is usually at 75% to 80% of the target heartrate zone and is designed to move at least to, and often beyond, the anaerobic threshold.

The **work-to-recovery ratio** is how long the high intensity (work) lasts in comparison to the moderate or low intensity (recovery). Most interval-training programs use a 1 to 3 or a 1.5 to 3 work-to-recovery ratio. This means 60 to 75 seconds of high intensity (anaerobic) are followed by three minutes of low to moderate intensity (aerobic) for each cycle. Some programs use a 1 to 2 ratio and others a 1 to 1 ratio. The most common is a 1 to 3 work-to-recovery ratio.

Equipment

Equipment generally is not used in interval training, unless it is part of a regular program for the recovery portion of intervals. For example, if gloves are used in the three-minute portion of the cycle, they can be left on during the high-intensity portion. In order to achieve the intensity required, aquatic equipment can be used if it can be added to the workout without interrupting or stopping it.

Water Depth

Water depth for interval training varies, depending on the type of training being done. Because the concept of intervals can be used in deep-water running, water walking, or water aerobics, different water levels are used. The depth commonly used for the regular program is the depth that should be used when intervals are added.

Comparison to Land Workout

Interval training can be achieved more safely and effectively in water than on land. Working against water resistance allows the exerciser to move into a high-intensity workout without the stress received in land-based interval-training programs.

Purpose/Benefits

The goal of interval training is to improve the cardiorespiratory system; thus, benefits will be seen not only in the fitness component of cardiorespiratory fitness but also in body composition because of the impact on caloric consumption. Muscular endurance also can be improved during the program; and muscular strength can be improved during the strength or toning portion of the class. Flexibility can be improved through the use of full range of motion and the final stretch.

Common Errors

Participants of interval-training classes need to be aware that while increasing the speed of the movements may elevate the heartrate and perceived exertion level, it may compromise the joints and connective tissues. Too many times, exercisers try to increase the intensity by only increasing the speed of the movements. Using equipment, increasing frontal resistance, increasing acceleration, and using long levers all can increase the workout's intensity. Moving through water also increases energy requirements.

Interval training, like all fitness programs, should work toward improving muscle balance. All major muscle groups should be worked and stretched during the workout.

Modifications can be made to the program to open participation to less-conditioned individuals. The 3-minute moderate-intensity portion can be followed by a 75-second low-intensity portion, while other participants are doing 75 seconds of high intensity. The 75-second part of the cycle can be the recovery portion for less-conditioned participants.

Deep-Water Exercise

Definition

Deep-water exercise refers to any type of water exercise program done in the diving well of the pool or in water depth above a participant's head. It is a completely nonimpact workout. With every footfall on land, the legs bear two to five times the body's weight; in deep water, the legs bear none.

Deep-water exercise usually falls into one of two categories—running or exercises. Deep-water running is simply running in deep water, using different strides. Deep-water exercises usually constitute a class that follows the format for an aerobic workout, usually including some

DIAGRAM 2-11 *Deep-Water Training*

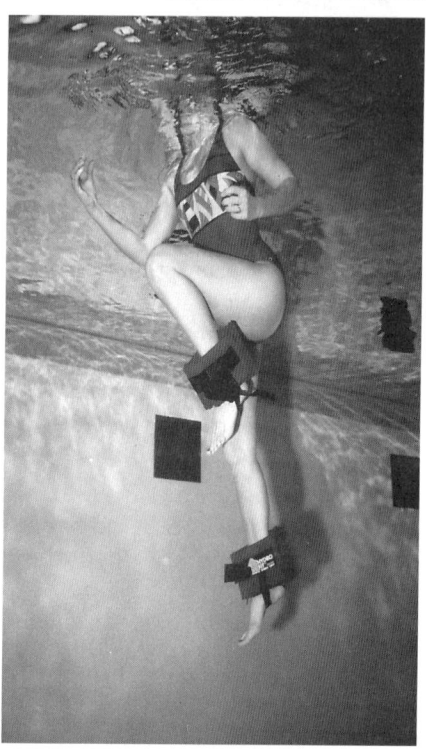

deep-water running. Deep-water exercises can be added to any program for variety.

Format

Many people get into the pool and start running immediately, but a well thought out program takes the runners through a complete warm-up segment before beginning the run, and finishes with cooldown and flexibility segments after the run. Deep-water exercise programs should always follow the format for a safe, effective cardiorespiratory workout. (The format is reviewed at the beginning of this chapter.)

Exercises done in the shallow end can be done in deep water with one precaution—all movements should be bilateral. Rather than kick one leg forward, a deep-water exerciser should kick one leg forward while kicking the other back. Rather than kick one leg out to the side, the deep-water exerciser should match the movement on the other side with the other leg. In order to keep good balance and alignment in deep water, every move needs to be balanced by an opposite move.

Equipment

All participants in deep-water exercise should use flotation belts or vests. An AquaJogger, Wet Vest, Hydro-Tone, Sprint/Rothhammer and J & B Foam's belt all work to keep the exerciser afloat. Even good swimmers and floaters should wear flotation devices so they can concentrate on performing the exercises correctly, rather than on treading water.

The workout intensity can be increased by using equipment like Hydro-Fit or Aqua Jazz that not only keeps the participants afloat but also increases the resistance. These kinds of equipment use the concepts of both buoyancy and resistance, rather than just buoyancy. As with all equipment designed to increase intensity, the principle of progressive overload should be followed.

Water Depth

Although most deep-water training occurs in water 8 to 12 feet deep, shallower water can be used. With the proper buoyant equipment, exercisers can do deep-water training in water three to four inches less than their heights. For example, a 5-foot, 4-inch individual can deep-water train in water five feet deep.

Comparison to Land Workout

Long-distance runners are told to put in one hundred miles a week during training. Deep-water exercise makes that obsolete. With three or four deep-water workouts a week, long-distance runners can cut their mileage up to 50%. A Clemson University runner whose personal best for the mile was 4 minutes, 18 seconds trained in the water for four weeks and was able to run a 4-minute, 3-second mile (Murphy, 1985).

Purpose/Benefits

The purpose of deep-water exercise is to improve cardiorespiratory fitness. Other benefits include improvements in body composition, flexibility, and muscular endurance. Deep-water exercise is especially suited to the well-conditioned participant but it also works well for injured, older, and obese adults who cannot tolerate any impact. Other advantages to deep-water exercise include reduced pressure on joints and bones, elimination of neuromuscular trauma, and an increased speed and endurance.

Common Errors

The most common mistake in deep-water exercise is poor alignment. Most exercisers lean forward, backward, or to the side during different exercises. Poor alignment makes the exercises easier to do but keeps from working the proper muscles. Leaning forward while running through the water makes it easier to cover more space, more quickly. Keeping the body in an upright, vertical, aligned posture creates more frontal resistance and, therefore, increases the intensity. This keeps the body in good alignment during training, causes cocontraction in the abdominal and back muscles, strengthens them, and allows the muscles that are being used to properly work, contract, and elongate.

Circuit Training

Definition

Circuit training is an aerobic workout that combines strength training and aerobic conditioning. It uses the aerobic and anaerobic energy systems. Circuit training takes place during the aerobic portion of a cardiorespiratory workout. The program follows the format for all cardiorespiratory workouts defined earlier in this chapter. The complete warm-up (thermal, stretch, and cardio) is followed by a 20- to 40-minute circuit-training aerobic portion. Participants work one muscle group, usually with equipment, for 30 to 60 seconds, and then move to aerobics for 1 to 3 minutes. Following the aerobic interval, participants work another muscle group. This is continued until all major muscle groups have been used for 20 to 40 minutes. The cooldown follows, with the poststretch or flexibility segment at the end.

DIAGRAM 2-12 Circuit Training

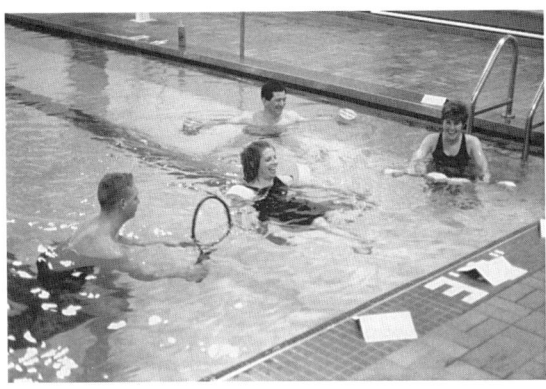

Format

Strength circuits usually are set up in stations around the edge of the pool so students can move to a different station during each strength segment. This is called the **self-guided method.** Only students who are well motivated and understand how to perform the moves at each station will achieve good results. If all the participants need more help and there is enough equipment, everyone in the class can move to the edge of the pool and do the same strength move together. This allows the instructor to give the group motivational hints, correctional cues, and information on the muscle being used. This is called the **group-travel method.** People at all fitness levels are able to participate in circuit-training programs by personally modifying the intensity level of the strength and aerobic portions of the workout.

Equipment

Many different kinds of equipment can be used during circuit training. SPRI tubing, Dynabands, buoyant devices (such as Nuvo Sport Spa Bells, J & B Foam, B-Wise Fitness Bars, Hydro-Fit, and Sprint/Rothhammer), resistant devices (such as Nuvo Sport Spa Bells and Hydro-Tone), weights, and the Aquarius Water Workout Station all help create the overload needed on the muscles during the strength circuits. The equipment should be simple to put on, and it should be left on throughout the entire workout to be sure the training intensity level is not lost.

Water Depth

Circuit training can be done at the shallow (midriff to armpit) end of the pool or in the diving well. If deep water is used, participants should wear flotation vests or belts.

Comparison to Land Workout

Circuit training in water compares well to land-based circuit training. Done in water, the exercises cause less stress and less muscle soreness than land-based exercises. Similar results will be achieved in both water- and land-based circuit training.

Purpose/Benefits

The goal of aquatic circuit training is to achieve both cardiorespiratory fitness and improved muscular strength. Body composition, muscular endurance, and flexibility also improve during a circuit-training program. Both strength trainers who want to add cardiorespiratory training to their workout and aerobics students who want to add some strength training to their workout benefit from circuit training. Circuits add variety to the workout and help students avoid burnout and exercise plateaus. The minor components of physical fitness (coordination, power, agility, and balance) all improve. People at all fitness levels are able to participate in circuit-training programs by personally modifying the intensity level of the strength and aerobic portions of the workout.

Since circuit training has become popular, other kinds of circuits have also been developed. Sports circuits using sports-conditioning moves at different stations can be done. Motor-skill circuits, calisthenic circuits, and interval-training circuits also can be done.

Common Errors

A common mistake made during circuit training is losing continuous movement and, therefore, aerobic training effect. Students who tire during the strength stations need to be reminded to keep moving even if they have to slow down. Students also can lose aerobic conditioning while moving to the pool edge if they do not move quickly. Picking up or putting on equipment is another time when students may stop continuous movement. If continuous movement is not stressed, the workout loses many of its benefits.

Strength-training moves should be full range of motion, slow, and controlled. All major muscles should be used during a circuit-training class. (Read the Strength Training segment, earlier in this chapter, for more information on speed of moves and muscle balance.)

Alignment is important. Students' hips, shoulders, and ears should be in a straight line if viewed from the side. Proper postural alignment helps prevent injuries in the exercise program.

The strength-training moves should be powerful, putting as much muscle as possible behind each rep. Power, not speed, should be encouraged.

Plyometric Training

Definition

Plyometrics has become popular as a training technique to improve power, speed, and jumping abilities in athletes. **Plyometric training** involves a series of jumping, bounding, and hopping moves. The program begins with the easiest type of exercise (inplace jumps) and progresses to the most demanding (bench jumps). Plyometrics is an anaerobic training program that is used by highly conditioned athletes whose sports involve power, speed, or jumping. It can be incorporated into a water aerobics class for the well conditioned. Plyometric moves work well in sport-specific-training, circuit-training, and interval-training programs.

Inplace jumps (described in Chapter 9) used in plyometrics include scissor jumps, jumping-jack jumps, and tuck jumps. Inplace jumps begin with two feet and progress to one-foot jumps.

Hops are the next progression and include skipping, hopping, and hopping up steps. Participants begin in place and gradually move forward, backward, and sideways. During these hops, the athlete jumps up with complete plantar flexion of the ankle joint.

Bounding is the next progression. It involves both inplace jumps and hopping, covering as much distance as possible.

Bench jumps are the final progression. These involve jumping on and off benches that are 10 to 20 inches high (depending on the conditioning level of the participant) using tuck jumps, long jumps, and side jumps.

Format

Participants begin with about 12 reps of each jump and progress to about 20. A total of 100 jumps per workout for a beginning program and 300 jumps per workout for an advanced program is average. Maximum effort should be expended during each move. A rest period of one to two minutes between exercises is required.

Equipment

Equipment is unnecessary for beginning students but can be added as students progress. Resistant equipment, such as Hydro-Tone and Nuvo Sport Spa Bells, increases drag and enhances intensity. Other equipment, like aqua gloves by Sprint/Rothhammer and Hydro-Fit, can improve distance jumps while using upper-body muscles.

Water Depth

Ideal water depth is midriff to armpit. Armpit depth is better for strong participants and those who cannot tolerate heavy impact. Waist to midriff depth is good for weak students if they can tolerate the impact.

DIAGRAM 2-13 Plyometrics

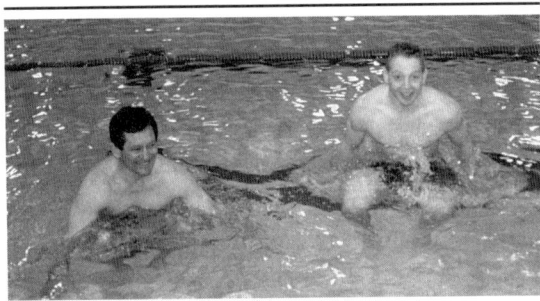
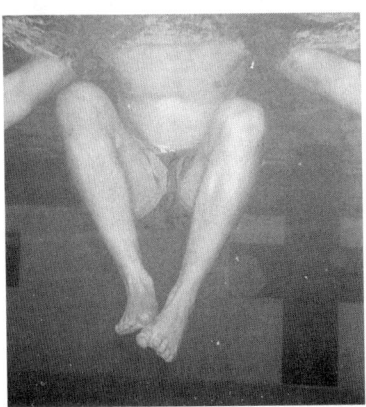

Comparison to Land Workout

Plyometric training done in water allows the exerciser to work out with less incidence of injury because of water buoyancy. The exerciser is challenged more in water than on land because of water resistance.

Purpose/Benefits

The purpose of plyometric training is not to achieve aerobic conditioning but rather anaerobic conditioning. Benefits include increased aerobic capacity, increased muscular strength and endurance, and improved body composition.

Common Errors

The most common error made in classes using plyometric moves is allowing students to slow down and not use maximum effort. Participants should make an all-out effort all the time.

Relaxation Techniques

Purpose

Relaxation techniques frequently are used to augment or add variety to aquatic exercise classes. Some of the techniques discussed can be done while in the water; others need to be done on the deck. It is possible to use just portions of any of these relaxation techniques during a two- to three-minute relaxation period at the end of class.

Exercise participants often are unconsciously tense or tight because of stressful situations in their everyday lives. As the specific muscles that are tense or tight get tired of being continually contracted, they "give notice" by feeling sore and being stiff and aching, freezing, or going into spasm. The muscles that are habitually contracted by tension are being forced to work when no work is required. This tends to shorten these muscles, which contributes to muscular imbalance, which in turn causes aches or pains and further tightening. Relaxation techniques can assist participants in improving muscle balance.

Types

There are two basic types of relaxation techniques. Muscle-to-mind approaches use muscular contraction and release to make the entire body—including the mind—relax. Mind-to-muscle techniques use the mind and its abilities to relax the entire body, including the muscles.

Muscle-to-Mind. Breath awareness is one example of a muscle-to-mind relaxation approach. Breathing techniques are the simplest tools for promoting relaxation. Simply being aware of each inhalation and exhalation begins the relaxation approach. Participants are encouraged to feel that fresh, clean air is entering the body during the inhalation and that impurities are leaving the body during exhalation. Participants also are asked to pay attention to the time between inhalation and exhalation; some count to any number between 4 and 10 during each inhalation and exhalation.

Progressive relaxation is another muscle-to-mind relaxation technique. Participants contract specific muscles in the body and then relax them to "let go." The progression generally goes up through the body, beginning with

DIAGRAM 2–14 Relaxation

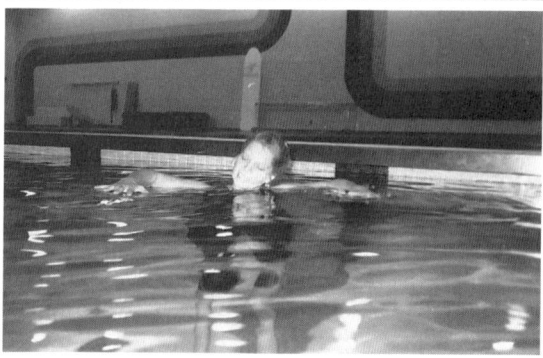

the feet. The progression also can work down, beginning with the head. Each muscle group is contracted approximately 5 times for 10 seconds each time. The first one or two contractions are strong all-out contractions. The following two contractions use only half the tension, and the last contraction is barely strong enough to be felt.

Mind-to-Muscle. Meditation is a form of mind-to-muscle relaxation technique. It focuses one's attention on a single syllable or sound. The participant attempts to totally clear his or her mind from any interfering thoughts or distractions.

Benson's relaxation response is another mind-to-muscle technique. A Harvard cardiologist named Herbert Benson brought some of the concepts and principles of Eastern forms of meditation to the West (Riposo, 1985). His relaxation response technique is similar to meditation. The environment must be comfortable and quiet. Benson uses words, such as *one* and *relax* as the syllable or sound to be repeated. He recommends that participants have a passive attitude during meditation, allowing thoughts to come into the mind, gently pushing them back out, and refocusing on the word or sound.

Imagery or visualization is a relaxation technique frequently used by aerobics instructors. Research shows that by imagining themselves in successful situations, people can enhance their own success. This concept is used in imagery and visualization relaxation. The instructor often verbally guides the class into a relaxing environment, such as a beach or mountain retreat. The relaxing environment is then described by the instructor in more detail, while the participants relax and visualize the new setting.

Autogenic training is a form of relaxation in which the body is trained to produce sensations of heaviness and warmth. The learning process is based on techniques similar to meditation and visualization, with concentration focused on the sensations. There are six stages of application for the technique:

1. heaviness in the arms and then the legs
2. warmth in the arms and the legs
3. heartrate regulation
4. breathing-rate regulation
5. warmth in the solar plexus
6. coolness in the forehead

Instructors using imagery and visualization talk students through this type of relaxation technique, going through each of the six stages gradually.

CHOOSING AN AQUATIC FITNESS PROGRAM

Choosing a program can be confusing. Cardiorespiratory fitness and body composition change are the goals of most participants. Many want to lose weight, which can be done best by burning calories through cardiorespiratory or aerobic training. Most want to look good, which comes from having a good lean-to-fat mass ratio, or good body composition. That is achieved best through cardiorespiratory training with some strength training. Match the goal with the purpose of the class.

The instructor should be adequately trained to create an aquatic fitness program. **Instructor certification** programs are offered by the Aquatic Exercise Association. Certification shows that the instructor has studied for and passed a training program of basic standards to teach aquatic exercise. The instructor should accept all persons in class, make modifications for special situations, and be prompt, courteous and motivating. For more information on specific knowledge necessary, see Chapter 12.

Heartrate or perceived exertion should be checked during an aerobics class to be sure cardiorespiratory conditioning is taking place.

All classes should begin with a warm-up before getting into the actual work segment of the class. All classes should end with a cooldown and final stretch segment. All classes also should include balanced workouts in terms of muscle groups used.

Finding programs that meet specific needs can be challenging but also rewarding. Fitness goals can be met easily with the right class or mix of classes.

KEY WORDS

Warm-up
Thermal warm-up
Prestretch
Cardiorespiratory warm-up
Respiration
Intensity
Cardiorespiratory workout
Mode
Duration
Frequency
Toning
Flexibility
Body alignment
Muscle balance

Water walking
Shallow water jogging
Water aerobics
Water toning
Repetitions
Lactic acid
Muscle contraction
Sets
ACSM resistance guidelines
Flexibility training
Static
Ballistic
Stretch-reflex

Aqua-power aerobics
Sport-specific workouts
Bench aerobics
Interval training
Cycle
Work-to-recovery ratio
Deep-water exercise
Circuit training
Self-guided method
Group-travel method
Plyometric training
Relaxation techniques
Instructor certification

SUMMARY

— The format of aquatic exercise programs varies depending on their goals.
— Water aerobic classes usually begin with a thermal warm-up.
— A prestretch segment after the thermal warm-up is designed to prevent injury during the workout.
— The cardiorespiratory warm-up includes moderate intensity moves and follows the prestretch.
— The aerobic portion, following the cardiorespiratory warm-up, is the "calorie-burning" segment.
— The cooldown uses large, rhythmical movements.
— Toning or strength work usually follows the cooldown.
— The water aerobics class always should end with a poststretch or flexibility section.
— The ACSM has made recommendations regarding the mode, duration, intensity and frequency of a quality training program.

— Water walking is simply striding in waist-to-chest-deep water.
— Shallow-water jogging is done with bounding or leaping steps.
— Water aerobics includes a wide variety of dance and calisthenic moves.
— Water-toning programs are created specifically to improve muscular endurance.
— Strength training in water is a program aimed specifically at body building.
— Flexibility-training participants stretch different muscle groups to improve their long-term flexibility.
— Aqua-power aerobics is a program that combines cardiorespiratory conditioning, strength training, and muscle toning in the aerobic portion of the workout.
— Sport-specific workouts are aerobic workouts that are designed to assist sports enthusiasts in developing the muscle strength and flexibility, skills, agility, balance, and coordination needed in their sport.

- Bench workouts are aerobic workouts that achieve cardiorespiratory conditioning through stepping up and down on a bench.
- Interval training is an exertive exercise program usually reserved for well-conditioned athletes.
- Deep-water exercise refers to any type of water exercise program done in water depth above the participant's head.
- Circuit training is an aerobic workout that combines strength training and aerobic conditioning.
- Plyometric training is a popular training technique to improve power, speed, and jumping abilities in athletes.
- Relaxation techniques frequently are used to augment or add variety to aquatic exercise classes.
- Match the goal of the participant to the purpose of the class when choosing a fitness program.
- Be sure the instructor is qualified.

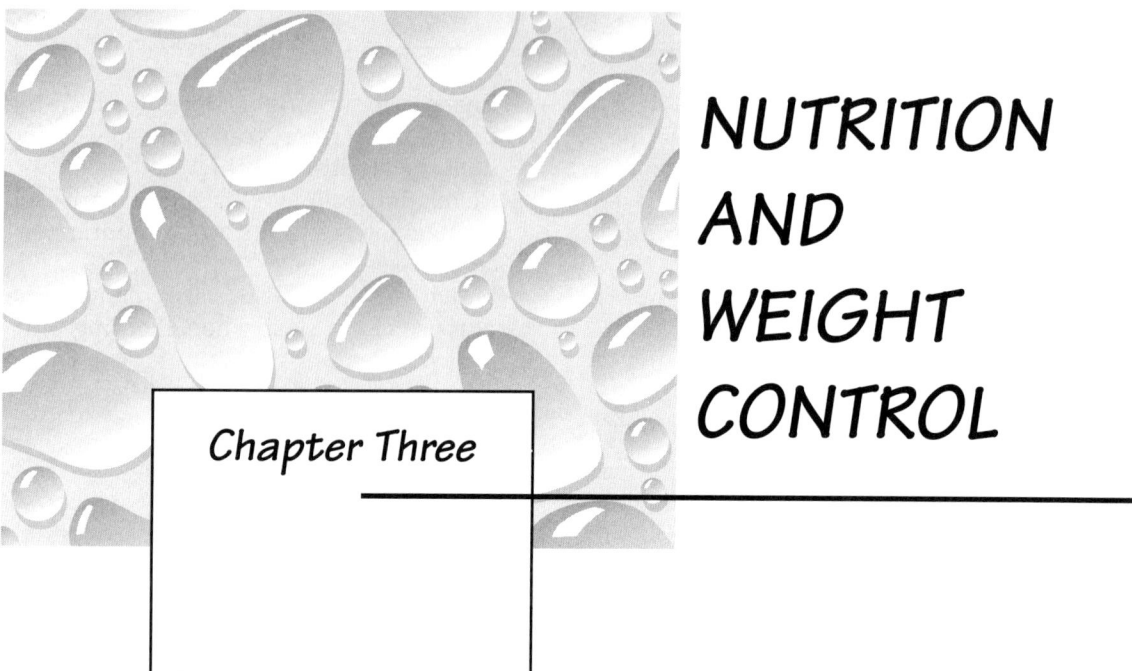

NUTRITION AND WEIGHT CONTROL

Chapter Three

NUTRITION

The most important thing a student can do to enhance his or her state of health is maintain proper **nutrition.** The body cannot function well without a proper supply of nutrients and energy. Students need to know the basics of good nutrition to ensure their diets supply the best possible balance of nutrients for good health and adequate calories to meet their energy requirements.

Water

Water is the most essential nutrient and also probably the most important in relation to physical performance. Approximately 60% of body weight is water that comes from three sources: (1) fluids we drink, (2) water in foods (lettuce and celery are over 90% water, bread is about 36%), and (3) metabolic water, which is the by-product of numerous chemical reactions in the body.

Under normal circumstances, about two quarts of water are lost each day. Water leaves the body in urine and feces, in exhaled air, and through the skin. Kidney function maintains the crucial and delicate balance of water in the body.

During exercise, water is needed to control body temperature. This is achieved through the production and evaporation of sweat through the skin. In addition to water, sweat contains *electrolytes*—the **minerals** sodium, potassium, and chloride—which are important for fluid balance and nerve and muscle function. Inadequate water intake before and during exercise adversely affects athletic performance and heat tolerance, possibly leading to heat cramps, heat exhaustion, and heatstroke.

Cardiovascular performance also can be impaired. Fluid depletion lowers blood volume, leading to decreased stroke volume and a corresponding increase in heartrate at the same workload. As temperature and humidity increase, so does the need for water.

Drinking water is the safest way to replace lost sweat. It is important to be aware that during heavy exercise, thirst is not a good indicator of the need for water. It is a good practice to drink water before, during, and after exercise.

Guidelines for Good Nutrition

In 1979, the U.S. Food and Drug Administration developed four broad classifications of foods, based on certain key **nutrients** (Riposo, 1990). The groups include fruits and vegetables, grain products, milk and milk products, and meats and meat substitutes. While recommendations for the number of servings per day from each group vary, based on age and growth development, a recommended average diet includes the following:

- Fruits and vegetables, 4 servings daily
- Grain products (breads and cereals), 4 servings daily
- Milk and milk products, 2 servings daily
- Meats and meat substitutes, 2 servings daily

The recommended servings from the basic four food groups furnish approximately 1,200 to 1,500 calories per day and adequate amounts of essential nutrients, provided a variety of foods are selected.

In 1977, the Senate Agricultural Subcommittee on Nutrition set the following dietary guidelines to improve Americans' health and quality of life:

1. Avoid becoming overweight by consuming only as much energy (**calories**) as can be expended. If overweight, decrease energy intake, and increase energy expenditure.
2. Eat enough complex **carbohydrates** and naturally occurring sugars to account for about 40% of energy intake. Do this by eating fresh fruits, vegetables, whole grains, and products made with stoneground flour. Restrict the intake of refined sugars and fruits that contain sucrose, corn sugar, and corn syrup.
3. Limit overall fat consumption to approximately 30% of your energy intake. Restrict consumption of saturated fats by choosing meats, poultry, fish, and dairy products that are low in saturated fat. Restrict consumption of saturated fats to about 10% of the total energy intake, with polyunsaturated fats accounting for 20%.
4. Maintain **cholesterol** consumption at about 300 mg per day by controlling the amount of milk products, eggs, and butter fat consumed.
5. Limit intake of sodium to less than 5 grams per day by controlling consumption of salt and processed foods.
6. Reduce consumption of artificial colorings, artificial flavorings, thickeners, preservatives, and other food additives. (Riposo, 1985)

In 1979, the Department of Agriculture and the Department of Health and Human Services published "Nutrition and Your Health, Dietary Guidelines for Americans," which is the source of the following recommendations:

1. Eat a variety of foods daily, including selections of fruits; vegetables; whole-grain and enriched breads, cereals, and grain products; milk, cheese, and yogurt; meats, poultry, fish, and eggs; and legumes (dry peas and beans).
2. Maintain acceptable body weight by losing any excess and improving eating habits. To lose weight, increase physical activity, eat less fat and fatty foods, eat less sugar and sweets, and avoid too much alcohol. To improve eating habits, eat slowly, prepare smaller portions, and avoid seconds.
3. Avoid too much fat, saturated fat, and cholesterol. Choose lean meat, fish, poultry, dry beans, and peas as **protein**

sources. Moderate consumption of eggs and organ meats (liver). Limit intake of butter, cream, hydrogenated margarines, shortenings, coconut oil, and foods made from such products. Trim excess fat off meats. Broil, bake, or boil rather than fry. Read labels carefully to determine both amounts and types of fat contained in foods.
4. Eat foods with adequate *starch* and *fiber*: Substitute starches for fats and sugars, and select foods that are good sources of fiber and starch, such as whole-grain breads and cereals, fruits and vegetables, beans, peas, and nuts.
5. Avoid too much sugar. Use less of all sugars, including white sugar, brown sugar, raw sugar, honey, and syrup. Eat less food containing these sugars, such as candy, soft drinks, ice cream, cake, and cookies. Select fresh fruits or canned fruits without sugar or in light syrup rather than heavy syrup. Read food labels for clues on sugar content. If the ingredients *sucrose, glucose, maltose, dextrose, lactose, fructose,* or *syrups* appear first, the product contains a large amount of sugar. And remember: How *often* you eat sugar is as important as how *much* sugar you eat.
6. Avoid too much **sodium.** Learn to enjoy the unsalted flavors of foods. Cook with only small amounts of added salt. Add little or no salt to foods at the table. Limit intake of salty foods, such as potato chips, pretzels, salted nuts, popcorn, condiments (soy sauce, steak sauce, garlic salt), cheese, pickled foods, and cured meats. Read food labels carefully to determine amounts of sodium in processed foods and snack items.
7. If you drink alcohol, do so in moderation. Refrain from sustained or heavy drinking (more than two drinks per day).

WEIGHT CONTROL

When considering the issues of body weight and body fat, it is useful to think of the body as being composed of two distinct parts: (1) lean body mass, and (2) fat body mass. The *lean body mass* is the fat-free component, which consists of water, electrolytes, minerals, glycogen stores, muscle tissue, internal organs, and bones.

Fat body mass, or **body fat,** is composed of two parts: essential fat and storage fat. *Essential fat* is necessary for normal physiological functioning and nerve conduction. It makes up approximately 3% to 7% of total body weight in men and about 15% in women. *Storage fat,* which is also called *depot fat,* constitutes anywhere from a few percent of total body weight on a lean individual to 40% to 50% of body weight on an obese person. For most people, concerns about being overweight actually are concerns about being overfat. Body-fat standards for men indicate that lean is 5% to 10%, ideal is 18%, and obese is 20% and over. Body-fat standards for women show lean as 10% to 20%, ideal as 22%, and obese as 30% and over.

Fads and Fallacies

Current social standards call for the slim-and-fit look. The weight-control industry has cashed in on this ideal; it is bigger than ever, with annual sales over $220 million. Unfortunately, some weight-control regimens and products make exaggerated claims and are grossly misleading. Whatever weight loss they produce usually is a reduction in lean body tissue or in body water. The only proven way to reduce body fat is to make lifestyle changes that include different eating behaviors and increased levels of physical activity.

Spot Reduction

Spot reduction is not possible. Individuals cannot lose fat from a specific location on the body. In one study, subjects did 5,000 sit-ups over a 27-day period; afterward, fat biopsies showed no preferential loss of fat in the abdominal area (Riposo, 1990). Exercises for specific parts of the body may strengthen the muscles there, but they have no effect on fat. Fat that is burned during exercise comes from all over the body in a genetically predetermined pattern.

Saunas and Steambaths

Saunas and steambaths produce weight loss by using heat to induce sweating. Since only water weight is lost, the pounds are regained quickly when fluid is restored by drinking.

Saunas and steambaths may be dangerous for the elderly and people suffering from diabetes, heart disease, or high blood pressure. Risks increase with the use of alcohol, drugs, and certain medications.

Body Wraps

In some reduction programs, bandages are soaked in a "magic" solution and wrapped tightly around the body. While this may compress the skin and move body fluids around, the change in body size is temporary. There is no actual weight loss.

Nonporous Sweatsuits

Plastic or rubberized garments produce temporary weight loss by inducing sweating. Again, however, this is water weight being lost; it will be regained quickly. When worn during exercise, such garments increase the risk of dehydration and heat-related injury.

Vibrating Belts

These and other passive mechanical devices, such as motor-driven toning machines and bicycles, do not induce weight loss or contribute to fitness. Vibrating belts may even be harmful when used on the abdomen, especially by women who are pregnant, menstruating, or using an IUD.

Diet Pills

Most diet pills sold over the counter contain phenylpropanolamine (PPA), which is a chemical relative to amphetamines or speed. Diet pills temporarily decrease appetite; typically, any weight loss is rapidly regained when the user stops taking them. Besides the danger of dependency, diet pills with PPA cause a sharp, potentially dangerous increase in blood pressure, and heart abnormalities also have been reported.

Fasting

Diet programs that severely restrict caloric intake should only be undertaken under direct medical supervision. **Fasting** results in the loss of large amounts of water, minerals, and lean body tissue, such as muscle. It also results in a minimal amount of fat loss. Prolonged fasting may cause dizziness and fainting, gout, anemia, kidney damage, hair loss, muscle cramping, reduced physical capabilities, emotional disturbances, and even death. Most people who reduce by fasting or through very-low calorie diets tend to regain much or all of the weight lost.

A change in dietary habits or physical activity aids in weight control and weight loss. A combination of diet and exercise is the ultimate weight-loss program.

Approaches to Weight Loss

Diet

Controlling diet by itself results in weight loss, even when daily caloric restriction is fairly modest. For example, if a dieter were to eat consistently over a long period of time 100 fewer calories a day (the equivalent of one bran muffin, one tablespoon of peanut butter, or one Bartlett pear), he or she would have a 700-calorie-per-week deficit. Since a deficit of 3,500 calories is needed to lose one pound of body fat, the dieter would lose a pound every five weeks, or ten pounds in a year.

Unfortunately, few people are patient enough to accept such a gradual weight loss. Instead, most are likely to restrict caloric intake substantially when beginning a diet. While they may have initial success, the weight usually is regained in the long run for several reasons.

First, it is difficult to stay on a low-calorie diet for a long period of time, and also it is unhealthy. Adequate essential nutrients may be lacking in diets that furnish fewer than 2,000 calories a day. Initial weight loss is a result of the depletion of carbohydrate stores in body fat and is quickly regained if normal eating resumes.

A second set of problems with dieting has to do with the "energy-out" side of the equation. The body "spends" at least two-thirds of its energy on basal metabolism, which includes all the processes that go on inside the body to support life, such as heartbeat, breathing, nerve and muscle impulses, and metabolic activity of cells. The remainder is spent on physical activity, or if unneeded, stored as fat.

The body has an internal mechanism to protect itself against starvation. When food intake is restricted, physiological changes cause a decrease in **basal metabolic rate (BMR).** In other words, the body automatically conserves energy, which causes a less effective diet. Over a period of time, weight loss by diet alone can cause a significant loss of lean body mass (LBM). Since LBM is more active metabolically than fat, the effect is to reduce BMR even further.

And finally, since dieters often feel tired and lethargic, they also tend to decrease physical activity, further lowering the output side of the equation.

Exercise

Exercise by itself also produces weight loss. A 150-pound person who walks at a normal pace for one-half hour, five times a week, burns 810 calories a week and achieves a weight loss of about 1 pound (a 3,500-calorie deficit) in about 30 days. If food consumption remains the same, this modest exercise program results in a loss of 12 pounds in a year.

The best exercise program for weight loss involves aerobic, endurance-type activities. With regular exercise, some of the factors that tilt the energy balance toward the deficit side are:

1. *Increase expenditure for physical activity*—Not only are more calories burned during physical activity, but energy expenditure has been shown to remain elevated for several hours afterward.
2. *Increase BMR*—Aerobic exercise increases the use of fatty acids for fuel in the muscles and speeds up the release of fat from storage. Exercise also increases bone mass and muscle density. The result is a change in body composition. Since LBM is more metabolically active than fat, exercise increases BMR, even at rest.
3. *Reduce appetite*—Moderate aerobic exercise has been shown to slightly depress the appetite.

Diet and Exercise Combined

By combining diet and exercise—reducing calorie intake by 100 calories a day and walking for 30 minutes, five times a week—our hypothetical 150-pound person could lose 22 pounds per year. People who incorporate regular aerobic exercise in a weight-loss program lose more weight than those who do not.

Combining diet and exercise also protects against the loss of lean tissue, eliminates the constant hunger and psychological stress of food deprivation, and allows for flexibility in a weight-loss regimen.

Set-Point Theory

The **set-point theory** states that the body has an internal regulating mechanism that strives to maintain a certain biologically determined body-fat level. In other words, when body-fat stores drop below a certain level, or set point, either because of dieting or starvation, the body automatically reacts to conserve energy by lowering BMR and increasing appetite. When fat stores are above the set point, the body will seek to lower them by decreasing appetite and increasing BMR, or by "wasting" energy. This theory purports to explain why so many people who lose weight by dieting tend to gain it back, and why other people can eat large amounts of food and remain slim.

Heredity, activity level, cigarette smoking, eating habits, and other factors combine to determine an individual's set point. While food deprivation tends to elevate the set point, exercise appears to lower it. Though many other factors are involved, the set-point theory implies that exercise, rather than calorie restriction, should be the first line of treatment for the overweight.

KEY WORDS

Nutrition
Nutrients
Minerals
Calories
Cholesterol
Sodium
Protein
Fiber
Body fat
Spot reduction
Fasting
Carbohydrate
Basal metabolic rate (BMR)
Set-point theory

SUMMARY

— The most important thing a student can do to enhance his or her state of health is maintain proper nutrition.
— Water is the most essential nutrient and also the most important in relation to physical performance.
— The U.S. Food and Drug Administration developed four classifications of foods: fruits and vegetables, grain products, milk and milk products, and meats and meat substitutes.
— The recommended servings from the basic four food groups furnish approximately 1200 to 1500 calories per day and adequate amounts of essential nutrients if a variety of foods are selected.
— When considering the issues of body weight and body fat, think of the body as being composed of two distinct parts: (1) lean body mass, and (2) fat body mass.
— It is not possible to lose fat from a specific location on the body.
— A combination of diet and exercise results in the ultimate weight-loss program.
— The set-point theory states that the body has an internal regulating mechanism that strives to maintain a certain biologically determined body-fat level.

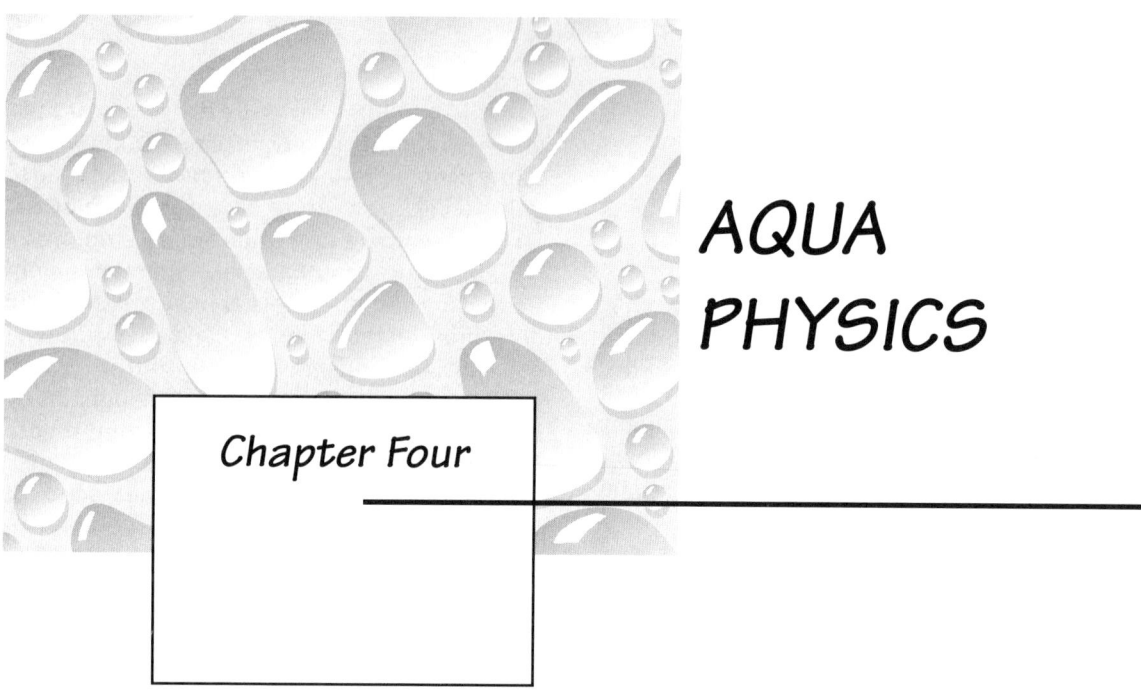

AQUA PHYSICS

Chapter Four

GENERAL INFORMATION

Because of water's unique properties, water-based exercise provides somewhat different benefits than land-based exercise. To allow for those properties, modifications need to be made before using land-based exercises.

Water Resistance

Water resistance is the power of fluid to oppose an exercise movement. Water has approximately 12 times the resistance of air. That resistance may slow the exerciser down, but it gives him or her some tremendous benefits.

Movement Speed

Movement speed refers to the quickness of an exercise motion. When moving in the water, exercisers need to modify the pace of movements to allow for water resistance. The speed must be adjusted so movements are accomplished without jerking or compromising alignment and use a full range of motion. Movements always should be controlled. If the exercise being done causes the body to move out of alignment in an uncontrolled fashion, it is too fast. The speed at which one would jog on land is not the speed at which one should jog in water. Likewise, the speed of kicks done on land should not be the same for kicks done in the water. Moving through the water with ballistic, land-based speed movements can cause injuries to the joints and ligaments.

Toning Potential

Water resistance, while slowing an exerciser down, also provides excellent benefits. When moving through water, one not only receives cardiovascular benefits (by pushing the heartrate or perceived exertion level up into the target zone); one also receives toning benefits not available on land. Water resistance acts with equalized pressure on all submerged body parts. Any time a limb is moved through the water, additional toning occurs because of water resistance.

Muscle Balance

Muscle balance is another benefit of working in water. Almost all joints in the body have some muscles that flex them and other muscles that extend them. The two muscles that work a joint (flex and extend) are generally thought of as a pair, or muscle pair. The **flexors** almost always are stronger than the extensors. The **extensors** generally work with gravity, which does the work for them; thus, extensors usually are not well developed. If exercise programs contribute to naturally occurring muscle imbalance, injury could result, especially if those joints are weight bearing.

When participants exercise in water, they receive equalized muscle balance that is not available through any other medium. Due to the flotation effect of water, a person working in water uses the iliopsoas (hip flexor) muscles when lifting (kicking forward) the leg and gets the additional benefit (not received on land) of using the gluteals and hamstrings when lowering the leg back through the water. The same is true with the bicep and tricep muscle pair and most other muscle pairs in the body. The tricep gets virtually no work during arm extensions in land-based exercises (gravity does the work). Water resistance, however, forces the tricep to work when doing arm extensions. Muscle balance is a tremendous benefit of water exercise.

Energy Expenditure

A water workout gives a greater **energy expenditure** than a similar land-based exercise. When walking on land, each step recruits a certain amount of muscle fibers. Each muscle fiber needs a certain amount of oxygen to keep it going. **Oxygen consumption** correlates with energy and caloric consumption. When the same walking is done in water, more muscle fibers need to be recruited for each step taken. That means more oxygen is used, and there is greater energy and caloric expenditure.

Water-based exercise achieves a workout intensity similar to that of land-based exercise with less heart stress. One function of the heart is to help the body dissipate heat. If the heart has to work at dissipating heat at the same time it is working to deliver oxygen to muscles, it can become overloaded and work at a higher rate (beats per minute) than necessary for cardiovascular fitness. If the body is cooled by water and the heart does not have to work at dissipating heat, it can concentrate on simply supplying oxygen to the muscles. Thus, a similar workout intensity is achieved while maintaining a lower heartrate.

Arm Movements

Arm movements in aquatic exercise can be used in much the same way they are used on land: for variety and fun, for balance, for coordination improvement, and for adding intensity to the workout. In addition, arm movements can be used for other purposes more particularly suited to aquatic exercise.

Arm movements can help the body move through water. By pressing the hands from front to back, the exerciser is propelled forward. By starting with the arms to the right and sweeping left, the participant slides to the right. If the hands are pushed straight down, the body will spring up. Each of these movements can be reversed for the opposite effect.

The benefit of using arms to assist with movement in the water becomes apparent when the body presents a large surface area and is, therefore, resistant to the movement. For example, when a participant is facing straight forward and attempts to jump ahead through the water, the frontal resistance of the body is at its greatest. It is extremely difficult to accomplish this movement without using the arms. As one jogs through the water, more territory can be covered if arms are added to the movement to help pull the body forward.

Changing directions can produce swirls of water, which make movement more difficult. Appropriate arm movements can assist the body in accomplishing direction changes.

In the water, when the body is at a standstill, it takes more effort to put it into motion than it does to maintain a standstill. Upper-body movements can add to the total effort and make it possible to overcome this resistance.

All the while arms are being used in the water for balance, coordination, movement assists, or fun, they are also developing upper-body muscular endurance and strength. Pushing, pulling, sweeping, flicking, and lifting all work muscles in the upper and lower arms, the shoulders, the chest, the abdominals, and the upper and lower back. If arms are kept submerged while executing the movements, the potential for gains is greater, because water resistance acts like weights or bands to increase the difficulty of the exercise. Although some land-based movements are advantageous for the students and assure that joints move through a full range of motion, the benefits of using arms in the water to increase the workload should not be overlooked.

The position of the hands and upper body can increase or decrease the intensity of various exercises. Because swimming programs train people to move efficiently in water, it is sometimes difficult for students to learn to purposely increase water resistance for a more difficult workout.

Presenting a small surface area against the water makes it easier to perform arm movements. For example, turning the hands so they slice through the water requires less upper body effort than if the hands are flattened to the direction of the movement. By choosing the appropriate hand position for each movement, aquatic exercisers can do one movement but develop different degrees of conditioning, depending on the workload they place on the muscle.

In addition to affecting the particular muscles in use, arm movements can affect the cardiorespiratory demands on the body during exercise. Greater demand is placed on the heart and lungs as they work harder to meet the muscles' need for oxygen, nutrients, and waste removal. This is accomplished simply by adding arm movements rather than letting arms hang in the water. Cardiorespiratory conditioning can be boosted even further by cupping or flattening the hands as the arms move through the water.

Water Buoyancy and Cushioning

The cushioning effect is another benefit of exercise in the water. Because of the 90% apparent weight loss in shoulder-depth water, participants can exercise with less biomechanical stress during each footstrike or **impact.** This allows them to exercise longer and more frequently and to gain more benefits without the likelihood of injury.

KEY WORDS

Water resistance
Movement speed
Muscle balance

Energy expenditure
Oxygen consumption
Water buoyancy

Flexors
Extensors
Impact

SUMMARY

—Water has approximately 12 times the resistance of air.

—When moving in the water, exercisers need to modify the pace of movements to allow for the water resistance.

—Water resistance, while slowing an exer-

ciser down, also provides excellent benefits.
- Muscle balance is a benefit of working in water.
- A water workout can give a greater energy expenditure than a similar land-based exercise.
- Water-based exercise can achieve a workout intensity similar to that of land-based exercise with less heart stress.
- Arm movements in the aquatic exercise can be used in much the same way they are used on land: for variety and fun, for balance, for coordination improvement, and to add intensity.
- Arm movements also can be used for purposes more particularly suited to aquatic exercise.
- Because of the 90% apparent weight loss in shoulder-depth water, participants can exercise with less biomechanical stress during each footstrike or impact.

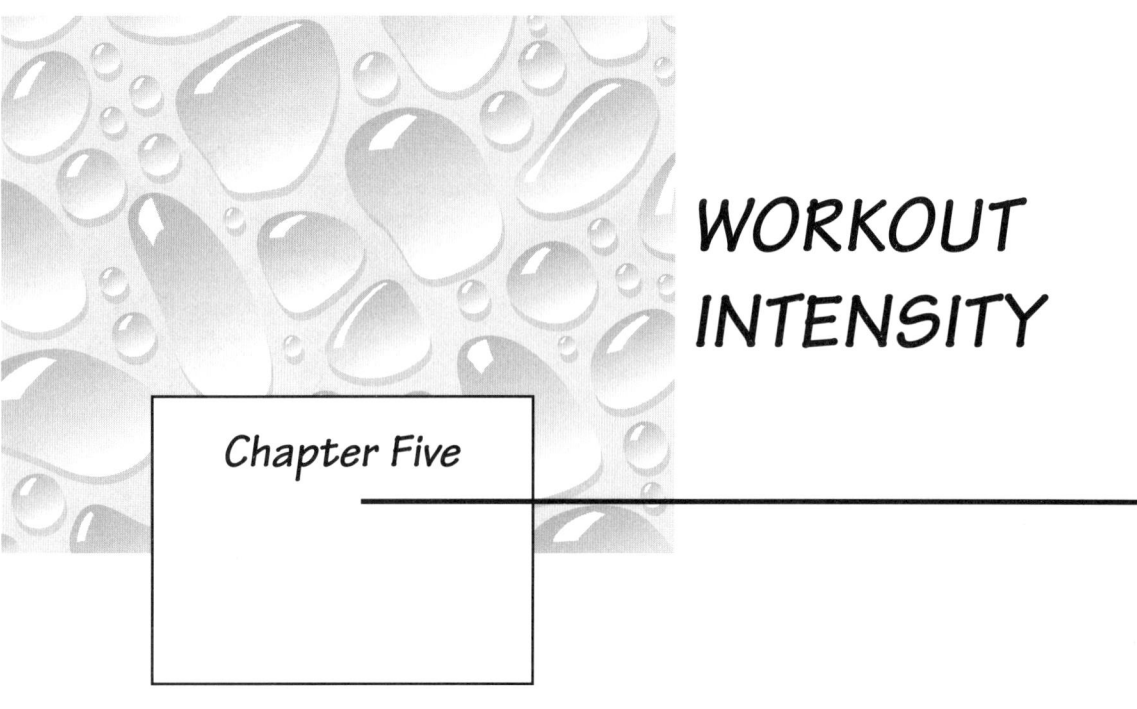

WORKOUT INTENSITY

Chapter Five

USING HEARTRATE TO MEASURE INTENSITY

The relationship between **heartrate** and workout intensity always has been an enigma. Program guidelines advise checking exertion levels during class. However, checking heartrates often seems counterproductive. Many students—especially fit ones—are disappointed to learn that their heartrates usually remain lower than the target range recommended for aerobic improvement. Checking perceived exertion does not seem to work either, because students often do not feel that they work as hard in a water exercise class as they do outside running or in a land-based aerobics class.

What is a participant to do? Exertion levels need to be checked, but doing so sometimes leads them to think that water workouts are wimpy. To solve this dilemma, students must have a thorough understanding of heartrates and their significance in aquatics classes.

Terms and Definitions

Several different terms are used to characterize heartrates:

- Resting heartrate (RHR)
- Maximal heartrate
- Working heartrate range
- Minimum working heartrate
- Maximum working heartrate
- Optimum working heartrate
- Target zone
- Recovery heartrate

Resting Heartrate

The **resting heartrate (RHR)** is the number of times the heart beats per minute when the body is at rest. This heartrate usually is counted over 60 seconds. The RHR should be measured before getting up in the morning or after sitting quietly for 20 minutes. To ensure an accurate RHR, the exercise participant should measure the resting heartrate on three separate occasions and take the average.

Maximal Heartrate

The **maximal heartrate** is the greatest number of times per minute the heart is capable of beating. It is the highest heartrate a person can attain during heavy exercise. An accurate measure of the maximal heartrate can be determined by a graded exercise test called a *stress electrocardiogram*. Exercise leaders who do not have access to, or the training necessary to do, a stress electrocardiogram often calculate maximal heartrate by subtracting the participant's age from 220. This number is the general estimation for the maximal heartrate.

Working Heartrate Range

The **working heartrate range** is the zone within which an individual needs to work for aerobic training to take place. It is the area between, and including, the minimum working heartrate and the maximum working heartrate. When the exercising heartrate remains in this zone, cardiorespiratory conditioning is likely to occur. The training intensity range often varies from as little as 50% to 85% of maximal oxygen consumption. A linear relationship exists between heartrate, oxygen consumption, and workload or workout intensity in most land-based exercise situations. Because of that, the *target zone* (target heartrate range or training zone) is used to determine when cardiorespiratory conditioning is occurring during exercise.

Several formulas currently are in use to determine the working heartrate range. The most common (discussed later) is the *Karvonen formula*.

The top of the target zone, which would be the upper limit of suggested exercise intensity, is the highest percentage. The low percentage is used to determine the minimum threshold to improve cardiorespiratory fitness. Students who are unfit or just beginning exercise should use the low percentage or work at or above the minimum working heartrate. As conditioning occurs, students can work at a more comfortable intensity in the middle of the zone. Many internal and external factors affect a participant's heartrate. This zone is merely a guideline. Heartrate varies from person to person and situation to situation.

Minimum Working Heartrate

Minimum working heartrate is at the low end of the working heartrate range. This is the minimum number of times the heart should beat per minute during exercise for cardiorespiratory training to take place. It is sometimes referred to as the *threshold for aerobic training*. Students should know this number so they can work toward it during exercise.

Maximum Working Heartrate

The **maximum working heartrate** is at the upper end of the working heartrate range. This is the maximum number of times the heart should beat per minute during exercise for cardiorespiratory training to take place. Working at a higher level can be dangerous to individuals with known or unsuspected cardiorespiratory disease, and it does not promote efficient use of fats for fuel. Working at a rate higher than the maximum working heartrate is considered an anaerobic workout. The maximum working heartrate is often called the *anaerobic threshold*.

Optimum Working Heartrate

Optimum working heartrate is the ideal number of beats per minute for cardiorespiratory training to take place. There are different optimum working heartrates for different fitness goals. The optimum working heartrate always falls between the minimum working heartrate and the maximum working heartrate.

Target Zone

Target zone is another term for the working heartrate range.

Recovery Heartrate

The **recovery heartrate** is the number of times the heart beats per minute when monitored 5 to 10 minutes after vigorous exercise. It reflects how quickly the cardiorespiratory system returns to its preexercise condition. A more fit person recovers faster than a less fit person. The recovery heartrate often is used as an indicator of cardiorespiratory fitness.

Participants who do not recover to a normal range after five minutes have probably exercised too vigorously and are not conditioned enough to maintain that level for future exercise. They should be cautioned to exercise at a lower intensity during future exercise sessions.

Using Heartrates

It is important to understand heartrate terminology and formulas. Review the previous sections thoroughly to reinforce understanding of these concepts.

Scientists have found that the exercising heartrate often correlates closely to **oxygen consumption** (Pollack et al., 1982). Based on this correlation, a formula was developed for land-based exercise by a scientist named Karvonen that calculates the heartrate an individual must achieve in order to get desired benefits. The formula is adjusted for age and conditioning level. Aquatic exercisers also have begun to adapt it for their fitness programs.

Heartrates can be monitored easily by periodically taking the pulse during an exercise session and then adjusting the exercise intensity to bring the heartrate to the recommended level.

In order to use the formula, exercisers must be taught to monitor their heartrates. Begin by lightly pressing the index and middle fingers on the throat along the carotid artery. Some exercisers prefer to place the fingers on the wrist at the radial pulse. At either site, the exerciser counts the pulsations while the instructor keeps track of time. While counting, the exerciser should be sure to continue to exercise by walking or jogging in place so that the heartrate does not slow down. The thumb should never be used to count pulsation, since it has a pulse of its own.

Formula for Determining Heartrate

Karvonen. The **Karvonen formula** is a scientific formula commonly accepted as the safest way to calculate the appropriate exertion level for land-based aerobic exercise. It is a relatively accurate and popular method of determining target heartrate. The Karvonen formula has an error rate of plus or minus 10 beats per minute when used on average individuals in land-based exercise. It is recommended by the American College of Sports Medicine (ACSM).

Actually measuring the maximal heartrate requires special equipment and trained personnel, whereas, the Karvonen formula uses

DIAGRAM 5-1 Karvonen Formula

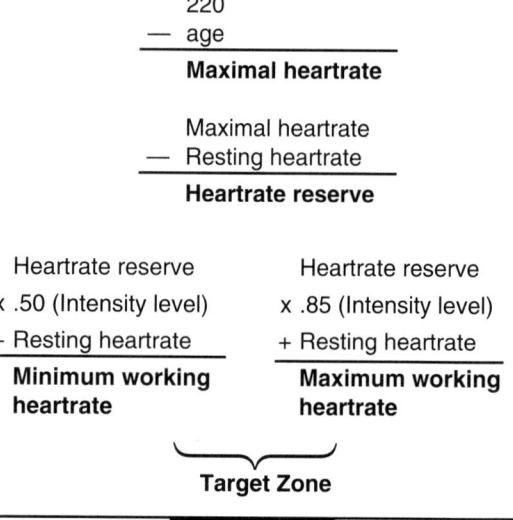

an age-predicted heartrate formula to arrive at the maximal heartrate. The formula is:

220 − age = Maximal heartrate

The age-predicted maximal heartrate formula estimates that 220 is the approximate maximal heartrate of a baby and that each year this rate decreases by one beat. For example, a 20-year-old person would have an estimated maximal heartrate of 200 beats per minute (220 − 20 = 200). A 40-year-old would have an estimated maximal heartrate of 180 (220 − 40 = 180). Although this is a commonly used formula, maximal heartrates often vary by plus or minus 10 beats per minute at any given age.

The Karvonen formula then goes on to calculate the heartrate reserve, which is the difference between the resting heartrate and the maximal heartrate. This portion of the formula is:

Maximal heartrate
− Resting heartrate
Heartrate reserve

For example, a 40-year-old with a resting heartrate of 60 beats per minute would have a heartrate reserve of 120 (220 − 40 = 180; 180 − 60 = 120).

Once the heartrate reserve has been calculated for each participant, the Karvonen formula becomes simple. The target heartrate equals the heartrate reserve times the percentage of intensity plus the resting heartrate. The training intensity range used in the Karvonen formula is 50% to 85% of maximal heartrate reserve.

For example, a 40-year-old whose resting heartrate is 60 beats per minute is just beginning to exercise regularly and needs to know his or her minimum working heartrate. The heartrate reserve is multiplied by the intensity level, which in this case is 50%, to determine the minimum working heartrate plus the resting heartrate of 60 beats per minute (120 x .50 + 60 = 120). The minimum working heartrate for this exerciser is 120 beats per minute. The maximum working heartrate is determined in the same fashion, but 85% is used for intensity level (120 x .85 + 60 = 162). The maximum working heartrate for this exerciser is 162 beats per minute. The target zone for the exerciser is from 120 to 162 beats per minute.

Heartrate, Oxygen, and Caloric Consumption

Some students in aquatics classes feel they do not get as good a workout in water as they do on land. They definitely are wrong. They need education on heartrate, oxygen consumption, and caloric consumption.

Many students judge the intensity of a workout and, thus, the value of a class by the heartrate they achieve. If their heartrate is up, they are getting a good workout; if it isn't, they are not. Their mistake is assuming that heartrate is always an indication of workout intensity. This is not necessarily true. **Target heartrates are valid indicators of intensity only if they correlate with oxygen consumption.** Because we are aerobic beings, physiologists measure workout intensity, or energy expenditure, by measuring how much oxygen is utilized by the body during a given activity compared with how much oxygen is used at rest.

A given pace of exercise requires a specific amount of oxygen utilization. One quart of oxygen utilization equals 5 calories. If a participant wants to work at a 10-calorie-per-minute pace, he or she needs 2 quarts of oxygen per minute. The average outdoor walker uses 5 calories per minute, which would be 1 quart of oxygen per minute. The average outdoor jogger uses 10 calories per minute or 2 quarts per minute.

This information can make it simple for students to understand that **caloric consumption** is tied to oxygen consumption or utilization, not to heartrate. Heartrate is not always indicative of the amount of calories being burned. If caloric consumption is the exerciser's goal, he or she should increase his or her oxygen consumption, not necessarily his or her heartrate.

Unfortunately, oxygen consumption is measured with expensive, technical, cumbersome equipment that is attached to the exerciser with a breathing apparatus. It is impossible for exercisers outside a laboratory to check oxygen consumption.

That brings us back to heartrate. Heartrate is checked instead of oxygen consumption simply because everyone can do it easily. Formulas have been devised to correlate heartrate almost exactly to oxygen consumption if all conditions are ideal. Many land-based exercises, like running, biking, and aerobics, have almost ideal conditions and can use heartrate as their guide for workout intensity level.

Aquatic Heartrate

Students who participate in both land- and water-based exercise often find their heartrates lower from water exercise than land exercise, yet they receive the same benefits. There are no conclusive studies as to why this happens. There are, however, several commonly accepted theories under investigation.

Theories for Variations

1. **Heat dissipation**—When exercising, the body creates excess heat. The body gets rid of the heat through evaporation (sweat) and radiation (transferring heat to the skin, where it is radiated out to the environment). Because water dissipates heat more effectively than air, it is easier and, therefore, less stressful for the body to get rid of the excess heat in the water than on land. Moreover, less stress on the body results in a lower heartrate.
2. **Gravity**—Water lessens the effect of **gravity** on the body. Not only is it easier to spring up high in water, it also is easier for the blood to be pumped uphill and back to the heart. This lessens the strain on the heart, resulting in a lower exercising heartrate.
3. **Compression**—Water acts like a compressor on the body, lending support. This extra compression is not limited to the superficial skin. It also penetrates to the deeper layers and organs of the body, including the blood vessels. This subtle compression on veins and arteries facilitates bloodflow while exercising, reducing stress on the heart and resulting in a lower working heartrate.
4. **Partial pressure**—Gases enter liquids more easily under pressure. Thus, oxygen is absorbed more easily into the blood during exercise. More efficient oxygen transfer may reduce the workload of the heart.
5. **Dive reflex**—A primitive reflex associated with a nerve found in the nasal area is called the dive reflex. When the face is submerged, this reflex lowers heartrate and blood pressure. This reflex is stronger in some individuals than others. Some research suggests that the face does not need to be in the water for the dive reflex to occur.

To compensate for the observed reduction in heartrate during water-based exercise, a variety of techniques are used. A study done at the Human Performance Lab at Adelphi University found that even though water-based heartrates were reported to be 13% lower than the land-based minimum and maximum counts, the cardiorespiratory benefits were the same as those produced by land-based exercise (Lindle, 1989). The Institute for Aerobics Research in Dallas, Texas, deducts 17 beats per minute from their projected heartrates for water exercise (Windhorst and Chossek, 1988). The 17-beat deduction was also verified in horizontal water exercise and documented by McArdle, Katch, and Katch in

Exercise, Physiology, Energy, Nutrition, and Human Performance (McArdle, 1986).

While observation has shown that heartrates generally are lower in aquatic exercise, clearly more studies are needed. Until then, heartrate information must be accepted as a basic guide rather than a hard-and-fast rule for measuring exercise intensity.

Applying Variations to the Karvonen Formula

Applying this information to the Karvonen formula, consider once again a prospective exerciser who is 40 years old and has reported a resting heartrate of 60 beats per minute (see earlier examples). The final target zone of working heartrates for *water exercise* would be from 103 to 145 beats per minute. This range is determined by subtracting 17 from the original land-based figures for minimum and maximum working heartrates. Namely, the minimum working heartrate for land-based exercise was 120 beats per minute and the maximum, 162 beats per minute.

Methods of Taking Pulse Checks

Although heartrate often is discussed in terms of beats per minute, it is not actually accurate to take exercise pulse counts over a full minute, because the heart begins to slow down as soon as exercise diminishes or stops. Instead, one-minute heartrates typically are monitored by counting the beats for 6 seconds and then adding a 0 (i.e., multiply times 10).

For example, during class, the instructor would alert students of a **heartrate check** by saying, "Heartrates, go." Students would be timed for 6 seconds, at which point the instructor would say, "Stop." If a student counts 12 pulsations, that is equivalent to 120 beats per minute. A 6-second count of 16 is equivalent to 160 beats per minute. By making this simple conversion and by knowing the target zone, students can know quickly if the exercise intensity is too high or too low for them to earn cardiorespiratory benefits.

Heartrate typically is checked up to 4 times during a 45- to 60-minute class. The first check is made after the cardiovascular warm-up, when the rate might be 100 to 110 beats per minute. During the aerobic segment, working heartrates typically range from 103 to 145 when adjusted for water. A final (recovery) heartrate should be taken 5 to 10 minutes after the vigorous segment or after the cooldown. Heartrates of 110 or lower are considered safe for resuming normal activities.

When students first join, heartrates should be checked every 5 to 10 minutes simply to get participants used to the procedure and to help them understand the heartrate at which they usually work. As students become more familiar with finding the heartrate site, counting the pulse, and understanding the meaning of the resultant number, heartrates can be

DIAGRAM 5–2 Karvonen Formula for Water Exercise

```
         220
       — age
    Maximal heartrate

     Maximal heartrate
   — Resting heartrate
    Heartrate reserve
```

Heartrate reserve	Heartrate reserve
x .50 (Intensity level)	x .85 (Intensity level)
+ Resting heartrate	+ Resting heartrate
Minimum working heartrate (land-based exercise)	**Maximum working heartrate** (land-based exercise)
Minimum working heartrate (land-based exercise)	Maximum working heartrate (land-based exercise)
— 17 beats per minute	— 17 beats per minute
Minimum working heartrate for aquatic exercise	**Maximum working heartrate for aquatic exercise**

Target Zone

checked less frequently. When students are comfortable with the procedure, a heartrate check every 10 to 15 minutes is recommended.

Common Errors

The most common errors in checking heartrate are miscounting and taking too long to begin counting. It is crucial to begin the heartrate check while still exercising vigorously. If students slack off slightly while locating a watch or clock or waiting for the sweep second hand to reach a certain place, the monitoring loses accuracy.

To remedy these problems, students should wear a stopwatch or position themselves where a clock is easily in view. The student should be in the habit of starting the monitoring from any position of the sweep second hand or purchase a stopwatch to eliminate the problem completely. Students should remind themselves to continue vigorous movement throughout the pulse count to keep it as accurate as possible.

Participants should know ahead of time when heartrates are going to be checked and should continue moving while they are checking their pulses. Stopping completely to check a pulse may cause the blood to pool in the extremities, which results in fainting, dizziness, or lightheadedness.

Student Variations

Common sense must prevail when monitoring heartrate. There is a percentage of students for whom the technique and formula will not be accurate. This may be due to medications or specific disease conditions, both chronic and acute. Students should familiarize themselves with other subjective measures of exercise intensity, such as the perceived exertion scale, the "talk test," and respiration rate so that they can be used in place of heartrate monitoring. Instructors should observe each student for signs of overexertion, such as shortness of breath, excessively red or splotchy skin color, excessive sweating, or excessive fatigue. If these symptoms are observed, exercise should be stopped by gradually cooling down, and the student should be referred to a doctor.

Sometimes the conditioning of the skeletal muscles proceeds more slowly than the conditioning of the cardiorespiratory muscles and systems. When this happens, the student will not have the strength to elevate, use longer levers, or make the body more resistant in the water. The converse also can be true. The student in either case must be encouraged to proceed slowly as the different systems catch up to each other in their conditioning levels.

When the heartrate is below the target zone and the student feels comfortable working harder, he or she can add more elevation to the movements, use longer-levered movements, and/or make body parts more resistant to the water to increase the intensity of the workout. When the heartrate is higher than the student's target zone, he or she can take the elevation out of the movements, use shorter-levered movements, and/or make the body more streamlined in water.

Target heartrates may have to be adjusted for students who lose training effects by exercising irregularly, who return to class after an illness, and who change fitness levels.

If a student's working heartrate is extremely low, but he or she feels weak and dizzy, he or she should not work at a higher level. Instead, the student should notify his or her doctor and seek medical advice.

Recovery heartrates following exercise are considered safe when recorded at 110 beats per minute or lower. If a student's heartrate is still above 110, he or she should continue exercising at a low level and check the heartrate again after a few minutes. A student should not leave the pool or be left unsupervised until the heartrate is below 110 beats per minute.

If a student consistently takes a long time to recover from aerobics, he or she should use a slightly slower, less strenuous pace throughout the workout. Continue to check the recovery heartrate. If the pattern continues, the student should notify his or her doctor.

Comparison of Land and Water Exercise Intensities

Many studies have been done comparing the heartrate responses during land- and water-based exercise. Most of the studies done in chest-deep water show that water exercise heartrates often are lower than those produced by comparable workouts on land. Adelphi University's study showed that heartrates were 13% lower for aquatic exercisers than for exercisers doing the same program on land (Lindle, 1989).

Other studies have compared different training responses and parameters of physical fitness. A study done for Indiana University and the National Institute for Fitness and Sport on the effect of water exercise on various parameters of physical fitness found that after a 12-week water exercise program, no change was found in participants' **VO$_2$ max,** total cholesterol, HDL, resting heartrate, or resting systolic blood pressure (Wigglesworth et al., 1990). There also was no change in weight. However, a significant decrease in thigh skin fold was found.

Another study comparing selected training responses to water aerobics and land-based, low-impact aerobics done by personnel from Boise State University, Indiana State University, and the Idaho Sports Medicine Institute concluded that both groups demonstrated significant improvements in treadmill time, estimated VO$_2$ max, percentage of body fat, flexibility, and knee and shoulder strength (Spitzer, 1989). A significant decrease in resting heartrate also was found in both groups. The water aerobics group experienced greater strength gains than the land-based, low-impact aerobics group.

A study done by Birger Johnson from California State University with a research team at the Norwegian College of Physical Education and Sport in Oslo, Norway, found that both heartrate and **oxygen uptake** were greater during exercises in water than on land (Johnson et al., 1977). Arm and leg exercises were found to require significantly more oxygen when performed in water than on land.

The type of aquatics program, the depth of the water, and the water and air temperatures all affect the heartrate response during research testing. It is evident that more research needs to be done with greater controls.

AEA Heartrate Chart

The Aquatic Exercise Association (AEA) has acknowledged, but does not endorse, the use of lower heartrate response in average (82° Fahrenheit) water temperature and chest-deep water. Diagram 5-3 is a copy of the AEA's aquatic heartrate chart that has been modified for water exercise.

DIAGRAM 5-3 Aquatic Exercise Association Aquatics Heartrate Chart

Age	Minimum Working Heartrate	Maximum Working Heartrate
20–29	124	179
30–39	119	161
40–49	114	152
50–59	108	143
60–69	103	134
70+	98	125

Checking Heartrates

Take pulses after vigorous exercise to determine how hard the heart has worked.

1. As soon as exercise ceases, place the tips of the index and middle fingers lightly over one of the blood vessels on the neck (carotid arteries) located to the left or right of the Adam's apple.
2. Count the pulsations for six seconds, add a zero to the number, and refer to the chart.
3. If the pulse is below the target zone, exercise a little harder next time. If it is above the target zone, exercise should be lightened. If it falls within the target zone, exercise is taking place at the correct intensity.

Source: AEA, Port Washington, Wisconsin

ALTERNATE INTENSITY EVALUATION METHODS

Clearly the discussion in the first part of this chapter illustrates that many factors—from exercising in shallow water or high humidity to wearing restrictive clothing to taking medications—increase heartrate. Unfortunately, students often try to use these factors when trying to increase the intensity of a workout. But so often in aquatic exercise, the true intensity of the workout (oxygen consumption) and heartrate do not correlate at all. Because of this, students should be familiar with alternative methods of evaluating exercise intensity, which include subjective measurements such as perceived exertion, respiration rate, and the "talk test."

Rate of Perceived Exertion

While heartrate is not always a good indicator of intensity, exercisers are. Exercise physiologists working with a scientist named Gunnar Borg discovered that exercisers are able to sense their own intensity levels (Consistent Training, 1989). Participants are asked to label their activities as "Very, very light;" "Very light;" "Fairly light;" "Somewhat hard;" "Hard;" "Very hard;" or "Very, very hard." Participants are able to closely approximate their heartrate readings by how hard they perceive themselves to be working.

Based on Borg's **rate of perceived exertion (RPE)** chart (see Diagram 5–4), most exercisers should be working in the "Somewhat hard" to "Hard" range. "Very, very light" describes feelings of exertion at total rest, and "Very, very hard" describes feelings just before collapsing of exhaustion. The numbers in the left-hand column correspond to a 6-second land-based exercise heartrate.

Pollock, Wilmore, and Fox found that ratings of 12 to 13 are equal to about 60% of maximal heartrate reserve, while 16 is equal to about 90% of maximal heartrate reserve (Pollock et al., 1984). Participants working in the "Somewhat hard" to "Hard" range during the aerobic phase of the class will be working in the 60% to 90% range of maximal heartrate reserve.

Borg found that the RPE scale correlated very highly with heartrate, **ventilation,** oxygen consumption, and blood lactate concentration (Borg, 1982). Since it has already been shown that heartrate is not a very reliable measure of exertion in aquatic exercise, it seems that the RPE method may work well not only for aquatic exercisers but also for special populations using medications.

The ACSM revised the RPE scale in 1986 making it simpler for participants to use (see

DIAGRAM 5–4 Borg's Rate of Perceived Exertion (RPE) Chart

6	
7	Very, very light
8	
9	Very light
10	
11	Fairly light
12	
13	Somewhat hard
14	
15	Hard
16	
17	Very hard
18	
19	Very, very hard
20	

Source: Borg, G. A. V. (1982). Psychophysical Bases of Physical Exertion. *Medicine and Science in Sport and Exercise, 14,* 344–387. Used with permission.

DIAGRAM 5-5 American College of Sports Medicine (ACSM) Rate of Perceived Exertion (RPE) Chart

0	Nothing
0.5	Very, very light (just noticeable)
1.0	Very light
2	Light (weak)
3	Moderate
4	Somewhat hard
5	Heavy (strong)
6	
7	Very heavy
8	
9	
10	Very, very heavy (almost max)

Source: Consistent Training, 1989

Diagram 5-5). This scale goes from 0, which is "Nothing," to 10, which is "Very, very heavy." It provides more verbal descriptions for participants to rate their exertion levels.

Participants in water exercise sometimes perceive their exertion to be somewhat lower because of the cooling effect and the enjoyment of the water. This is not the case, however. The RPE method can be a reliable guide to measuring intensity in cardiovascular activity. In fact, some exercise professionals find it the most useful indicator of workout intensity. Some aquatic exercise instructors combine heartrate response and RPE methods. They have participants get used to taking a pulse during exercise and relating how they feel during that workout. After a few weeks of pulse checks, participants are able to perceive their own levels of intensity without checking pulses.

Respiration Rate

In order for an exerciser to get extra oxygen, he or she must take more breaths per minute. If the **respiration rate** (or breaths per minute) during activity does not increase, the exercise is not intense enough. Measuring respiration rate is a technique to determine just the lower limit (minimum working heartrate) of intensity. Using respiration rate to determine exercise intensity normally is done in conjunction with another method, such as heartrate or RPE, for monitoring intensity.

"Talk Test"

The so-called **"talk test"** is very simple: If participants cannot talk when they are exercising, it means they are working too hard. If they are working out so strenuously that they cannot visit with the person next to them, it means the exercise is no longer aerobic. Participants should be able to breathe comfortably and deeply during the entire workout. If they are short of breath, panting, or gasping and are unable to talk, their workout is too intense. Rather than burning fat and carbohydrate calories, they are burning protein. The "talk test" monitors only the top end of the target zone (maximum working heartrate).

Increasing Intensity

Participants often think they are getting a great workout in warm, shallow water, with their arms overhead and the sun shining. As most instructors know, heartrates are probably elevated only because of heart stress, not increased oxygen or caloric consumption.

Many of the conditions discussed above increase heartrate. If exercisers are too concerned with achieving a specific heartrate, they may injure themselves in an effort to burn calories. And ironically, they actually may not burn as many calories as they would with a more sensible program and a lower heartrate or perceived exertion rate. In these instances, the heartrate may not be in an average target range, but the oxygen consumption may be at a level high enough to burn calories, as if the heartrate were in the target range. This is what was found with the research discussed earlier.

If participants feel they are not working hard enough, they can increase their intensity level by experimenting with a few of the concepts listed below. They can tell what makes them "huff and puff," namely, increasing oxygen consumption. If they are not breathing harder and deeper after the warm-up, they're not working hard enough. (Kicks are used as an example, since almost all programs include them during a workout.)

1. Put a big bounce between every kick. Students should push up off the bottom of the pool as hard as they can to get the body high out of the water.
2. Delete the bounce completely. Have students use only muscle power to kick the leg as high as they can and then return it from the kick. The rest of the body should stay in good postural alignment. The top part of the body should barely move. This will increase the demand for oxygen in the leg muscles.
3. Move through the water during the kicks. Participants can move forward and backward or to the corners and back. Moving the body through the resistance of the water increases the body's oxygen demands.
4. Move further through the water than usual. If students usually can move four feet forward in eight kicks, challenge them to move five feet forward in eight kicks. This forces more muscle fibers into action and, therefore, increases oxygen consumption.
5. Lift the kicks higher. Push participants to achieve the largest range of motion possible in the time allotted for each kick. These should be done without jerking at the joint, moving out of alignment, or leaning forward.
6. Add some force or muscle power to the arm movements that are used with the kicks. The more muscles involved, the more oxygen will be required. Students also should get their arms working.
7. Do the kicks faster. Increasing the speed while still maintaining a safe, upright body alignment increases intensity. Students should not, however, compromise the joint by increasing the speed too much. If there is any joint stress, skip this hint and use only numbers one through six and eight.
8. Do the kicks slower. Slower kicks (again, done only with good postural alignment) will allow students to use a fuller range of motion (higher kicks) and concentrate on using muscles on the lifting and lowering portions of the kick.

Students need to challenge themselves personally at each class. The instructor's job is to offer a safe, effective, muscle-balanced workout and to help motivate each student. The student's job is to accept the challenge and do a little more at every class. Without adequate effort on the part of the individual, no exercise program will work.

KEY WORDS

Heartrate
Resting heartrate (RHR)
Maximal heartrate
Working heartrate range
Minimum working heartrate
Maximum working heartrate
Optimum working heartrate
Target zone
Recovery heartrate
Oxygen consumption
Karvonen formula
Caloric consumption

Heat dissipation
Gravity
Compression
Partial pressure
Dive reflex

Heartrate check
VO_2 max
Oxygen uptake
Rate of Perceived Exertion (RPE)

Ventilation
Respiration rate
Talk test

SUMMARY

- The relationship between heartrate and workout intensity has always been an enigma.
- Several different terms are used to discuss heartrates: resting heartrate, maximal heartrate, working heartrate range, minimum working heartrate, maximum working heartrate, optimum working heartrate, target zone, recovery heartrate.
- Scientists have found that the exercising heartrate often correlates closely to oxygen consumption.
- The Karvonen formula is a scientific formula commonly accepted as the safest way to calculate the appropriate exertion level for land-based aerobic exercise.
- Students who participate in both land- and water-based exercise often find their heartrates lower from water exercise than land exercise, yet they receive the same benefits.
- Although observation has shown that heatrates generally are lower in aquatic exercise, clearly more studies are needed.
- The most common errors that occur in checking heartrate are miscounting and taking too long to begin counting.
- Many studies have been done comparing the heartrate responses during land- and water-based exercise.
- Many factors—from exercising in shallow water or high humidity to wearing restrictive clothing to taking medications—increase heartrate.
- Exercisers can sense their own intensity levels.
- To get extra oxygen, an exerciser must take more breaths per minute.
- If participants cannot talk when they are exercising, it means they are working too hard.
- Students need to challenge themselves personally at each class.
- Without adequate effort on the part of an individual, no exercise program will work.

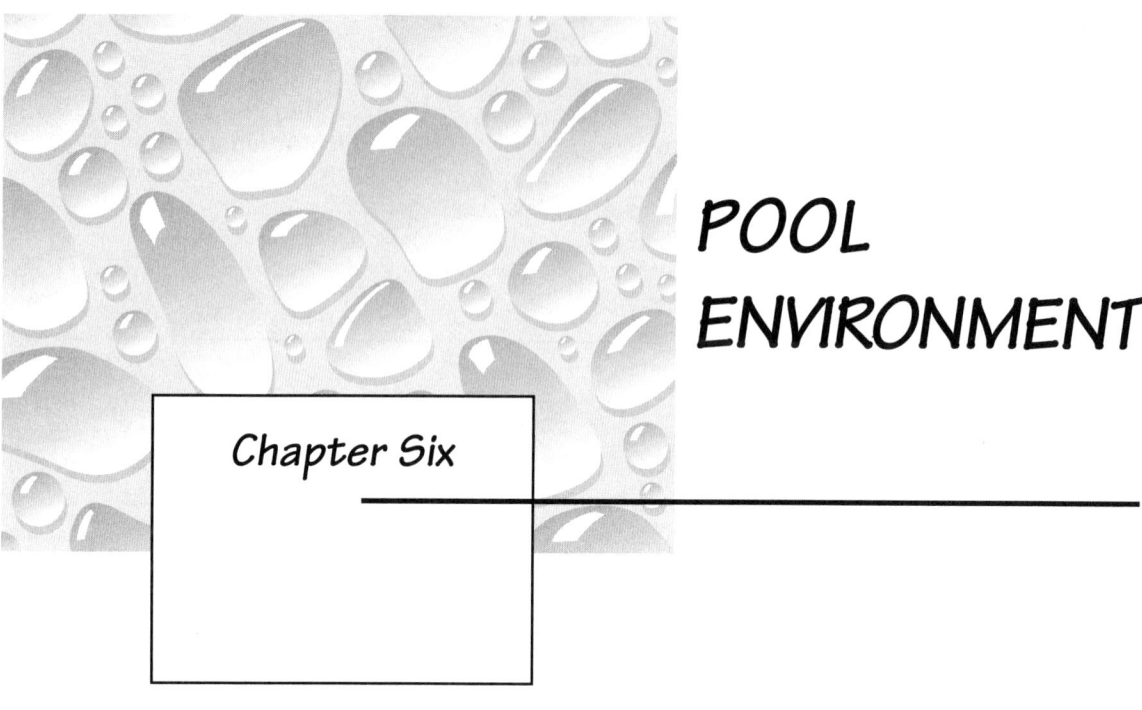

POOL ENVIRONMENT

Chapter Six

POOL CONDITIONS

Knowledge about the area where water exercise classes meet helps ensure a safe program for participants. Different programs are suited ideally to different pool environments. Being aware of the factors that are *not* ideal allows the instructor or student to modify conditions and compensate for inadequacies. **Pool conditions,** such as the surface of the pool bottom, the water temperature, humidity, sun exposure, and water depth all affect the safety of a workout.

Pool Bottom

While aquatic exercise is virtually stress and injury free, the type of pool bottom can affect the likelihood of injury. Slippery pool bottoms can easily cause injuries. Participants whose feet slide out from under them while exercising can injure muscles and ligaments in their legs and backs. Painted pool bottoms, or pools done completely in tile or fiberglass, or with tile lane markers are especially slippery. Exercisers encountering a slippery pool bottom should wear some type of footwear that provides traction, such as the Omega Reef Runner or Warrior. The Aquatic Consulting Services suggest .6 as a **minimum friction coefficient** for pool bottoms (Osinski,1990).

A **pool bottom** should have a smooth but nonslippery surface. It should be marked plainly and conspicuously to indicate depth, with specific markings at break points. The proper grate on the drain cover should be screwed in.

Rough pool bottoms often can cause undue wear and tear on the skin of the feet. Exercisers should use some type of protective footwear in the pool if they are losing more than a superficial layer of skin from the bottoms of their feet. Exercisers whose feet have open sores from a rough pool bottom should not be allowed back into the pool until their feet have healed.

Sloped pool bottoms often are dangerous because they create an imbalance in the exercising body, which in turn creates poor postural alignment. Having one foot slightly higher than the other or having either the toes or heels higher can lead eventually to an overuse injury. Pools with extreme slopes should not be used or should be used only for deep-water exercise. If an exerciser has to work in a pool with a mild slope, he or she should move to new areas of the pool, and he or she should turn in different directions so that the footstrike is not always off balance in exactly the same way. Most pools of depths of 5 feet or less are sloped at ratios of 1:8 (a one-foot slope for every eight feet of pool bottom) or 1:12, depending on state codes. Depths of over five feet usually have a slope ratio of 1:3.

Water Temperature

The average indoor pool temperature ranges from the high 70s to the low 90s (degrees Fahrenheit). Outdoor pool temperatures can range from the 40s to over 100 degrees.

Water temperature is of utmost importance. For high-intensity workouts with healthy, fit individuals who need to dissipate heat, ideal pool temperatures should be 80 to 83 degrees Fahrenheit. In water below 80 degrees, participants should increase the time spent in the warm-up phase before moving on to full-range-of-motion, high-level aerobic activity.

Even when it is within the ideal temperature range, pool water is cooler than body temperature, and it causes certain physiological reactions to occur: the blood vessels near the surface of the skin will become much smaller; **circulation** (movement of blood) occurs in the deeper vessels of the body in an attempt to conserve body heat; the muscles will automatically contract; and the participant may begin to shiver. Because of these natural reactions, it is essential that exercisers begin moving immediately upon entering the water. The thermal warm-up should have participants bouncing, jogging, and jazzkicking from the moment of immersion. Continuous motion must be maintained as the workout progresses and the exerciser begins to burn nutrients; this compensates for the heat that is lost to the cool water enveloping the body.

A body in water cools down approximately four times faster than a body in air. Even during a brief pause, the body's temperature can drop enough to cause muscle tightening. During leg, gluteal, and hip-flexor stretches, the arms should continue moving to generate body heat. While the exerciser stretches the upper body, the feet should keep marching or jogging. Because of these physiological responses to cool water, some instructors prefer to do the poststretch on the pool deck.

On occasion, the pool temperature will be too cold to enable participants to warm-up adequately and participate safely in an aquatic exercise program. Although the exact water temperatures will vary with different types of students, water temperature in the low 70s and under likely provides an unsafe exercise environment.

While cool temperatures present one set of difficulties, pools with temperatures over 85 degrees present another potential risk, that of overheating. Overheating may result when warm water interferes with heat dissipation, the body's ability to radiate excess heat to a cooler environment. *Caution is needed.* Some therapeutic pools are heated to over 90 degrees. These pools should not be used for aerobic activities.

Water temperature minimums and maximums sometimes are set by state, county, or city bathing codes. The temperature should be conducive to the types of activities being offered in the pool.

Water Depth

When choosing appropriate water depth, different considerations should be made regarding the exerciser's body type and the goal of the program: whether upper-body toning is a priority (if the arms are submerged, more upper-body toning will occur); how much control of movements is possible; whether a good sense of balance can be achieved; and how much safety from impact can be ensured.

The ideal **water depth** for most aquatic exercisers is midriff or armpit level. This water depth allows participants to use their arms, which provides additional body toning. They also experience enough body weight to control their movements, keep a good sense of balance, and maintain reasonable footing during the exercises. Midriff to armpit water depth also allows the exerciser to experience enough body weight to make the workout a challenge and achieve the intensity needed to produce cardiovascular benefits. At that depth, however, participants can experience enough buoyancy to protect their joints, ligaments, and tendons from the stress of high impact.

Sun Exposure

Instructors and students who work in outdoor pools are placed at unusually high risk for skin cancer if they are regularly exposed to the sun's direct or indirect rays. The American Cancer Society says that the risk is compounded by the fact that exposure is both to sunlight and potent UV reflections off the water surface (American Cancer Society, 1988). Skin cancer is almost entirely preventable if participants and instructors take necessary precautions. Wearing a wide-brimmed hat, using sunscreen or sunblock, and working out before 11 A.M. or after 2 P.M. helps protect the skin from sun exposure.

Eye safety also is an important consideration for exercisers working outdoors. They should wear protective eyewear to prevent **corneal sunburn.**

KEY WORDS

Pool conditions
Pool bottom
Minimum friction coefficient
Water temperature

Blood vessels
Circulation
Heat dissipation

Water depth
Sun exposure
Corneal sunburn

SUMMARY

— Knowledge about the area where water exercise classes meet helps ensure a safe program for participants.
— While aquatic exercise is virtually stress and injury free, the type of pool bottom can affect the likelihood of injury.
— For high-intensity workouts with healthy, fit individuals who need to dissipate heat, the ideal pool temperature should be 80 to 83 degrees Fahrenheit.
— A body in water cools down approximately four times faster than a body in air.
— On occasion the pool temperature will be too cold to enable participants to warm-up adequately and participate safely in an aquatic exercise program.
— While cool temperatures present one set of difficulties, pools with temperatures over 85 degrees present the risk of overheating.
— When choosing appropriate water depth, different considerations should be made regarding the exerciser's body type and the goal of the program.
— The ideal water depth for most aquatic exercisers is to the midriff or the armpit.
— Skin cancer is almost entirely preventable if participants and instructors take necessary precautions.

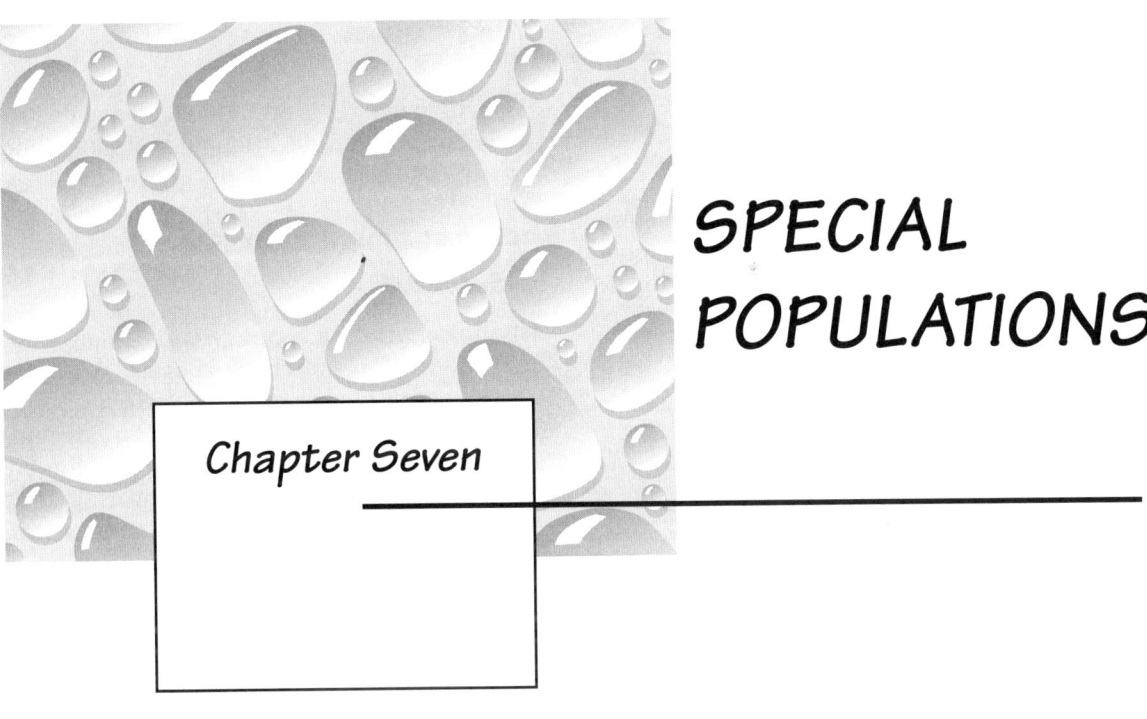

SPECIAL POPULATIONS

Chapter Seven

Because of the relative weightlessness of participants, water exercise is an excellent low-impact aerobic activity for people with some physical difficulty. With every footfall on land, the legs bear two to five times the body's weight. A participant exercising in water has very little body weight (60% to 90% less) and very little impact due to the lessened effect of gravity. Since exercisers are protected by the **cushioning** effect of water, injuries and stress are far less likely than with land-based aerobics.

This makes water aerobics the exercise of choice for millions of people who are overweight or pregnant; who suffer from arthritis, other joint problems, or back or knee pain; or who need rehabilitation or therapy after recent surgery or childbirth. In all of these cases, an instructor must be certain to lead participants through an extended warm-up phase. Full, controlled movements should be substituted for choppy, jerky ones. Progressive overload should be extremely gradual.

BASIC PRECAUTIONS

Health History and Physician's Approval

Although water exercise is one of the safest ways to work out, participants should be advised that this is an exertive program. All participants should inform their physicians of their intention to take part in aquatic exercise. An exerciser with a **health history** of any type of medical problem should obtain his or her **physician's approval,** along with possible suggestions to adapt the program to his or her individual needs.

65

Overexertion

If exercisers experience pain during any workout, they should stop exercising, walk slowly in place, and inform their instructor. Instructors should look out for participants who display any of the following signs of **overexertion:**
- nausea
- extreme weakness
- profuse sweating
- a red face
- breathlessness
- excessive fatigue
- chest pain or discomfort
- lightheadedness or dizziness
- focused musculoskeletal discomfort
- ataxic (unsteady) gait
- confusion

It is important that the aquatic exerciser understands the sources of fatigue so that the symptoms listed above can be eliminated.

Hyperthermia

Hyperthermia is the overheating of the body, which can happen in warm water or pool environments with very little circulation. The participant feels an overall loss of energy.

Glycogen Depletion

Glycogen depletion causes graduated and overall fatigue. Participants should keep the workout at low to moderate intensity for short periods and gradually overload to avoid glycogen depletion.

Musculoskeletal Fatigue

Musculoskeletal fatigue often is recognized by pain in a bone, joint, or muscle. Overdoing any one exercise movement can cause musculoskeletal fatigue.

Lactic Acid Accumulation

Lactic acid accumulation comes on relatively quickly and usually is focused in one particular muscle group. It can be avoided by reducing workout duration and intensity and by varying the exercise.

SPECIAL POPULATIONS
Older Adults

Olympic marathon runner Kenny Moore said, "You don't stop exercising because you grow old. You grow old because you stop exercising" (McWaters, 1988). The Aerobics Research Institute in Dallas, Texas, has drawn a similar conclusion: "Scientists are discovering that the true fountain of youth can be found within our own genes and cells and enhanced by our lifestyle choices" (Research Abstracts, 1990).

Programs should be designed to include stretching to improve or maintain range of motion and flexibility. Exercises to improve general postural alignment also benefit the older adult. **Older adults** tend to have increased joint stiffness and decreased flexibility. Joint surfaces degenerate with age. The amount and thickness of **synovial fluid** (the lubricant of the joint) also decreases with age. Regular exercise has been shown to increase joint flexibility and decrease joint pain in most adults.

Muscles tend to lose their strength with age. This decrease in the size of muscle fibers can be slowed with regular resistive exercise. Exercising in water offers the resistance older adults need.

Past studies have shown that muscular response (how fast a muscle reacts) slows with age due to shrinkage of the brain cells that control the movement. A study of 70-year-old women who exercised three times a week for 15 years found that they had the same response times as inactive college women (Research Abstracts, 1990).

An exercise program at the Hebrew Rehabilitation Center for the Aged in Boston had six women and four men doing strength training at 80% of one repetition maximum (Strovas, 1990). One repetition maximum tests the ability of muscle to exert great force in a single effort. The 10 participants in the study were between 90 and 96 years of age and considered in the "old old" classification. They had an approximate average of 4.5 chronic diseases per person and 4.5 daily medications. Seven had osteoarthritis, six had coronary artery disease, six had suffered stress fractures from osteoporosis, four had high blood pressure, and seven regularly used a cane or other walking device. The individuals took an average of 2.2 seconds to stand up from sitting in a straight chair, and eight of the ten had a history of falls related to muscular weakness.

After eight weeks of training, researchers from several Boston-area universities and hospitals concluded that a "high-intensity weight-training program is capable of inducing dramatic increases in muscle strength in frail men and women up to 96 years of age" (Pitts, 1990c, p. 12). A strength gain of 174% in eight weeks was realized, muscle size was increased, and mobility was improved.

In addition to physiological benefits, older adults can experience psychological and social benefits as by-products of regular vigorous exercise. These benefits include improved self-confidence and self-esteem, a better ability to handle change, an improved sense of well-being and independence, and decreased feelings of anxiety, tension, and isolation.

The class format for an older adult program should follow that of the traditional aerobics class. The older adult may need to spend more time warming up in order to release synovial fluid in joints and deliver oxygen to muscles. Everyone should be comfortably warm in the water before the vigorous, high-intensity workout begins. The intensity of the workout should be modified according to individual fitness levels. The program format also should include time for socializing while exercising, touching (some older adults who live alone no longer have anyone close enough to them to touch them), and working on balance or coordination activities.

Major muscle groups and fine-motor skills should be included in the programming. Exercise instructors often spend time working only major muscle groups. The older adult also needs to work the smaller muscles in the body to improve fine-motor skills. (Simply opening and closing the hands is an example of a fine-motor skill.)

Programs for older adults should use music from their era. Older adults enjoy music, such as Big Band, ragtime, and Broadway hits. They like the subtle rhythms from their time more than the pounding rhythms now heard. Avoid using excessively high volume with the music. Some older adult classes prefer not to have any music for background during their class, as it interferes with hearing the instructor.

The older adult who is unfit should begin exercise at the low end of the target zone or perceived exertion chart. Heartrates often are affected by medications. Progressive overload should be extremely gradual in terms of frequency, duration, and especially intensity.

New participants in class who are unaccustomed to water may want to stay in the shallowest portion of the pool and hold onto the edge. Gradually, they can move a little deeper and support themselves. They should always be encouraged to stay in the portion of the pool where they feel safe and secure. Water depth for the average participant should be midriff to armpit.

Older adults tend to appreciate warmer water more than younger adults and swimmers. If possible, water temperature in the 86- to 88-degree Fahrenheit range is recommended.

Equipment that does not require excessive gripping is recommended, since joint problems and arthritis can be exacerbated by prolonged gripping. Hydro-Fit and Sprint/Rothhammer aqua gloves seem to work exceptionally well. Other types of equipment can all be successful if they are used only for a portion of the class and in adherence to the concept of progressive overload. For toning, a ballet bar approximately four inches beneath the water surface and the Aquarius Water Workout Station often are beneficial for older adults.

Obese Individuals

Obesity is defined as being above 23% to 25% body fat for men and 30% to 33% percent body fat for women. The average body fat for men is approximately 15%, and the average for women is 25%.

Being **obese** and being overweight often are confused. Being overweight is a condition in which an individual exceeds the population norm or average, which is determined by height and frame size. Obesity is characterized by excess body fat, frequently resulting in significant impairment of health.

Not only do modifications need to be made because of the amount of weight with which a participant is exercising, but also because obesity predisposes participants to other medical problems: diabetes, high cholesterol, high levels of LDL cholesterol, and a high risk of coronary artery disease and hypertension. An obese person also is predisposed to a greater likelihood of musculoskeletal injuries and overexertion. The cardiovascular demands of exercise are much greater for an obese person because of the mass being moved and the likelihood of atrophied muscles due to inactivity.

To help the body burn fat, the program should be of low intensity and long duration. Workout heartrates should be near the bottom of the target zone, and perceived exertion should be at the minimum of the cardiorespiratory improvement segment. The exercisers should participate in a program at least three times a week, and they will see faster improvement if they participate four or five times per week as they adapt. Exercisers should not participate in class more than five times per week.

Water exercise is ideal for obese participants because it is extremely low impact. Nonimpact exercise in the deep area of the pool is an excellent consideration. Water walking in the shallow end of the pool, rather than a bouncing program, such as water jogging or water aerobics, is preferable. Obese individuals should experience as little impact as possible to eliminate the possibility of stress fractures or overuse injuries.

The obese often have poor coordination and balance, which is alleviated somewhat by water. Exercise patterns should be simple to follow. Some exercisers may prefer to hold onto the pool edge when first beginning class. To keep the impact as light as possible, an obese exerciser should move as deep in the water as possible without losing control of the motion. Deep water provides more buoyancy. Unfortunately, obese people usually are very buoyant. Moving too deep in the water to lessen the impact can cause floundering, loss of control of the exercise, and panic. Being too deep also often causes a person to exercise in a plantarflexed position (on tiptoes). This should be discouraged, because it can cause overuse injuries.

The obese person may want to wear cushioned aqua shoes such as the Omega Sun Runner to protect the bottoms of the feet from the abrasive pool. This also aids in absorbing impact during the program.

If the pool water, air temperature, or air humidity become high, obese participants are at high risk for heat exhaustion. Because of their weight, they have more difficulty dissipating heat. They also are more likely to experience hyperpnea and dyspnea (excessive or difficult breathing).

Obese individuals also have some movement restriction, limited mobility, and muscle weakness because of their body mass. Programming should take those concerns into consideration.

The format of the class for obese participants is modified only slightly. The warm-up is the same as for a regular aerobics class, but the aerobic portion should be at a lower intensity and of a longer duration. The cooldown may need to be increased in duration to ensure proper relief. The toning can be eliminated if the elongated aerobic portion demands it.

The average aerobics water temperature (78 degrees to 82 degrees Fahrenheit) seems comfortable for most obese participants. Water temperatures of 86 degrees and higher can trigger heat-stress syndromes.

Prenatal

Many theories have consider the effects of exercise on a pregnant woman and fetus. Research results are limited, divergent, and seem somewhat inconclusive. Generally, studies show that healthy pregnant women experience very few negative effects from moderate exercise.

Many special considerations factor into a prenatal exercise program. The **prenatal** woman experiences postural changes that alter the center of gravity and weight gains that may lead to lordosis and often kyphosis. **Lordosis** is an exaggerated anterior (forward) curvature of the lumbar spine (swayback), and **kyphosis** is an exaggerated sagittal curvature of the thoracic spine (rounded shoulders, dowager's hump). A pregnant woman often compensates for the excess weight carried in her abdomen by sticking her buttocks backward and her head forward. Plasma volume also increases during pregnancy, which can cause problems with circulation, such as swelling, cramping, and supine hypotension. Weight gains also can increase the workload on the heart, respiratory system, and joints.

In 1985, the **American College of Obstetricians and Gynecologists (ACOG)** set guidelines for exercise safety during pregnancy. The guidelines included information on the following:

- *Frequency*—Exercise should be done at least three times per week. Intermittent exercise should be eliminated.
- *Duration*—The aerobic portion of the exercise class should not exceed 15 minutes.
- *Intensity*—An intensity level of 50% to 60% of maximal functional capacity should be set. The maternal heartrate should not exceed 140 beats per minute.
- *Mode*—Exercises in the supine position should be eliminated after the fourth month of pregnancy. The Valsalva maneuver should not be used.

The ACOG also states that the maternal core temperature should not exceed 38 degrees Celsius (100 degrees Fahrenheit) and that caloric intake should be adequate to meet the extra energy needs of pregnancy and exercise. Many of these special precautions for the prenatal exerciser are listed because exercise and pregnancy both put stress on many of the same body systems (musculoskeletal, respiratory, circulatory, metabolic).

The format for a prenatal exercise program will vary from the traditional aerobics program in several ways. The warm-up and cooldown should be extended by two to three minutes each. The aerobic portion should not exceed 15 minutes. The entire class should be low impact or no impact at all. A water-walking or deep-water exercise class is recommended. The stretches during the stretching segment do not need to be held quite as long as usual and should never be ballistic (bouncing). The program should never be offered in hot, humid weather. Focus should be maintained on a pelvic tilt and good body alignment.

Arthritic Individuals

In the past, **arthritics** were cautioned to stay away from any movement or any type of exercise that might irritate the arthritic condition. New research shows that the pain and stiffness in arthritics' joints can be decreased through low- to moderate-intensity exercise. Movement releases synovial fluid, lubricating the joints and helping them to move more easily.

Any exercise that causes undue pain in the arthritic should be stopped immediately. Alternative exercises to accomplish the same goal should be used instead. Exercisers who are having an inflammatory episode, a flare-up, or who have hot joints should not participate in exercise without a physician's approval. The affected areas should be submerged beneath the water, since water naturally reduces **edema** (swelling). The exercise program should begin slowly and gradually progress. Intensity and duration of exercise should be decreased. The **"two-hour pain rule"** should be in effect for arthritis classes: That is, if it hurts after two hours, too much was attempted. The participant should do less next time.

Format changes for arthritic classes include an elongated warm-up period to allow the synovial fluid to enter the joints and prepare for more vigorous exercise. Range-of-motion exercises are extremely important in the arthritic class. In order to offer full-range-of-motion activities without ballistic moves, everything should be done slowly. Transitions should be fluid, with successive movements being made easily. All bouncing should be eliminated from the program. Water-walking and deep-water exercise are ideal for arthritic classes. The stretching segment should offer longer stretches, but only after the muscles have been adequately warmed. No full extensions or flexions should be incorporated into the program. While most exercise programs concentrate on using the large muscles and major joints (elbows, knees, and hips), the arthritic program should concentrate on the fine-motor skills and smaller joints (wrists, fingers, and ankles).

The ideal water temperature for arthritic classes is 88 to 92 degrees Fahrenheit. Many arthritic participants are able to exercise in 82-degree water but find that they are more comfortable in a full unitard, wetsuit, or windsurf suit.

Individuals with Low-Back Pain

Studies show that 90% of the American population will at some point in their lives suffer from **low-back pain.** Many participants come to aquatic exercise classes to take advantage of the impact-free workout afforded them. Programs need to be modified for those with low-back pain in order to ensure safety. Aquatic exercise instructors can only make modifications to alleviate the pain and protect the low back, however, since the cause of back pain can be so varied (poor posture, poor body mechanics, being overweight, poor abdominal strength, being sedentary, tight hamstrings and low back, weak gluteal muscles, tight hip flexors).

Any exercise that causes pain for low-back participants should be stopped immediately and replaced with a modified form of the movement or another movement that achieves the same results without pain. The "two-hour pain rule" applies to low-back pain participants: If they hurt after two hours, they probably attempted to do too much during the previous exercise session. They should do less next time.

Considerations in the format of the program for participants with back problems include specific strengthening and flexibility exercises. Abdominal-strengthening exercises should be used extensively, including isometric contractions while doing other moves. Mental cues regarding abdominals, such as "Hold the abdominals in, stand tall, remember the pelvic tilt, keep a slight flex in your knee, lift your ribs," help the participant. Strengthening gluteals also can assist. Special stretching exercises for the low back, hamstrings, and hip flexors should be incorporated. The Aquarius Water Workout Station offers excellent opportunities for stretching the low back, hamstrings, and hip flexors, as well as safely strengthening the abdominals. Bouncing should be eliminated completely from the program; water-walking or deep-water exercises are ideal. Arms should be used in the water, not overhead, since doing so while moving through the water can cause instability and lumbar hyperextension. The warm-up period can be slightly elongated. Moves that involve lateral flexion, forward flexion, and spinal rotation are tolerable if used singly. Spinal flexion and rotation should never be combined, nor should lateral flexion and rotation.

Individuals with Knee Problems and Chondromalacia Patella

Most participants in an aquatic exercise program who have knee problems are recovering from knee surgery or undergoing therapy for a knee injury or **chondromalacia patella.** Thus, protecting the knees is vital to a safe aquatics program.

Stair climbing, cycling, and step aerobics often can aggravate or compromise the knee, as can weight-bearing activities that require full flexion and extension. Any twisting moves with the feet planted also should be eliminated. The knee and foot should always be in the same longitudinal alignment, with the knee directly above the foot. This means that the knee and toes of the same foot should always be pointed in the same direction. This eliminates torque, twisting, or compromising the knee joint.

Even though water is extremely beneficial for participants with knee problems, well-cushioned shoes can decrease impact during the workout.

The format for an aqua-aerobics class should be slightly modified for participants with knee pain. Bouncing should be eliminated; this lessens the impact and alleviates some of the stress on the knees. Exercises strengthening the vastus medialus or quadriceps should be used; they involve knee extensions. Pain-free stretching of the quadriceps, hamstrings, and calves is important to keep participants injury free. This lengthens contracted muscles and tissues and increases blood supply.

Children

In comparison to adults' programs, children's programs should be modified in two ways. Namely, **children** differ from adults in their thermoregularity capacity and their anaerobic capacity. **Thermoregulators** regulate heat production and heat loss so that normal body temperature is maintained. Children, however, are slightly deficient in their ability to perspire, so instructors must take special care to discourage high-intensity workouts when the pool water, air humidity, or air temperature is high. Children also are deficient in their anaerobic capacity; again, high-intensity anaerobic exercise should be discouraged.

Children's aquatic fitness programs should follow the same format as traditional aqua-aerobics classes. Jacqueline Walters, of Fitness Productions, in her Children's Creative Movement seminar, suggests modifying the children's workout to involve the mind and body (Walters, 1990). Programming includes education involving the senses (rhythm, balance), emotions (movement designed to deal with feelings and body response), creativity (conceiving images, thoughts, actions), imagery (storytelling in workout-movement patterns), and relaxation training.

Children's aquatic programs should always involve interesting challenges to keep them enjoyable. Program activities should vary frequently.

All types of equipment can be used in children's aquatic classes, adding variety and challenge. Balloons, small balls, soccer balls, and beach balls can all be used, as can traditional aquatic equipment such as aqua gloves, B-Wise Fitness Bars, Hydro-Fit and Spa Bells. All bring variety and enjoyment to the program. Exercise bands and tubing, Frisbees, and sports equipment also have been used with success. When adding equipment to a children's program, gradual overload should be stressed to prevent injury.

KEY WORDS

Cushioning
Health history
Physician's approval
Overexertion
Hyperthermia
Glycogen depletion
Lactic acid accumulation
Older adults
Synovial fluid
Obese
Prenatal
Lordosis
Kyphosis
American College of Obstetricians and Gynecologists (ACOG)
Arthritics
Edema
Two-hour pain rule
Low-back pain
Chondromalacia patella
Children
Thermoregulators

SUMMARY

- Because of the relative weightlessness of participants, water exercise is an excellent low-impact aerobic activity for people who have some physical difficulty.
- If exercisers experience pain during any workout, they should stop exercising.
- In addition to physiological benefits, older adults can experience psychological and social benefits as by-products of regular vigorous exercise.
- Water exercise is ideal for obese participants because it is extremely low impact.
- Being obese and being overweight often are confused.
- Generally, studies show that healthy pregnant women experience very few negative effects from moderate exercise.
- Research has shown that the pain and stiffness in arthritics' joints can be decreased through low- to moderate-intensity exercise.
- Many participants with low-back pain come to aquatic exercise classes to take advantage of an impact-free workout.
- Participants recovering from knee surgery or undergoing therapy for a knee injury can often protect their knees in an aquatics program.
- Children differ from adults in their thermoregularity capacity and their anaerobic capacity.

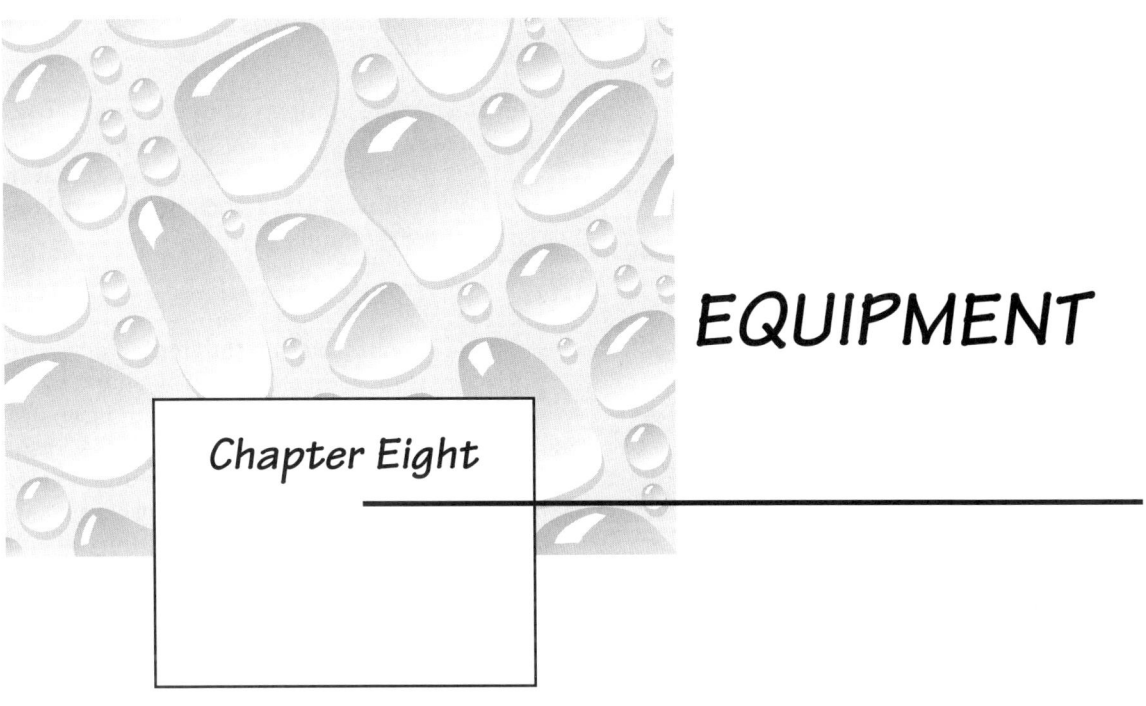

EQUIPMENT

Chapter Eight

In our society, from preschool age on up, we have become accustomed to learning in a fast-paced environment with frequent diversions. We enjoy instructors who are entertaining, and we like using learning tools. Equipment can fill that need in aquatic exercise and offer additional challenges for the bored or well-conditioned student.

EQUIPMENT INFORMATION

Equipment Principles

All equipment is based on one or more of three basic principles: **buoyancy, weight,** or **resistance.** Unless equipment is designed for therapeutic use or to keep a person buoyant in deep water, it is designed to inhibit movement (resistance), increase weight, or increase the force needed for a movement (buoyancy), thereby increasing the intensity. Weights increase impact, muscular endurance, and muscular strength. Buoyant equipment usually lessens impact and increases muscular strength and endurance. Resistant equipment does not affect impact but increases muscular endurance and strength.

Buoyancy

Buoyant equipment, attached to the wrist or hand held, increases the force needed to hold the arms beneath the water. The bulk of some buoyant equipment (Hydro-Fit) uses the concept of resistance with buoyancy to inhibit movement. Buoyancy increases the amount of force needed to hold the arms beneath the water and further increases resistance when the arms move through water. Buoyant equipment attached to the feet or ankles increases the amount of force needed to return the feet to the bottom of the pool after a kick or similar move. Buoyant leg attachments (such as Hydro-Fit) also increase intensity through resistance as the legs move through the water.

DIAGRAM 8-1 Buoyant Equipment

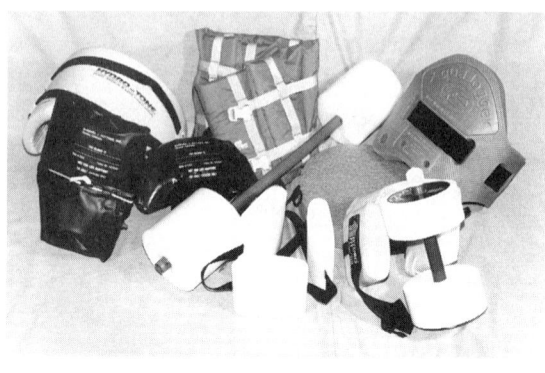

Buoyant belts and vests (such as J & B Foam's belt, Wet Vest, Hydro-Tone's belt, Sprint/Rothhammer's belt and AquaJogger) are designed to keep the body buoyant while working out in deep water, or to lessen impact while working out in shallow water. The buoyancy of a vest or belt is not intended to increase the intensity but simply to allow the exerciser to move freely.

Resistance

Resistance equipment is designed to inhibit limb or body movement through the water. Resistance equipment for the upper body includes webbed gloves, Frisbees, fitness paddles, Dynabands, and SPRI tubing. Lower-body resistant devices include Hydro-Tone boots and SPRI bands.

Weight

Equipment based on the concept of weight increases the weight of the limb moving through the water, therefore increasing the intensity. Wrist and ankle weights, weighted balls, vests, belts, and free weights are all used in water.

Adding weights to a water workout sometimes seems counterproductive. Many people exercise in the water for the buoyancy and lessened impact. Adding weights *increases* the **gravitational pull** and impact. Participants who are taking aquatic exercise because of the lessened impact should never use weighted equipment. Participants who are involved in water walking or other low-impact aquatic programs, such as toning or strength training, can use weights safely. Weights also can be used safely by a conditioned participant who enjoys the water and is not concerned about impact.

DIAGRAM 8-2 Resistance Equipment

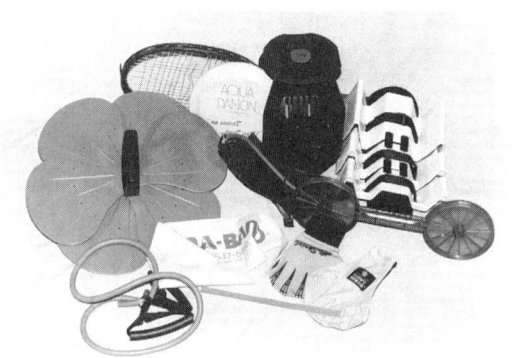

DIAGRAM 8-3 Weighted Equipment

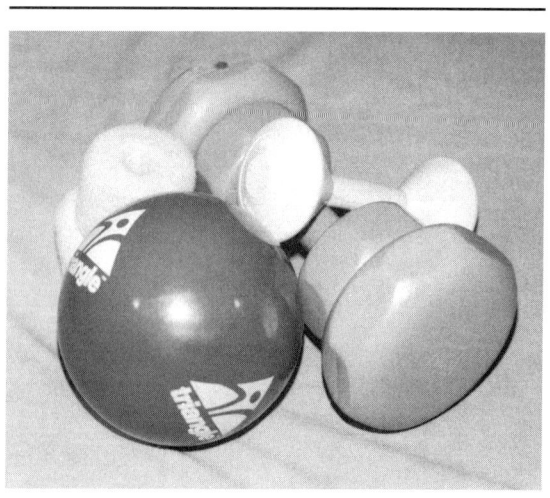

Precautions and Contraindications

Exercisers using equipment should follow specific guidelines, regardless of whether buoyant, resistant, or weighted equipment is used. The following are **precautions,** or measures to guard against injuries:

1. *Progressive overload:* When adding equipment, the concept of gradual overload should be applied in terms of intensity, frequency, and duration. Intensity can be increased in a number of ways. Using equipment, a participant should begin with a light piece and gradually progress to a heavy piece. An example would be to begin with webbed gloves, progress to Frisbees, and after adaptation occurs, progress to Hydro-Tone. In terms of duration, equipment should be added only for 5 to 10 minutes the first day. As students adapt to the equipment, time can be increased. In the beginning, equipment should be used only once or twice a week. Participants can increase the frequency gradually as adaptation occurs.
2. *Begin slowly:* Each time equipment is used, participants should begin slowly and gradually add more forceful movements. They also should begin using short levers and gradually progress to longer levers and more intense moves. Short levers also should be used for faster movements and long levers reserved for slower movements. Using long levers quickly can damage the soft tissue around joints.
3. *Muscle balance:* The muscles on each side of a joint should be worked equally to assure muscle balance during a workout. In order to ensure muscle balance, the exerciser should apply equal force in both directions of the movement.
4. *Keep joints "soft":* Full extensions of the knees, shoulders, elbows, and wrists should be eliminated. These joints should always be "soft," or slightly flexed, to prevent injury.
5. *Keep the equipment in the water:* Moves using aquatic exercise equipment should be accomplished completely in the water. Eliminate in-and-out-of-the-water types of moves, as they can severely compromise joints and muscles.
6. *Stretch what you strengthen:* While flexibility is important in all types of programs, stretching is even more vital when equipment is used. Any muscles that are worked with equipment should be stretched at the end of the program.
7. *Move toward and away from the body center:* To reduce strain on ligaments and tendons in the shoulders, elbows, knees, and hips, use moves such as bicep curls or sidekicks that move toward and away from the body center. Extensive movements on the periphery of the body, such as arm circles or leg circles, can cause strain.
8. *Always "place" the piece of equipment:* Participants sometimes fling equipment, especially if the movement is performed too quickly. Students should visualize where the piece of equipment will be at the end of the move and "place" it there. For safety purposes, participants should keep a firm grip on the equipment so it stays with them and does not hit other body parts or other individuals. Students should always know where the equipment is going.
9. *Use equipment only after the warm-up:* Before adding equipment, allow the body to warm up, supplying muscles with oxygenated blood and lubricating the joints.
10. *Use full range of motion:* Participants often cut movements short when they tire. If the movement is not brought back to its beginning position, it results in ineffective work and muscle

shortening. **Full range of motion** must be stressed.

11. *Use proper alignment:* Alignment is important in all programs and even more important when using equipment. Improper use of equipment can easily cause injuries to students. Exercisers should have complete control over movements with equipment.

Population Contraindications

Without a medical professional's guidance, some special populations should not use equipment. Participants with high blood pressure, heart disease, arthritis, or other joint problems should not use equipment. Participants with back or knee problems or pregnant women should have medical approval before attempting to use equipment that increases the intensity of the program.

EQUIPMENT TYPES

Weights

Weights are designed to increase the intensity of a workout. They can be used for the upper or lower body and can attach to the ankles or wrists or be hand held. They can be used during the toning or aerobics portions of classes and can also be used for specific programming, such as circuit training and strength training.

All weights currently on the market, with the exception of scuba weights, were created for land-based fitness programs. Many of these are not suitable for water and will leak or rust.

When using weights in aquatic exercise class, participants should be cautioned regarding the increased impact. Ankle weights are not recommended during the aerobic portion of class, unless it contains only basic moves such as walking and jogging. Weights should be used exclusively in shallow water.

Spenco weights were created for general fitness purposes and also work well in the water. They come in half-pound and one-pound increments. They are soft weights covered with terrycloth, and they can be used on either wrists or ankles. Aerobic Rings also are fitness weights that have transferred well to the water medium. They come in half-pound increments and are covered with a Lycra-nylon material. Scuba-diving weights come in a variety of sizes and attach with straps to ankles, waist, or wrists. Other weights made for aquatic exercise can be found in the catalog and equipment categories in the Resource section of this book (Chapter 13).

Water weights should be used in shallow water during the strengthening and toning portions of aquatic programs. Precautions should be taken to ensure their safe use. Weights range in price from $10 to $25.

Jugs

Empty Jugs

Empty milk, juice, or bleach jugs, either in half-gallon or one-gallon sizes, can be used to increase the intensity of a workout. They are popular because they are available free.

Empty jugs capitalize on the principles of buoyancy and resistance. They can be used for upper-body toning and also to assist in lower-body toning. They are hand held or attached with bands to the ankles. When used in lower-body toning, they are sometimes used under the armpits for flotation. Empty jugs should be used exclusively during the toning portion of class in deep or shallow water; they can be dangerous if used during the aerobic portion. The excessive buoyancy of empty milk jugs can cause shoulder impingement problems. Impingement is the squeezing of connective tissues in the shoulder and shoulder girdle muscles. Impingement eventually leads to pain and injury.

Partially Filled Jugs

Partially filled jugs are hand held and used in shallow water for upper-body toning. They capitalize on the principles of buoyancy, resistance, and weight. Partially filled jugs should be used only at or beneath the water surface. Using them overhead with the water sloshing around makes an extremely unstable, dangerous weight.

Cutout Jugs

Half- or one-gallon milk jugs that have the bottom third cut out can be used to increase intensity and muscular endurance for toning the upper body. They capitalize on the principle of resistance. They are hand held and should be used only in shallow water during the toning portion of class. If used during the aerobic portion, the amount of resistance could be too stressful for the upper body. If the milk jug is too resistant, the cap can be removed to reduce resistance.

Although many students find jugs useful in their aquatic workouts, they are not recommended. In short, jugs were not created as fitness devices and, therefore, should not be used as such. The use of such homemade equipment invites safety problems and, thus, liability.

Towels

Towels have been used to increase workout intensity. Based on the principles of resistance and weight, they are used for upper-body toning and can be hand held or strapped around the wrist or elbow. They should be used only during the toning portion of an aqua aerobics class but can be used during the entire aerobics portion of a water-walking or jogging class. They should be used in shallow water. The approximate price range is $2 to $10.

Towels are fairly safe because they cannot bump the body and cause bruising or injury. However, they were not created as exercise equipment and are not recommended for use during aqua aerobics classes.

Pull Buoys

Pull buoys are two cylindrical styrofoam pieces attached by a strap. They capitalize on the

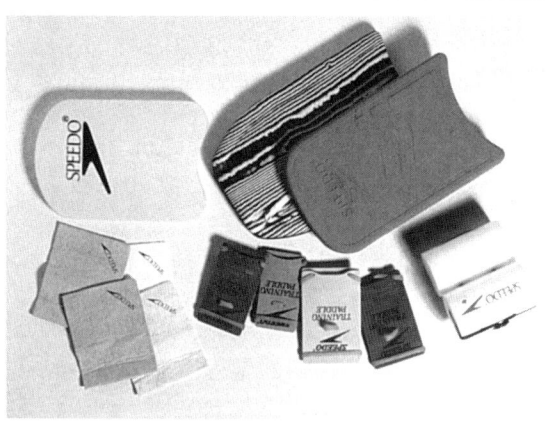

DIAGRAM 8–4 Kickboards, Hand Paddles, and Pull Buoys

principle of buoyancy and somewhat on the principle of resistance. They can be used for upper-body toning by holding the strap or slipping the hand between the two cylinders, and for lower-body toning by resting the heel of the foot between the two cylinders. They also can be attached to ankles with a Velcro strip. Pull buoys should be used in shallow water during the toning portion of class. They range in price from $2 to $5 each.

Pull buoys were originally designed for swimmers to keep their knees or ankles elevated, causing drag. Since they were not designed specifically for aquatic exercise, precautions should be taken to protect the skin from rubbing and to ensure a safe workout.

Water Wings

Children's inflatable water wings can be used to increase the intensity of a workout. They capitalize on the principle of buoyancy. Water wings can be used for upper-body toning in shallow water by slipping them over the wrists or above the elbows. They range in price from $2 to $7 per pair.

Water wings were not designed specifically for aquatic exercise, so precautions should be taken to provide a safe workout and protect the skin from rubbing.

Kickboards

Kickboards are based on the concepts of buoyancy and resistance. They can be used for upper-body toning by pressing them under the water and moving them from side to side. They can also be used as flotation devices for lower-body toning by using one under each forearm. They should be used only during the toning portion of the class in either shallow or deep water. They range in price from $5 to $12.

Kickboards were created as a swimming aid and not as aquatic exercise equipment. Precautions should be taken to ensure their safe use during class. Information on the Sprint/Rothhammer kickboard is included in Chapter 13.

Margarine Lids and Frozen Dinner Plates

Margarine lids and frozen dinner plates capitalize on the principle of resistance. They are hand held and used strictly for upper-body toning. Because of the inability to change the hand grip when using this equipment, they should be used in shallow water and only during toning, never during aerobics.

Like jugs, lids and plates were not created for use in aquatic exercise and they are not recommended.

Balloons, Balls, and Beach Balls

Balloons and balls, including beach balls, all capitalize on the principle of buoyancy and are used in shallow or deep water for upper-body toning. They are held with the hands and sometimes placed between the knees for isometric adductor contractions. To allow for muscle balance and adequate work of the upper-body muscles on the dorsal surface of the body, one ball should be held in each hand rather than holding one ball by both hands. These balls or balloons held in only one hand will, by necessity, be smaller but will be safer and offer greater benefits in the form of a better balanced program. Balls should not be used during the aerobics portion of the class, since their excessive buoyancy can cause shoulder impingement problems. The price range of balls is from $1 to $10.

Since balls, beach balls, and balloons were not created for aquatic exercise use, they are not recommended.

Mindy McCurdy Waterballs

Waterballs have handles attached and are based on both the buoyancy and resistance principles. They can be used in upper body strengthening and toning. They also are used for flotation during lower-body toning. Mindy McCurdy Waterballs retail for $35 to $40 per set. The Mindy McCurdy Waterballs were made expressly for aquatic exercise.

Deep-Water Vests and Belts

All equipment allowing participants to work out in the deep end of the pool capitalizes on the principle of buoyancy. Deep-water flotation vests and belts also can be used in chest-deep water to minimize footstrike.

The Wet Vest looks like a thin water-ski vest. It is slimmer so it does not impede movement in the water. It comes over the shoulders, covers the midriff, and has a "beaver" tail. It attaches with Velcro. The Wet Vest price range is $120 to $140.

The AquaJogger is a midriff flotation vest made of cushioned rubber. It is adjustable; one size fits all. The AquaJogger retails for approximately $45.

The Sprint/Rothhammer deep water belt is made of soft styrofoam discs. The price rage of this belt is approximately $10.

J & B Foam's belt has four buoyant styrofoam discs and attaches to the waist. The

DIAGRAM 8–5 Belts

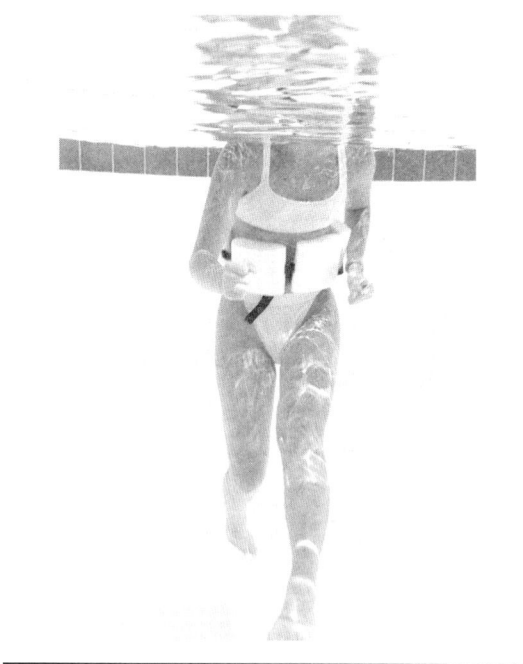

price range of the J & B deep-water belt is $5 to $10.

Hydro-Tone International makes a deep water belt also.

These deep-water vests and belts, and others not listed here, can be found in the equipment and catalog categories of the Resource section of this book (Chapter 13). These belts and vests were expressly created for aquatic exercise and can be used safely if manufacturers' guidelines are followed.

SpaBells

SpaBells are hand-held barbells that are both resistant and buoyant. The resistance can be adjusted by changing the attachments (power vanes) on the end compartment. The air chambers, which are dome attachments, provide the flotation factor. The domes can be water filled to create a weighted piece of equipment. Since SpaBells are resistant when moved through the water, they also capitalize on the resistance principle. They are used strictly for upper-body work in shallow water and can be used during the toning or aerobics portion of the class, if the aerobics portion moves slowly. They cost approximately $95.

SpaBells were created expressly for aquatic exercise and come with a laminated exercise sheet. Nuvo Sport Inc. is the manufacturer. Manufacturers' guidelines should be followed.

Hydro-Fit

A set of Hydro-Fit equipment includes buoyant ankle floats and buoyant barbells that are used in the deep water for a nonimpact workout or in shallow water for a light-impact workout. Hydro-Fit equipment is made from styrofoam and covered with a nylon fabric. It capitalizes on the principles of buoyancy and resistance and works both the upper and lower body. It can be used during the aerobic or toning portion of class and for specialized classes such as strength training and circuit training. The ankle floats or barbells can be used separately or as a set either in deep or shallow water. The barbells are hand held, and the ankle cuffs attach around the ankle. The approximate cost of a set of Hydro-Fit is $70.

Hydro-Fit was created expressly for aquatic exercise and comes with an instructional booklet describing various exercises in which it can be safely used. (Hydro-Fit ankle cuffs are shown in Diagram 2–11 in Chapter 2, Deep Water.)

Aerobic Workbench

The Aerobic Workbench was created for aquatic exercise bench or step programs. It is a full size bench weighing less than 20 pounds that comes in 6-inch, 8-inch and 10-inch heights. It is stackable, has side handle cut-outs for carrying, a non-slip surface, rounded corners, and a non-skid base that prevents shifting on the pool bottom. It should only be used in shallow water, and can be used safely in aquatic bench classes.

It is a single unit construction with no assembly required. The benches range in price from $45 to $55. Bench or step videos are available through the Aquatic Exercise Association listed in the Organizations section of Chapter 13. More information on the bench is available through Aerobic Workbench listed in the Equipment section of Chapter 13.

Spri Tubing, Bands, and Belts

Spri products are based on the concept of resistance. Although created for land-based fitness workouts, the equipment holds up well in water. It should be used in shallow water. The tubing is used for upper-body toning. Participants stand on the length of tubing and hold the handles of the tubing in their hands. The price range of the tubing is $5 to $10 per piece. Spri exercise bands are used for lower-body toning (placing them around the feet or ankles) or for upper-body toning. They cost $1 to $3 each. The Spri belt is a seatbelt-fabric belt with tubing and handles. The belt is attached around the waist and the hands are slipped into the handles of the tubing; it is used for upper-body toning during the aerobic portion of the class. The Spri belts retail for approximately $10 to $15 each. Using a belt and tube combination, the instructor can create a tether system for exercisers who run or swim in a limited space.

Again, although Spri equipment was created for land-based fitness classes, it has transferred well to aquatics programs. Special program instructions, precautions for use, and sample exercises are included with the aquatics package.

Hand Paddles

Hand paddles capitalize on the principle of resistance. Each is a flat, plastic disc, a little larger than hand size. Rubber tubing attaches to the wrist and fingers to hold the paddles on. Paddles are used in shallow water for upper-body work during the toning and sometimes the aerobic portions of classes. They range in price from $6 to $8 a pair.

Hand paddles were created for swimmers to develop strength and stroke techniques. They also can be used in advanced aquatics classes. Precautions should be taken to ensure their safe use. Hand paddles are available through the Sprint/Rothhammer catalog listed in the Resources chapter of this book (Chapter 13).

Dynabands

Dynabands are stretchy fabric bands that are comfortable to use and do not cut into the skin. They are based on the principle of resistance. Dynabands can be used for upper-body work, or the length of Dynabands can be tied together, forming a circle, and placed around the ankles or feet for lower-body toning. Dynabands should be used exclusively during the toning portion of the class and in shallow water. The approximate cost is $1.50 per Dynaband.

Dynabands, originally designed for land-based toning exercise, hold up in chemically treated water for approximately one to two

DIAGRAM 8–6 Spri Equipment

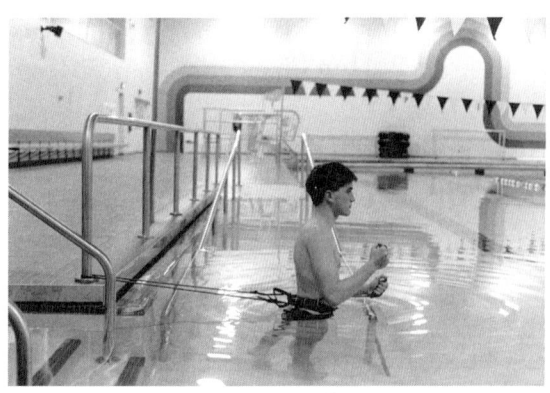

DIAGRAM 8-7 Dynaband

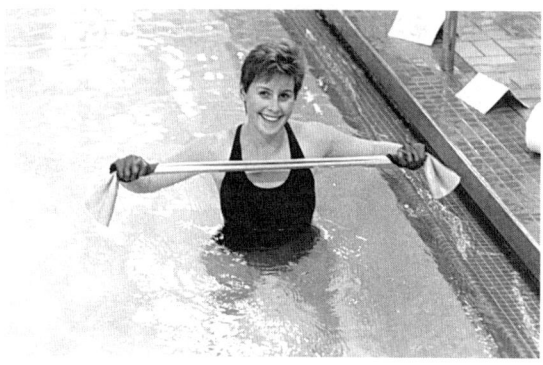

years, depending on frequency of use and general care. Dynabands are available through the Fitness Wholesale catalog listed in the Resources chapter of this book (Chapter 13).

Precautions should be taken to ensure their safe use during class.

Styrofoam Barbells

Styrofoam barbells capitalize on the principles of buoyancy and resistance and are used strictly for upper-body toning. They are hand held during the toning portion of class and used in shallow and sometimes deep water. Styrofoam barbells cost about $8 to $15 per pair.

These barbells were created expressly for aquatic exercise. They are available through J & B Foam, Sprint/Rothhammer and Hydro-Fit in the Resources chapter of this book (Chapter 13).

Styrofoam Discs

J & B Foam makes a disc-shaped piece of styrofoam that is based on the concepts of buoyancy and resistance. It can be used for upper-body toning and abdominal toning. It should be used in shallow water unless it is used as a kickboard. The approximate cost of the foam disc is $8 to $12.

The disc was created expressly for aquatic exercise to replace cumbersome kickboards.

Aqua Gloves

Aqua gloves are Lycra or rubberized gloves that have webbing between the fingers. They are based on the principle of resistance. The resistance can be varied by turning the hand into a slicing or flattened position. Aqua gloves can be used in shallow water for upper-body toning and throughout the aerobics portion of the class. The price range is $10 to $20 per pair.

DIAGRAM 8-8 Styrofoam Barbells

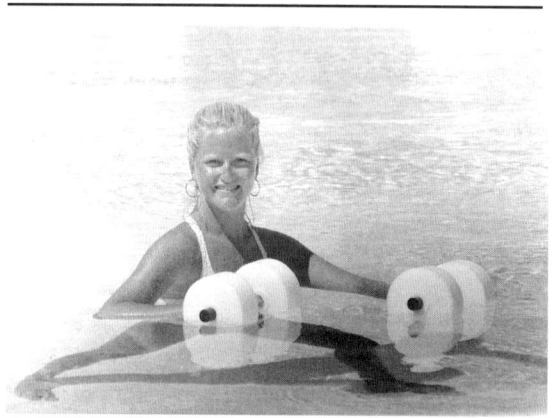

DIAGRAM 8-9 Aqua Gloves

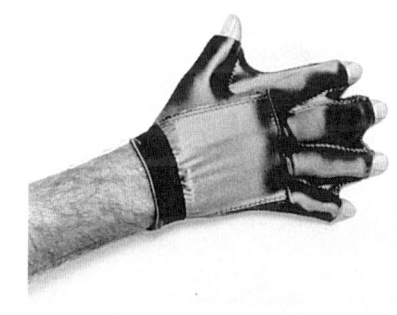

Aqua gloves were created expressly for aquatic exercise. They can be used both in beginner and advanced classes. Aqua gloves are available through Sprint/Rothhammer (water gloves) and Hydro-Fit (Wave Webs) in the equipment section of Chapter 13.

B-Wise Swim Fitness Bar

This buoyant polystyrene bar was created for aquatic exercise by B-Wise Enterprise, Inc. It can be used in shallow or deep water for upper body and midriff toning exercises. It can be used in deep water for lower body and midriff toning exercises. It is based on the principle of buoyancy. They are hand held with a padded bar between the two buoyant bells. The price is approximately $8 per bar.

Hydro-Tone

The Hydro-Tone set contains boots, made of scuba wetsuit material covered by hard, molded plastic fins, and a set of three-dimensional hard plastic bells. The boots attach with a back zipper, and the bells are hand held. The set capitalizes on the principle of resistance. They strengthen and tone both the upper and lower body. They can be used during the toning portion of a regular class and during the aerobics portion of a class for well-conditioned students. Hydro-Tone also can be used during specialized classes, such as strength training and circuit training. The equipment was created for use in shallow water but also is used successfully in deep water. The set of Hydro-Tone, complete with nylon mesh bag, video tape, and instructional sheet, retails for approximately $220.

Hydro-Tone was created specifically for aquatic exercise.

Aquatoner

Aquatoner paddles are made with a center hub, with three blades that can be adjusted so they overlap to various degrees. When they open completely, they provide a high degree of resistance. When there is space between the blades, there is less resistance. The Aquatoner paddles capitalize on the principle of resistance. They can be hand held, attached to the wrist, attached to the ankle, or attached above the knee. The paddles are used for upper- or lower-body work during the toning or strength-

DIAGRAM 8–10 Hydro-Tone

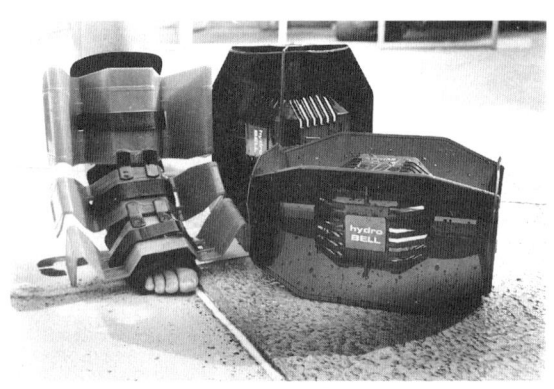

DIAGRAM 8–11 Aquatoner

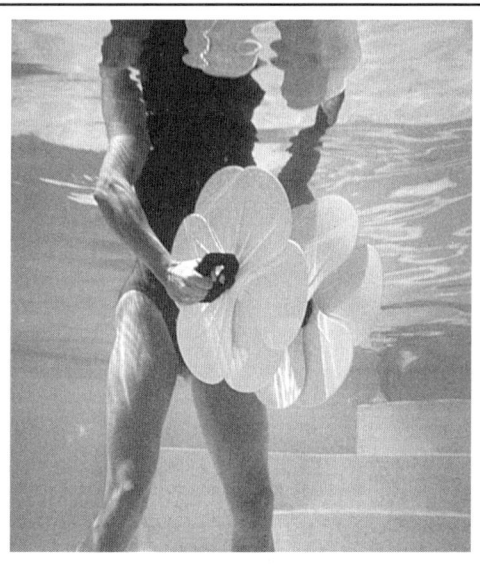

training portions of class. They also can be used in specialized classes such as circuit training and strength training. They should be used in shallow water. The approximate cost of one Aquatoner is $50.

Aquatoner paddles have been created especially for water exercise and therapy.

AQUATIC AIDS

Aquatic aids are pieces of equipment, toys, or props used to improve the quality or enjoyment of a workout.

Aquarius Water Workout Station

The Aquarius Water Workout Station is designed for those with sport injuries, low back pain, obesity, and some forms of arthritis. It has been used successfully in rehabilitation, cardiovascular conditioning, muscle toning, and general body strengthening. An illustrated exercise guide shows the exerciser how to do sit-ups, push-ups, leg-ups, etc. It also has been used effectively with the well-conditioned exerciser. The unit is manufactured by Aquatic Fitness Products and is listed in the Equipment section of Chapter 13.

Aquarius Rehabilitation Tank

The tank is a 1,600 gallon, totally self-contained, 8 foot by 8 foot by 42-inch high, free standing, marine grade, stainless steel rehabilitation tank with therapeutic ladder. The tank includes protocol for lower back pain, weakness on the lubopelvic girdle, abdominal and lumbar paraspinals and loading of pathological structures by gravity. The unit is manufactured by Aquatic Fitness Products and is listed in the Equipment section of Chapter 13.

Relaxation Tanks

A float tank resembles a large bathtub with a dome. These tanks are used exclusively in the medical and rehabilitation fields and are designed to enhance relaxation. Floating in a warm solution of Epsom Salts and water, free of restrictive clothing, shut off from light and sound and 90% of external sensory stimulation, allows the patient to focus on problems or behavior. Such therapy has been shown to decrease the need for medication and also to decrease pain.

Shoes

Aqua shoes generally have four purposes in pool use: (1) protect the skin on the feet; (2) assure good footing; (3) provide support; and (4) provide added weight.

If shoes are being worn to protect the skin, the style and quality of the shoe is irrelevant, as long as participants maintain good body alignment while wearing them. If the shoes are being worn to assure good footing, only the sole is relevant. The tread should have enough grid to keep the feet from slipping.

If shoes are being worn to provide support, consider the same factors as when buying them for land use. It is important to have good arch support. The fit, heel cup, flexibility, and cushioning also are important. People with knee and back problems and those who are

DIAGRAM 8–12 Aqua Shoes . . . All Brands

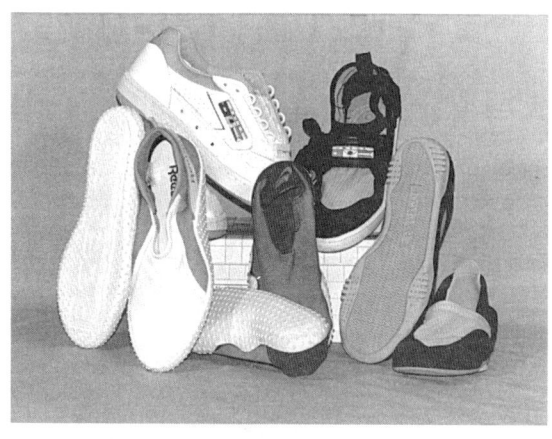

obese may want to use shoes to allow the cushioning to absorb impact.

If shoes are used to provide added weight, they should be absorbent. An absorbent shoe picks up more water weight and, therefore, adds more drag during the workout.

A variety of shoe manufacturers now make aquatic exercise shoes. While aqua shoes are not required in an aquatic exercise program, they are recommended for safety. Most accidents occur on the deck as a result of slipping. Aquatic shoes can eliminate that problem.

Choosing aquatic exercise shoes can be confusing. Above all, the student should look for a shoe that is comfortable. There should be no rubbing or tight spots. The perfect aquatic shoe has cushioning to protect against impact, good arch support, a stabilized heel, and a well-supported forefoot. The shoes should stay comfortably in place during exercise and be secure enough to resist the pull of the water's resistance. The shoes should be easy to put on and should dry quickly. (Sources for aquatic exercise shoes including the Omega Reef Warrior are included in the Resource section of this book, Chapter 13.)

Aquatic exercisers who want the more advanced cushioning and support of fitness shoes can purchase running, tennis, or aerobic shoes to wear in the pool. These are worn with or without socks, have nonmarking soles, and are used exclusively for water exercise.

Exercise Clothing

Aquatic exercise instructors and students are beginning to wear exercise clothing rather than swimwear to class. Most wear a leotard or swimsuit over a basic black or dark unitard or crop tight. There are several reasons for this.

1. *To see and be seen*—When instructors and students are all in the pool, the skin tones blend in with the water, pool bottom, and pool wall. Students have trouble seeing what the instructor is doing, and instructors cannot see if students are performing moves safely and correctly. With **aquawear**, both problems are solved because black or dark unitards or tights are easily visible in the water.

2. *Warmth*—Many students and instructors find the extra body covering provided by aquawear helps keep them comfortably warm during the cool times of class.

3. *The "exercise versus leisure" attitude*—Swim suits are regarded as leisure or sunbathing wear, not as strenuous exercise clothing. Instructors and students may want to have the exercise attitude subtly enforced by wearing aquawear. There is a psychological advantage to wearing clothes that look good and fit well. "You are what you wear" may not be true, but exercise clothes have a great deal to do with the way participants view themselves and their fitness regimen. Stylish, colorful clothing can contribute to feelings of enthusiasm, energy, and well-being.

4. *Comfort*—Aquawear eliminates cutting and creeping problems. Spaghetti straps, ties around the neck, and elastic around the legs on swimwear can cut and creep when students move in the water. Aquawear stays where it is supposed to and does not rub or cut.

5. *Support wear*—Men and women both have found that swimming suits alone do not provide enough support for the bouncing aquatic exercisers do in class. Aquawear allows for good support wear to be worn underneath

6. *Professionalism*—Students and instructors alike feel that aquawear makes the instructor look more professional. This likely has some inspirational effect on students.

Most aquawear is made of a Lycra and nylon blend; the fabric is usually chlorine resistant and holds up well in the pool. Cotton aquawear fades sooner, but some people find it more comfortable, than Lycrawear. Pool administrators and owners approve of both types of aquawear, as long as there are no loose or raveling threads.

Exercise clothing should be lightweight, comfortable, and nonrestrictive. The garments should be durable enough to withstand exercise movement and able to maintain their shape through frequent laundering. (Aquatic and exercise apparel manufacturers and catalogs are listed in the Resource section of this book, Chapter 13.)

MUSIC

Music is used in most aquatic exercise classes, even though the acoustics of most settings are far from ideal. Music can nourish the spirit while the body is being revitalized through exercise. It should elicit feelings of joy, fun, and excitement.

Making **music selection** (musical choices) for aquatics classes can be extremely confusing, since the science of music must be considered. Rhythm and tempo, dynamics, melody and lyrics, vibrational frequencies and pitch, and demographic composition are all factors. Fortunately, most instructors have an innate feeling regarding music that allows them to choose music that is right for their classes. Instructors not comfortable with music choice should find students who are and give them guidelines to help with selection.

The music should make participants want to move in a lively manner. It should allow them to concentrate on the exercise movements, and it should not be so complex or absorbing that participants become mentally disoriented. Music should promote joy, fun, excitement, and exuberance. The music used in class can be a powerful force that motivates students to peak performance or can make the workout a drudgery.

Sources

Finding appropriate music often is difficult for the aquatics instructor. Luckily, many sources are available. Newsletters discuss, recommend, and review new pieces of music. Some services supply complete music for the entire class; others create music especially to meet specific needs. Strom-Berg Productions is the only music service that produces aquatic specialty music. They are listed in the Music section of Chapter 13. Students, friends, and libraries are all sources of free music. Record stores often allow instructors to listen to music before buying it.

Mediums

Records are rarely used anymore, and record players in pool areas are a thing of the past. Cassettes and cassette players currently are the most popular form of music medium in aquatic settings. Compact discs and CD players are the newest medium.

Whatever medium is used, safety must always be kept in mind. Players should be away from the pool edge, and systems should be safely grounded. Batteries are recommended for most systems. Waterproof systems are preferable.

Tempo

Music tempo is measured in beats per minute (BPM). In aerobic exercise, the tempo of the music determines the intensity of the exercise because it dictates the speed of the movement: The faster the tempo, the greater the intensity. But in aquatic exercise, a slow movement is sometimes more exertive than a fast one. Thus, beats per minute should be considered in aquatics classes to provide a good workout, but tempo is not as vital to music choice as it is in land aerobics classes.

A tempo of 130 to 160 beats per minute works well in water if used at half time. A tempo of 120 beats per minute or slower can be used at full time. Participants with long limbs and those using equipment may have to move more slowly or use a shorter lever to keep up with the beat used for the rest of the class.

The tempo of the music should be exciting, not relaxing, during the aerobics portion. Relaxing music can be used during the final stretch.

Many cassette and compact disc players have pitch control, which allows the instructor to speed up or slow down the music by approximately 12%. Vocal music can be varied by up to 3% without sounding distorted.

Styles

Music should be chosen to reflect the interests of participants. African, Latin, New Age, and rap are the newest music styles to be used in land aerobics classes. They may appeal to younger students more so than older ones. Instructors with a mixed group of people may select music that mixes polka, rock and roll, bluegrass, Eurorock, religious rock, oldies, and soft rock.

Copyright

Music is copyrighted. The copyright owner has the right to charge a fee when his or her music is used in a public performance. All exercise and fitness classes are deemed *public performances.*

KEY WORDS

Buoyance
Resistance
Weight
Gravitational pull

Precautions
Full range of motion
Aquatic aids

Aqua shoes
Aquawear
Music selection

SUMMARY

- Equipment can fill the need in aquatic exercise for variety and challenge for the bored or well-conditioned student.
- All equipment is based on one or more of the three basic principles: buoyancy, weight, or resistance.
- Buoyant equipment increases the force needed to hold the item beneath the water.
- Resistant equipment is designed to inhibit movement of a limb or the body through the water.
- Weighted equipment increases the weight of the limb moving through the water and, therefore, increases the intensity.
- Exercisers should follow specific guidelines for safe equipment use.
- Without a medical professional's guidance, some special populations should not use equipment.
- When choosing equipment, participants should try to match the type of equipment to the purpose of the workout.
- Although many participants find "free" equipment useful, such equipment is not recommended. They were not created as fitness devices and, therefore, should not be used as such. The use of homemade devices invites safety problems.
- Aqua shoes can protect the skin on the feet, assure good footing, provide support, and provide added weight.
- Aquawear rather than swimwear allows the participant to be more comfortable and to wear necessary support garments underneath.
- Music used in aquatic exercise classes should elicit feelings of joy, fun, and excitement.

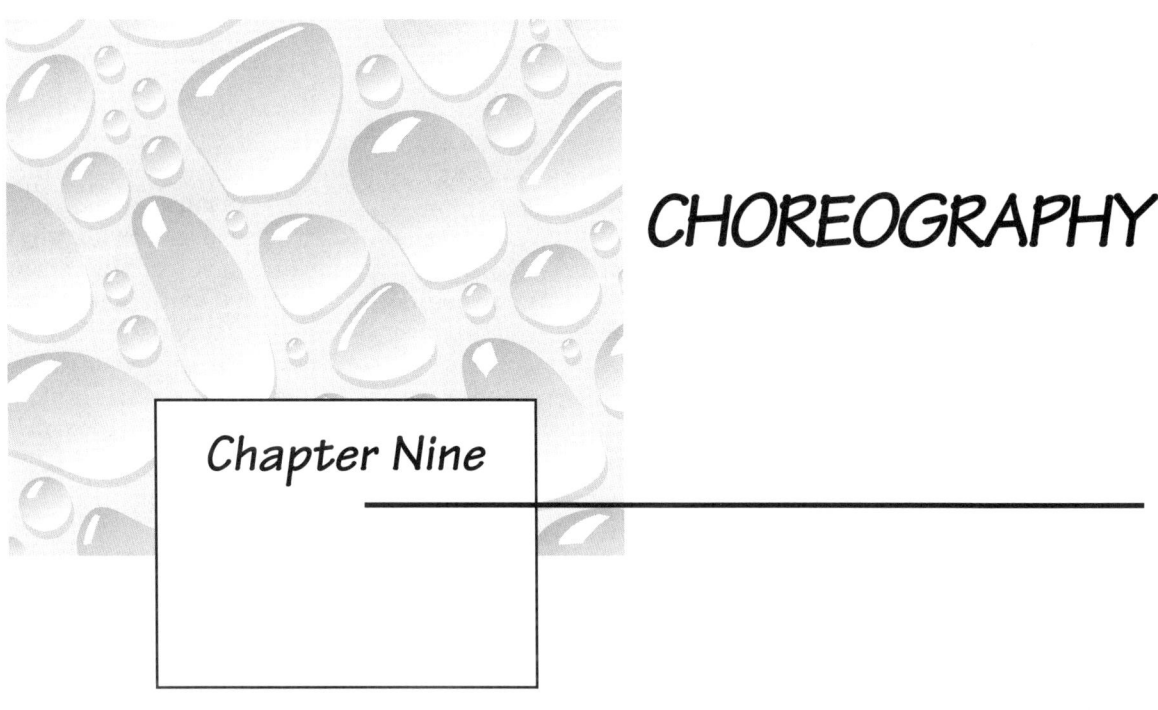

CHOREOGRAPHY

Chapter Nine

MUSCLE BALANCE

Muscle imbalances reflect differences in the relative strengths and flexibilities of the various muscles surrounding a joint or body part. Muscle imbalances occur when some body segments are much more developed than others. Besides adversely affecting shock absorption, muscle imbalances can predispose a person to spasm, pain, injury, and faulty coordination.

The human body is designed to be balanced in all ways. Muscle groups work in **muscle pairs,** *agonists* and *antagonists*. In daily living, a person frequently uses one **muscle group** more than its paired muscle group, resulting in muscular imbalance. Imbalance between agonist and antagonist pairs results in elongated, weak muscles across one surface of a joint and shortened, strong muscles across the other. This, coupled with the aging process, may limit function and cause much of the pain aging people experience. Eventually, this stresses the **skeletal framework,** leading to more frequent pain, injury complexities, and sometimes extensive disability.

Typical muscles that are shortened and strong include:

1. anterior chest wall muscles (pectorals)
2. back extensor muscles (erector spinae)
3. muscles of the front of the thigh (iliopsoas)
4. calf muscles (gastrocnemius)
5. anterior upper-arm muscles (biceps)

Often elongated and weak are the abdominals, the upper-back muscles (trapezius and rhomboids), the shin muscles (tibialis anterior), the buttocks muscles (gluteals), and the posterior upper-arm muscles (triceps).

Anterior chest wall muscles that are tighter or shorter than normal cause the shoulders to become rounded, which can result in poor posture, neck pain, and limited chest expansion. The combination of tight erector spinae with iliopsoas and weak abdominals and gluteals is a major cause of back pain. Muscle-balanced workouts can decrease these problems.

The most important factor, then, in successful aquatic exercise programming is a basic understanding of why each movement is used. An aquatic program should not be haphazardly thrown together but carefully planned to consider muscle balance and safety. Giving each move a purpose greatly increases the quality of an aquatic exercise program. Good programs also include movements that are simply fun. Nonetheless, aquatic instructors should examine fun moves to make sure they do not compromise muscle balance and safety.

When creating a program, **muscle balance** should always be considered. This means that each of the major muscle groups should be worked with two or three moves in every workout. Instructors should remember to work **opposing muscles** of a pair at least equally. If the program includes 16 bicep curls, it should also include 16 tricep extensions. If students are doing lots of kicks, kneelifts, and jogging with knees up, they will be strengthening and tightening the hip flexors. They should do an equal number of moves to work the gluteals.

The exception to equal work is when one partner of a muscle group is weaker than the other. Then it is accepted practice to use the weak muscle more extensively than the strong one. In other words, it is okay to use more moves that include the traditionally weaker muscles (triceps, abdominals, gluteals, and tibialis anterior) and fewer moves that use the traditionally stronger muscles (biceps, spinae erector, iliopsoas, and gastrocnemius). Instructors should make sure, however, the stronger of each pair is not ignored completely.

Since the stronger muscle in each pair is simpler to work, there is always the tendency to encourage existing muscle imbalance, doing only easy (kneelifts, jogs, jog arms) moves and trying to compensate in the toning section. Unfortunately, 10 to 15 minutes of toning cannot undo the muscle imbalance caused by everyday life. As a fitness professional, the instructor needs to assist students in overall health and wellness. In order to do that, the entire program should be well thought out in terms of why moves are used and if they assist in overall muscle balance.

Safety is another reason for knowing why a move is used. If an instructor is using movement to strengthen gluteals but finds that it may compromise the low back or is possibly a **contraindicated** move, he or she should modify it or replace it with a safer movement. Thinking about each move keeps the program top notch.

A CATALOG OF MOVEMENTS

Moves are listed in alphabetical order for convenience. Major muscle groups involved are listed in the description of each movement. Many moves begin in one of the basic positions listed here.

Starting Positions

- *Feet Together*—stand, with the feet lined up, neither foot forward of the other, and no more than six inches apart
- *Prone*—lie on the water surface in a face-down position
- *Stride Position*—stand, with the feet shoulder-width apart, toes and knees pointed forward
- *Supine*—Lie on the water surface in a face-up position

Arm Movements

Suggested arm movements are often listed for step movements, and step movements are often listed with arm movements. Arm movements may use the following terms:

- *Corresponding or Opposite*—Corresponding refers to movements in which the arm and leg on the same side of the body move together, in the same direction. *Opposite* refers to movements in which the arm on one side of the body moves in the same direction as the leg on the other side of the body.

A Catalog of Movements

— *Doubles and Singles*—*Doubles* indicates that both arms move together with the same movement, in the same direction. *Singles* indicates that only one arm is doing the movement.

All the moves listed in this section of the book can be used with all types of choreography (see end of chapter) and in any type of program (i.e., deep water, interval training, aerobics, sports conditioning).

Individual Moves

Abdominal Stretch
While standing, lift the ribs and push the rib cage forward. This will cause a slight hyperextension of the lumbar area of the spine. Use with caution.

— Abdominal Stretch

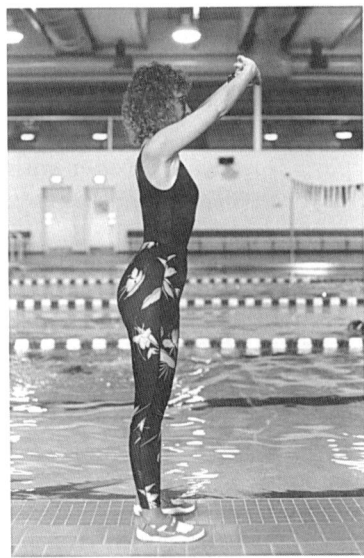

Abductor Stretch
While standing on one foot, pull the heel of the right foot toward the front of the hip of the left leg. Press the right knee in toward the left shoulder for the Abductor Stretch right. Reverse for Abductor Stretch left.

Adductor Stretch
Take a big step to the left, with the toes of both feet pointed forward. The feet will be more than shoulder-width apart. Bend the left knee, but keep the right knee straight. This will stretch the adductors in the right leg. If the water is too deep for this stretch to be effective, lift the right knee up and to the right to stretch the right adductor. Reverse to stretch the left leg adductor.

— Abductor Stretch

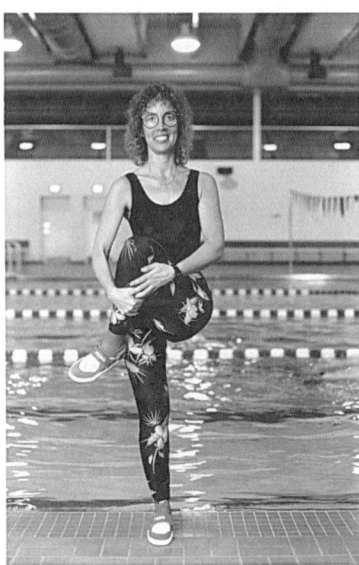

— Adductor Stretch (version 1)

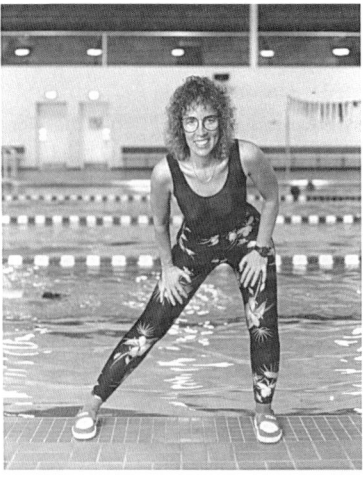

— Adductor Stretch (version 2)

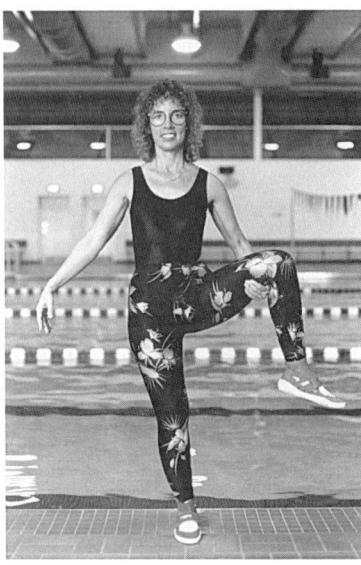

Anterior Deltoid Stretch

See Bicep, Anterior Deltoid, and Pectoral Stretch.

Anterior Tibialis Stretch

See Iliopsoas Stretch.

Armswing Forward

Begin with the arms down at the sides, palms back (pronated). Lift both arms forward through the water with force until the arms are extended in front of the body, just beneath the water surface. This portion of the move works the deltoids and pectorals. Keeping palms down, press both arms back to the beginning position. This portion of the move works the deltoids and latissimus dorsi. Proper body alignment should be maintained during the Armswings. This move can be varied by alternately swinging one arm forward and the other backward.

Armswing Forward Flexed

Begin with arms the down at the sides, elbows bent (flexed) at a 90- to 120-degree angle, and palms back (pronated). Lift both arms forward through the water, maintaining the original elbow flexion, until the arms are in front of the body, just beneath the water surface. This portion of the move works the deltoids, biceps, and pectorals. Keeping the palms down, press both arms back to the beginning position. This portion of the move works the deltoids, biceps, and latissimus dorsi. This move can be varied by alternately swinging one arm forward and the other backward.

Armswing Side

Begin with the arms down at the sides, palms back (pronated). Move both arms to the right and then up toward the water surface to the right. This is Armswing right. Return the arms to the beginning position. Move both arms to the left and then up toward the water surface to the left. This is Armswing left. Return the arms to the beginning position. This move can be varied in several ways. Armswing right with the right arm only and Armswing left with the left arm only is a Single (one arm only) Corresponding (the same side) Armswing right or left. The elbow can be slightly flexed to create variety. Palms can be pronated so hands slice through the water, or they can push through the water with the backs of the hands leading

— Armswing Forward

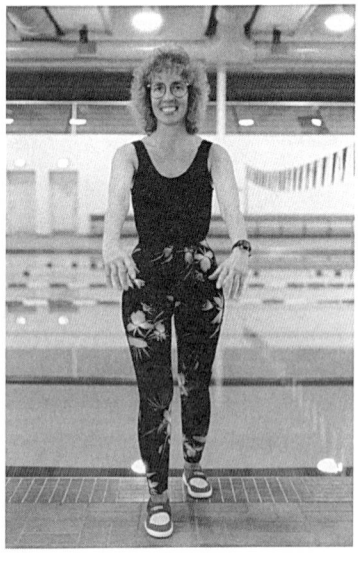

— Armswing Forward Flexed

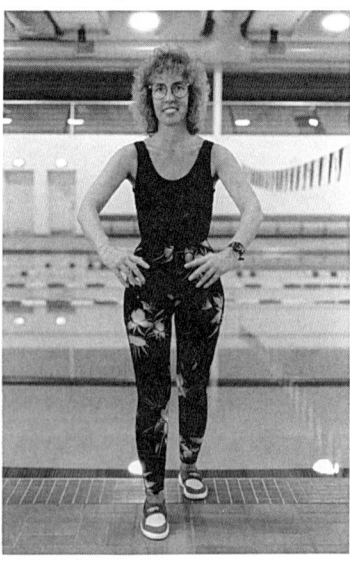

— Armswing Side

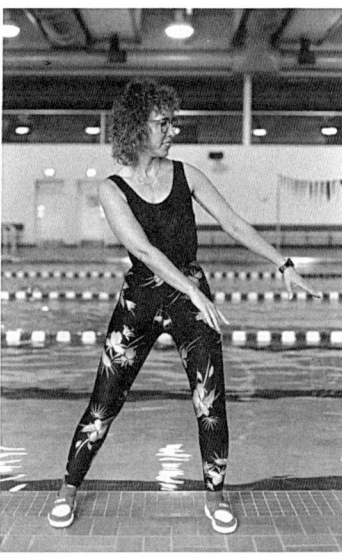

or with the palms cupped and leading for added resistance. Armswing Side works the deltoids, pectorals, and trapezius.

Back Kick

Begin with the feet in stride position, arms at the sides. Without flexing (bending) the knee, kick the right leg back (hip hyperextension). Return to the beginning position, and repeat the movement with the left leg. To protect the lower back, the right arm should swing forward, punch forward, or elbow press when the right leg kicks back. Both arms can swing, punch, or press forward when either leg kicks back. It is not advisable to move the arms back when the leg is moving back, since it may compromise the lower back. Back Kicks can be done slowly, with a bounce between each one, or quickly, kicking one out while the other returns. Another variation is alternating the kicks right and left or doing them in groups of two, four, or eight right before changing to the left leg. Back Kicks work the gluteals and iliopsoas.

Back-Kick Swing

Begin with the feet in stride position. Kick the right leg forward (hip flexion) for the first count, and swing it straight back to slight hip hyperextension for the second count. The Back-Kick Swing gives a larger range of motion while working the gluteals than the Back Kick. Abdominal muscles should be contracted while the leg is swinging back for back safety, and the work should be felt in the gluteals. The Back-Kick Swing works the iliopsoas and gluteals. It can be done alternating right and left legs or in groups of two, four, or eight with one leg before switching to the other. The left arm should swing forward as the right leg kicks forward, and the right arm should swing forward as the right leg swings back to avoid compromising the lower back.

Back Lunge

Begin with the feet in stride position, arms extended laterally (out to the sides), with palms facing forward. Step the right foot back, and shift the body weight to the right foot, keeping the left foot down in beginning position. During the step back, move the arms forward just beneath the water surface until palms almost

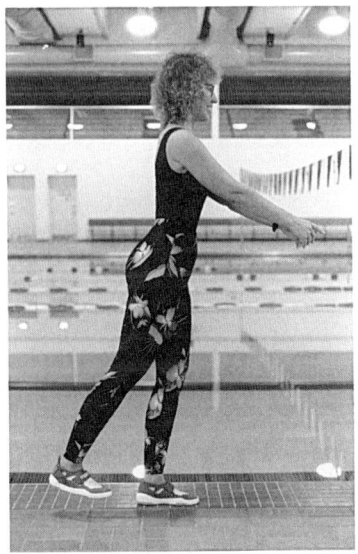
— Back Kick

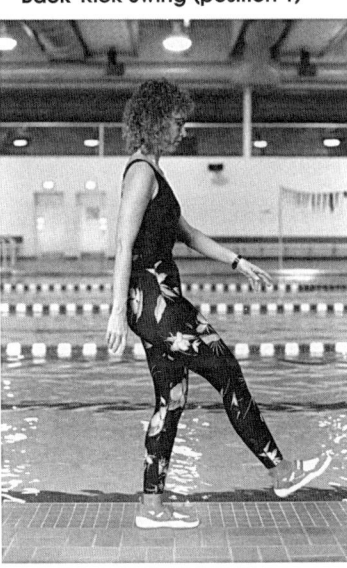
— Back-Kick Swing (position 1)

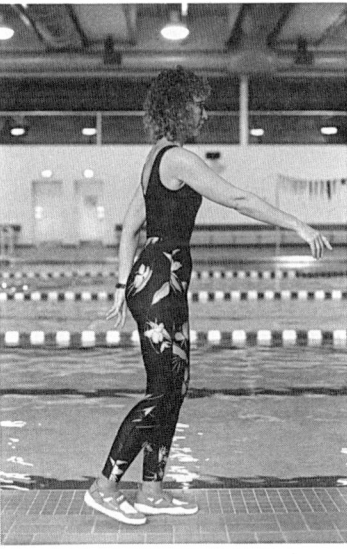
— Back-Kick Swing (position 2)

Back Lunge

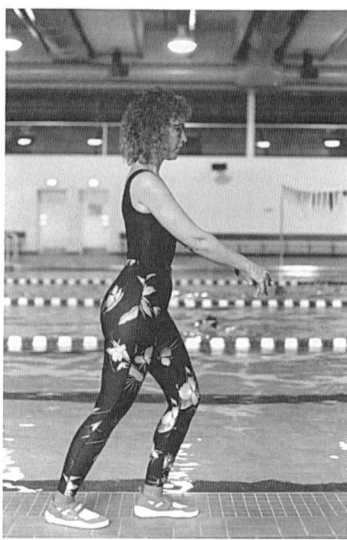

meet. Return the right foot to the beginning position, while pressing the arms back to the beginning position. Repeat with the left foot. This move works the gluteals, iliopsoas, pectorals, and trapezius.

Back Stretch

Begin facing the pool edge, with the hands and arms extended over it. Bring the knees to the chest, and hug them. See also Erector Spinae Stretch.

Back Touch

See Touch Back.

Backstroke

Begin with both elbows in at the waist and the forearms out to side for the **Short Backstroke**. With the palm supinated (facing forward) and the elbow flexed and staying in at waist, reach back with the hand, cup the water, and pull it forward (almost a complete circumduction of the elbow). This can be done alternating the right and left arms or using

Short Backstroke

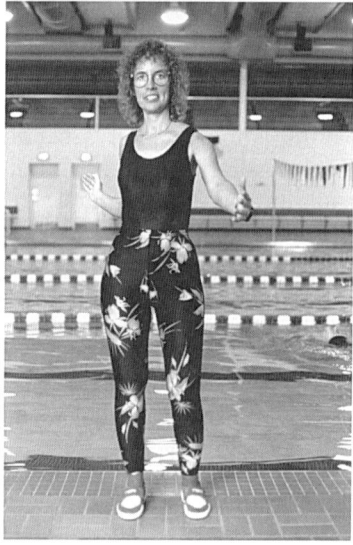

Long Backstroke

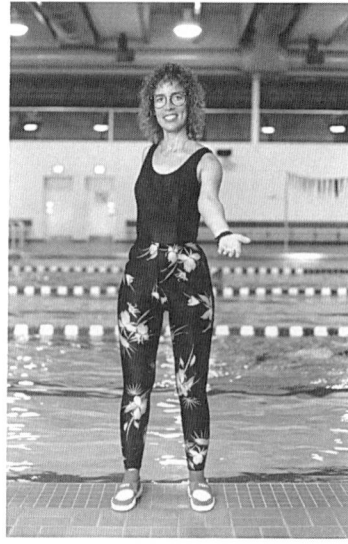

both together. The **Short Backstroke** works biceps and triceps. The **Long Backstroke** is the same move with arms extended. Both arms begin extended laterally, with palms down, just beneath the water surface. Reach back, turn the palm to face front, cup the water, and pull it down and forward. This move works the deltoids, trapezius, and pectorals. It can be done alternating the right and left arms or doing both at one time. Both backstrokes are excellent means of moving back through the water.

Backstroke Side

With the right arm extended just below the water surface, back to the right (behind the body), with a slight flex in the elbow and the palm facing right,

Backstroke Side

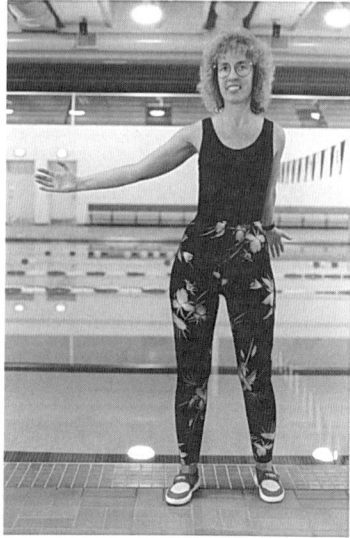

pull the right arm forward and left (still just below the water surface) until it is extended directly in front of the body. Return to the beginning position, and repeat with the left arm extended back to the left and moving forward. This move works pectorals, serratus anterior, deltoids, rhomboids, and trapezius. Performing the same move using the forearm only (the action will be in the elbow, not the shoulder) will work biceps and triceps. It can be performed using both arms at once in either manner. It works well with any ordinarily stationary move, either done in place or moving backwards.

Baseball Swing

Using both arms, swing back to the right and then forward, as though hitting a baseball. Repeat on the left side.

Basketball Jump

Bounce three times in a low, crouched position, mimicking bouncing a basketball. Push up and out of the water as far as possible, mimicking shooting a basketball.

Bicep, Anterior Deltoid, and Pectoral Stretch

With the fingers interlaced, low behind the back, turn the elbows in toward each other, and lift the arms up behind the back until a stretch is felt in the pectorals, anterior deltoids, and biceps. Keep the chest out, the chin in, and the back straight.

— Bicep, Anterior Deltoid, and Pectoral Stretch

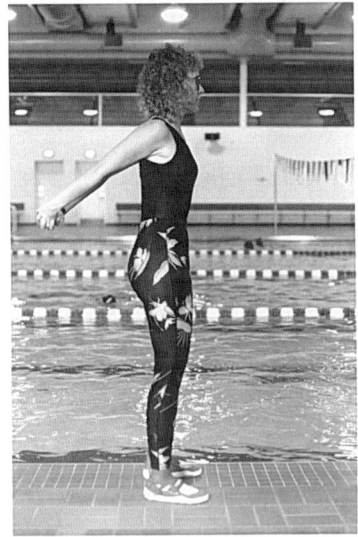

Bicep Curl

Begin with the elbows in at the waist and the hands down, palms forward (supinated). Bend the elbows (elbow flexion) to a 45- to 90-degree angle

— Bicep Curl

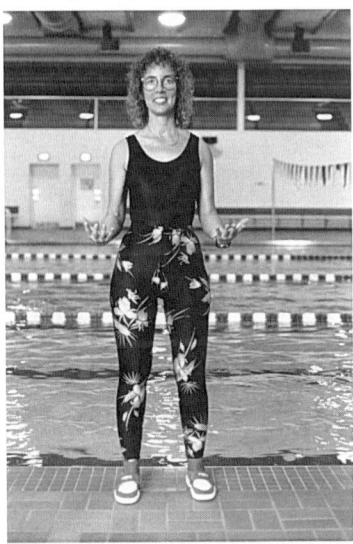

for the first count. Return to the beginning position for the second count. This is one Bicep Curl. Bicep Curls can be done singly (8 to 16 with one arm before switching to the other arm); this is often done during toning. They can also be done alternating right and left arms. Bicep Curls work the biceps.

Boogie

Begin with the feet in stride position. Step the right foot behind and to the left of the left foot, while the left foot remains stationary. The torso faces forward or may twist slightly to the left while the exerciser looks to the left. Reach the left arm down to the left diagonal; pull the right arm out of the water, and reach up to the right diagonal. This is the first count. Return to the beginning position for the second count. Step the left foot behind and to the right

— Boogie

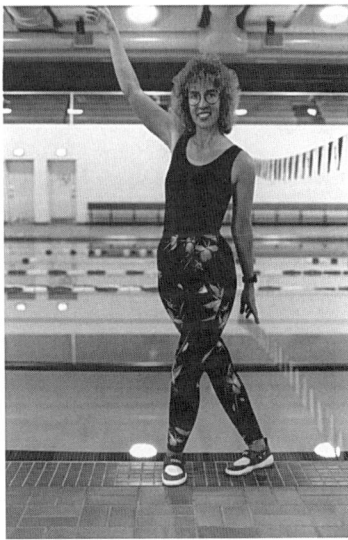

of the right foot. Look to the right and keep the torso either facing forward or slightly twisted to the right. Reach the right arm down to the right diagonal; pull the left arm out of the water, and reach up to the left diagonal. This is the third count. Return to beginning position for the fourth count. These four counts represent one set of Boogie. The Boogie works obliques, adductors, and gluteals. It can be done four or eight times with the right foot before changing to the left. The arm movements can be varied; keep them beneath the water surface by using Press Down Front arms.

Bow and Arrow

Begin with both arms extended laterally (out to the side) to the left side at shoulder level. Feet, knees, hips, and shoulders are pivoted to the left to allow the palms to begin together. With feet, knees, and hips stationary, pull the right elbow back until the right fist is near the right shoulder. (To eliminate the oblique work for people with back problems, allow the feet, knees, and hips to pivot with the shoulders.) Continue with several repetitions, using the right arm before switching to the left. Pectorals, deltoids, trapezius, and rhomboids are all involved with this move.

Buffalo Shuffle

The Buffalo Shuffle moves laterally, doing four or eight shuffles to the right followed by four or eight to the left. Begin in stride position. Step the right foot to the right, with the knees, toes, and torso facing forward; kick the left foot out slightly to the left side. Move the right arm out of the water, and point to the right diagonal; keep the left arm on the left hip. This is the first count. Step the left foot behind the right foot, while bringing the right knee up. Bring the right elbow down to the water surface. This is the second count. Repeat counts 1

— Buffalo Shuffle (position 1)

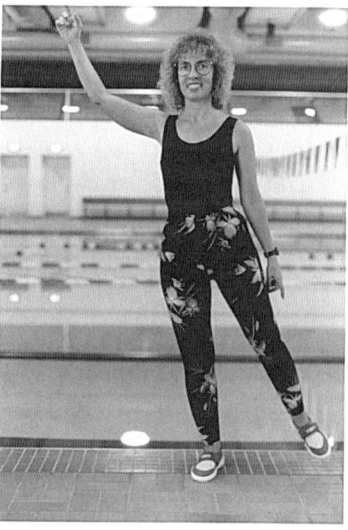

— Bow and Arrow (position 1)

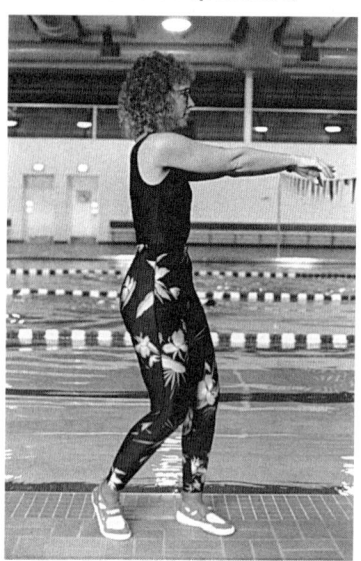

— Bow and Arrow (position 2)

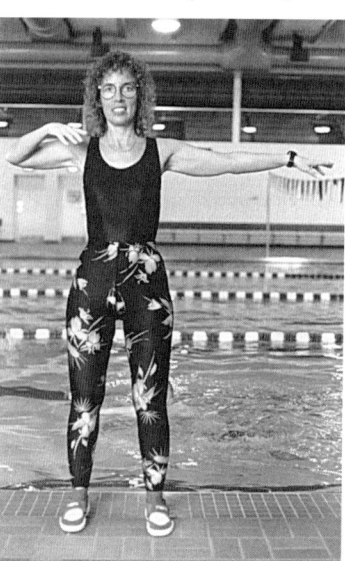

— Buffalo Shuffle (position 2)

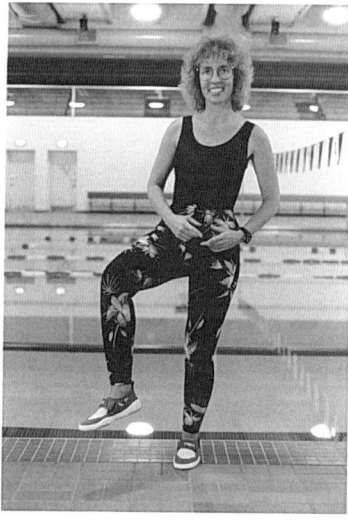

and 2 three or seven more times moving to the right.

For the Buffalo Shuffle left, step laterally to the left with the left foot while the knees, toes, and torso face forward; kick the right leg out slightly to the right. Move the left arm out of the water, and point to the left diagonal; keep the right hand on the right hip. This is the first count. Step the right foot behind the left foot, while bringing the left knee up. Bring the left elbow down to the water surface. This is the second count. Repeat counts 1 and 2 three or seven more times to complete a set of the Buffalo Shuffle left. The Buffalo Shuffle works adductors and abductors.

Calf Stretch

See Gastrocnemius Stretch.

Cross Kick

Begin with the feet in stride position, with the right hip slightly rotated externally (right toes will be pointed to the right diagonal). Cross and lift the right heel in front and to the left of the left ankle. Return to the beginning position. With the left hip slightly rotated externally (left toes will be pointed to the left diagonal), cross the left heel in front and to the right of the right ankle. Return to the beginning position. The Cross Kick works adductors and abductors. The move must be made with the heel leading through the water. If the hip rotates internally and the toes point to the opposite diagonal

– Cross Kick

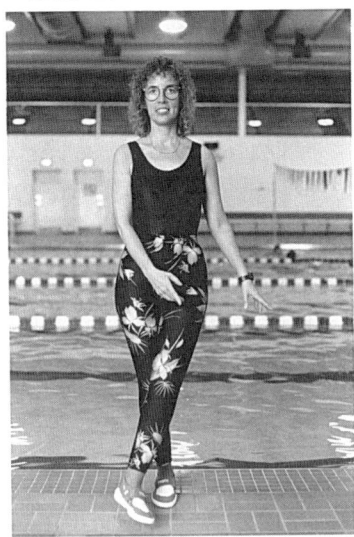

and lead the move, the iliopsoas will be involved. The torso should be kept facing forward. Lateral push to the right when the right leg is crossing to the left and vice versa.

Cross Rock

The Cross Rock is much like the Rocking Horse done with the legs in a crossed position. Begin with the weight on the left foot and the right leg lifted (hip flexion) slightly across the left leg. Step the right foot forward and across the left foot, leaning forward toward the left (over the right foot) but keeping the body straight. Avoid any spinal flexion that might cause the body to bend at the waist. Bring the left foot up, off the pool bottom, and kick back slightly to the right, shifting the weight to the right foot. This is the first count. Step the

– Cross Rock (position 1)

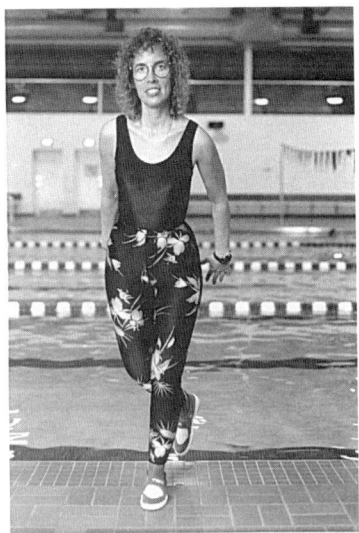

– Cross Rock (position 2)

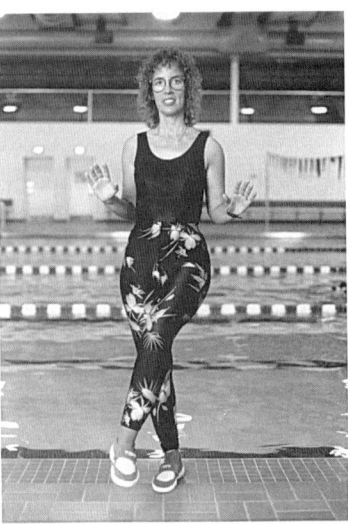

left foot back to the beginning position, and lean slightly back to the right, keeping the body straight. Avoid any spinal hyperextension that might cause the body to bend backward at the waist. Bring the right foot up, off the pool bottom, and kick forward to the left; shift the weight to the left leg. This is the second count. Repeat counts 1 and 2 three more times and then switch to Cross Rock left, with the left foot rocking forward and across the right foot and the right foot rocking back and to the left. The Cross Rock works iliopsoas, gluteals, obliques, and abdominals. Safe Arms, pushing back as the body leans or rocks forward and pushing forward as the body rocks back, work well with this move (see Safe Arms). This move can be varied to Cross Rock Doubles, Cross Rock in Three, or Cross Rock Seven and Up (as described in Rocking Horse sections) when done with a crossing rock.

Crossing Jog

The Crossing Jog moves laterally to the left in sets of four or eight and then returns to the right. Begin with the feet in stride position, hands on hips. Cross the right foot over and toward the left of the left foot; shift the weight to the right foot while lifting the left foot slightly off the pool bottom. This is the first count. Step the left foot to the left of the right foot; shift the weight to the left foot. This is the second count. Repeat counts 1 and 2 three or seven more times while moving sideways through the water to the left. Reverse by crossing the left foot over the right and shifting the weight to the left foot for the first count. Step the right foot laterally to the right of the left foot; shift the weight to the

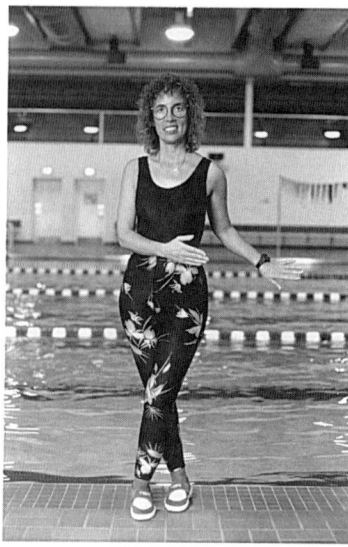

— Crossing Jog

right foot for the second count. Repeat counts 1 and 2 three or seven more times while moving right. The arms can stay on the hips or push laterally (to the right when moving left, to the left when moving right). Keep the torso facing forward to achieve the excellent oblique, adductor, and abductor work this move provides.

The Crossing Jog can also be done with the leading foot crossing behind instead of in front, as described above. While moving left, the right foot would step behind the left foot for the first count of each two-count segment. While moving right, the left foot would behind the right foot during the first count of each two-count segment. This is called Crossing Jog behind and also works the adductors and abductors. The Crossing Jog in front and behind can be combined to create a grapevine move. A two-count segment of Crossing Jog in front moving left would be followed by a two-count segment of Crossing Jog behind moving left; repeat twice before reversing to move to the right. This can be called a Crossing Jog Combo or a Grapevine. The cues would be "cross, step, back, step, cross, step, back, step."

Crossing Legswing

Begin standing, with the back to the pool edge. Lift the right leg (hip flexion) until it is at a 90-degree angle, with the knee slightly flexed (bent). Cross (horizontally adduct) the right leg toward the pool edge on the left side of the body. This is the first count. Return the leg to the beginning (forward) position for the second count. Swing the leg out (horizontally abduct) toward the pool edge on the right side of the body. This is the third count. Return it to beginning position for the fourth count. This is one Crossing Legswing. Repeat seven more times with the right leg before switching to the left leg for eight more. The Crossing Legswing works the adductors and abductors. **This move can severely compromise the stability of the weight-bearing knee**. If this move is used, the weight-bearing knee should be slightly flexed and never feel any twisting movement. The range of motion for the Crossing Legswing should be very small. The Kneeswing Cross-

— Crossing Legswing (position 1)

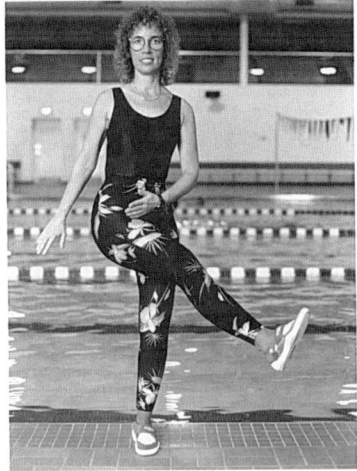

— Curl Down

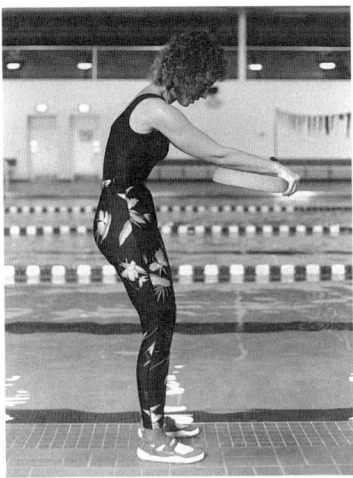

— Deltoid Lift

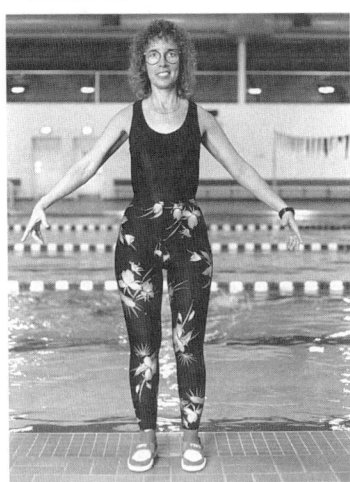

— Crossing Legswing (position 2)

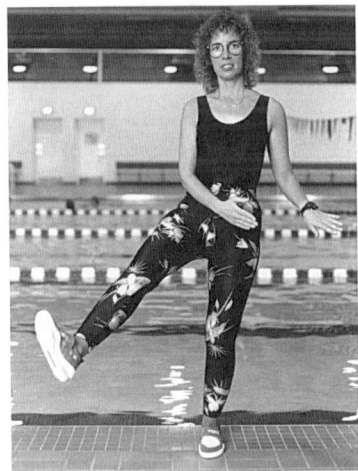

ing may be a better choice for adductor and abductor work.

Curl Down

Begin with the arms extended (shoulder flexion) straight in front of the body, just below the water surface. Bend forward (forward spinal flexion) at the waist, bringing the sternum and navel closer together. Return to an upright position. As the spine bends forward, keep the shoulders and elbows tight; the arms will be forced down, deeper into the water. The arms themselves should not do the moving (avoid any shoulder extension) but only move because of the spinal flexion. The arms will create a drag and force the abdominal muscles to work during the flexion. Students should be cautioned not to bend at the hips, as this will work the already strong iliopsoas muscles. The bend or flexion should occur only at the waist. Holding a buoyant device (milk jug, kickboard, ball, etc.) in the hands will increase the difficulty of the abdominal work. (See Chapter 8 on equipment.)

Deltoid Lift

Begin with both arms down at the sides, palms in at the thighs (supinated). Lift the arms with force to the sides and up (abduct). This portion of the move focuses on the deltoids. To reverse the move, press both arms down through the water. This portion of the move works the latissimus dorsi.

Deltoid Stretch (Medial)

Begin with a Neck Stretch (see Neck Stretch). When the head is tilted to the left side, reach behind the back with the left arm, and pull gently on the

— Deltoid Stretch (Medial)

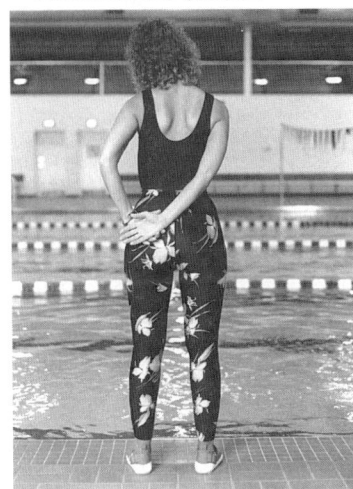

right wrist. Reverse for the Deltoid Stretch left.

Deltoid Stretch (Posterior)

With the right arm at shoulder level, pull the right elbow in toward the chest with the left hand, and bend the right elbow to feel the stretch in the posterior deltoids. Reverse for the Posterior Deltoid Stretch left.

– Deltoid Stretch (Posterior)

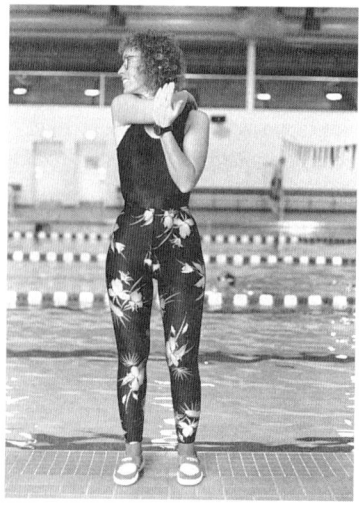

Diagonal Kick

See Kick Corner.

Elbow Press

Begin with both arms out to the sides (extended laterally). The elbows are flexed to 90 degrees, with the forearms straight up from the elbows. Lower the arms into the water. Begin the move in this position.

Press the elbows and hands toward each other (shoulder adduction) until they almost

– Elbow Press

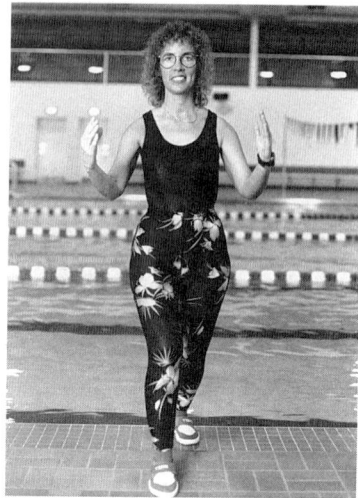

touch. Pull them apart to return to the beginning of the move. The press works the pectorals and serratus anterior, while the pull works the rhomboids and trapezius. Jogging, Mule Kicks, and Heel Tilts all work well with these arm movements (see Mule Kick and Heel Tilt). Be sure the arms are kept below the water surface, if possible.

Elbow Press Single

Begin with both arms out to the sides (extended laterally). The elbows are flexed to 90 degrees, with the forearms straight up from the elbows. Lower the arms into the water. Begin the move in this position. Press the right elbow across the body (shoulder adduction) to the left elbow, which has not moved. Stop and pull the elbow back to the beginning position (shoulder abduction). Repeat with the right arm, if desired, and then

– Elbow Press Single

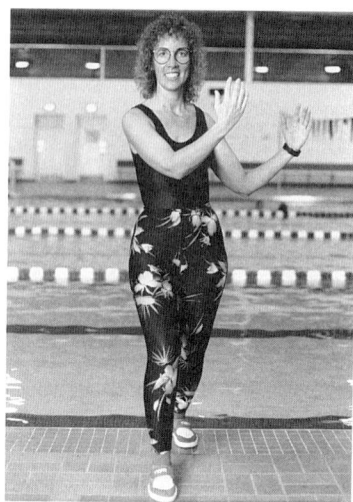

with the left arm. Swing Twists work well with these arms (see Swing Twist).

Elbow Press with Forearm Down

Begin with both arms out to the sides (extended laterally). The elbows are flexed to a 90- to

– Elbow Press with Forearm Down

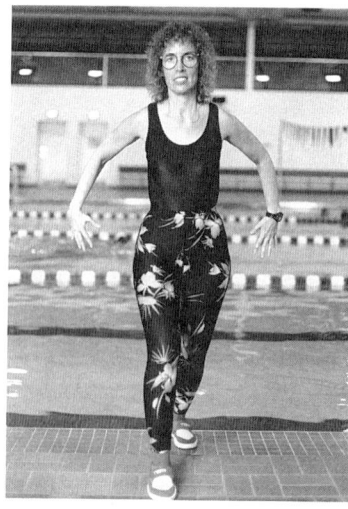

140-degree angle with the forearms straight down from the elbows. This will cause forward (anterior) shoulder rotation in most people. Widen the angle until no shoulder stress is experienced. Begin the move in this position. Press the elbows and hands back toward each other, reaching behind the body. This works the rhomboids and trapezius. Bring the arms forward to return to the beginning position.

Erector Spinae Stretch

With the toes and knees pointed forward and the feet shoulder-width apart, put the hands on the front of the thighs. Pull the abdominals in, and arch the back to feel the stretch. If the water is too deep, the stretch can be done with the hands interlaced and pushing forward.

— Erector Spinae Stretch

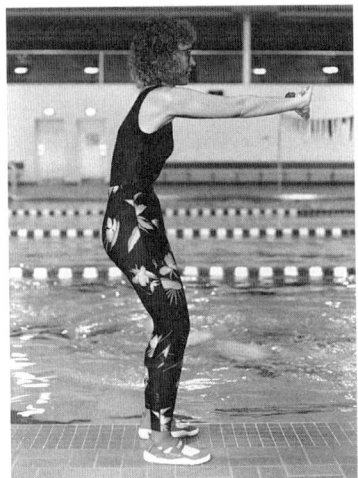

Flag Arms

Begin with the hands on the hips and the elbows out to the

— Flag Arms

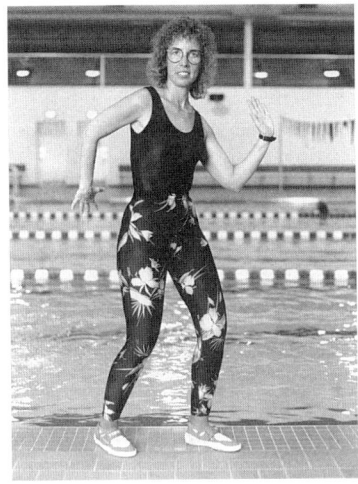

sides. While keeping the elbow in position, lift the forearm forward and up until it points straight up. The fingertips should be just beneath the water surface. This rotates the right shoulder externally. The left forearm moves down and back while the left elbow retains position. The left forearm should point straight down. This internally rotates the left shoulder. This is the first position of Flag Arms. Reverse by pressing the right forearm forward and down (internally rotating the shoulder) and lifting the left forearm forward and straight up (externally rotating the left shoulder). This is the second position of Flag Arms. Repeat positions 1 and 2 to work the shoulder rotator cuff, deltoids, and trapezius.

Flick Kick

Begin with the weight on the left leg and the right hip externally rotated (turned out). Flex the right knee and extend (bend and straighten) four times. This is Flick Kick–4. Repeat with the left leg. The Flick Kick works the quadriceps and hamstrings. To increase the work on the quadriceps, move forward to the right or right diagonal during the Flick Kick right. To increase the work on the hamstrings, move back.

— Flick Kick (position 1)

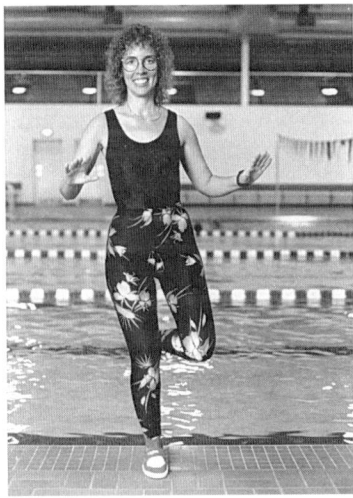

— Flick Kick (position 2)

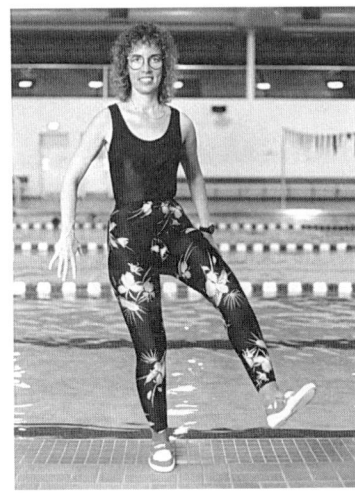

Fling

Begin with the weight on the left leg and the right hip externally rotated (turned out). Flex (bend) the right knee to about a 90-degree angle. Begin the move in this position. Lift the right heel forward as high as possible, while maintaining the knee flexion, hip flexion, and proper body alignment. The left (opposite) arm can come out of the water and reach overhead or stay underwater and press from abduction (arm straight out to the side just beneath the water surface) toward the right heel. Step the right foot down, and repeat with the left foot and right arm. The Fling can be done slowly, with both feet bouncing together between each move, or it can be done quickly, with the left heel lifting while the right one is returning, and vice versa. The Fling can also be done in groups of two, four, or eight right before switching to the left leg.

Fling Kick

Begin with the weight on the left foot and the right hip externally rotated (turned out). Flex (bend) the right knee to about a 120-degree angle. Begin the move in this position. Lift the right foot forward as high as possible, while maintaining the knee flexion, hip rotation, and proper body alignment. Step the right foot down, and repeat with the left leg. This move is much like a Kick with the toes pointed out (see Kick). To ensure adductor work, the heel and instep should lead. The Fling Kick can be done slowly, with both feet bouncing together between each kick, or quickly, with the left foot moving forward while the right foot is returning. It can be done in groups of two, four, or eight with the right leg before switching to the left leg. The Fling Kick works adductors and abductors. (See the Fling for optional arm movements.)

Flutter Kick

This move is usually done in a floating position with kickboards, jugs, or other buoyant devices under the arms (see Chapter 8 on equipment). It is also frequently done in a prone position (lying on the stomach) with the hands on the pool edge. With knees locked in at about a 5-degree flexion (bend), flex and extend (bend and straighten) the hip. The right leg kicks forward as the left leg kicks back, and the left leg kicks forward as the right leg kicks back. This move works iliopsoas and gluteals. **This move can compromise the lower back (lumbar area of the spine) if done in a prone position with the face out of the water.**

Forward Lunge

Begin in stride position, with the arms extended forward (shoulder flexion) and the palms facing out (away from each

— Fling

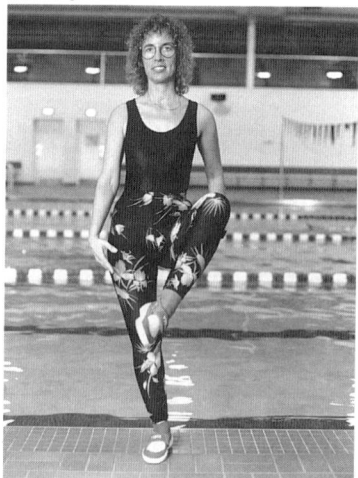

— Fling Kick

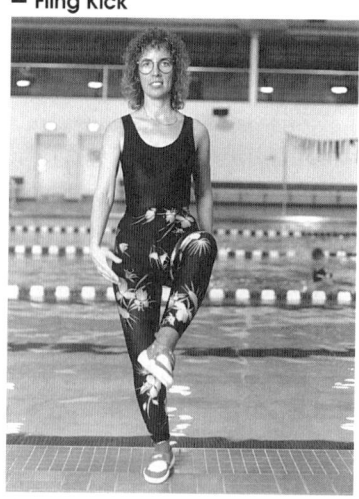

— Forward Lunge

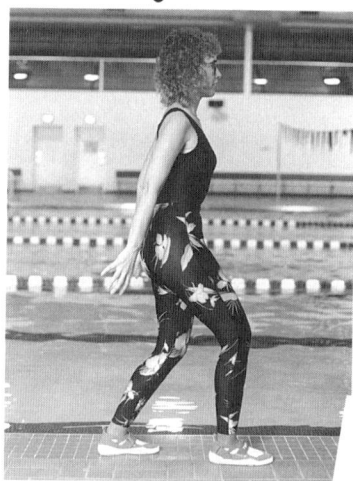

other). Step the right foot forward, and shift the body weight to the right foot while bending the right knee as the arms push straight back (as in Safe Arms). This is the first count. Step the right foot back to stride position, as the arms return to the beginning position. This is the second count. Repeat counts 1 and 2 with the left foot. This move works quadriceps, hamstrings, pectorals, rhomboids, and trapezius.

Forward Touch
See Touch Forward.

Forward Train
Begin with the feet in stride position, with arms forward, just beneath the water surface, and the palms back. Step the right foot forward and shift weight forward, while bending the right knee and pushing the arms back until they're extended laterally (out to the sides). Lift the left foot off the pool bottom, behind the left leg. This is the first count. Step the left foot back into the beginning position, while lifting the right knee and returning the arms to the beginning position. This is the second count. Step the right foot back and shift the body weight back onto the right foot, while lifting the left knee and pushing the arms forward and together. This is the third count. Step the left foot forward to the beginning position, while lifting the right knee and returning the arms to the beginning position. This is the fourth count. This is one Forward Train with the right foot leading; repeat three more times. Then do Forward Train four times with the left foot leading. Forward Train works pectorals, rhomboids, trapezius, iliopsoas, and gluteals.

— Forward Train (position 1)

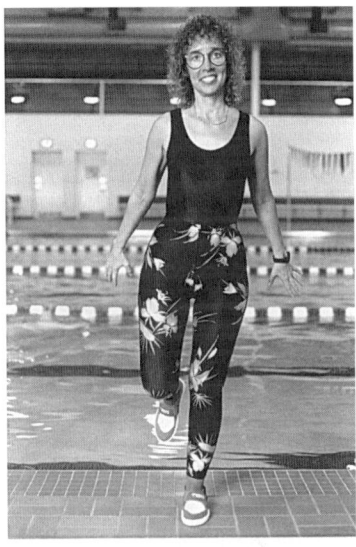

— Forward Train (position 3)

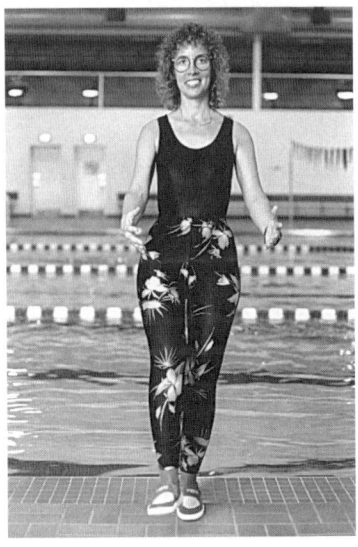

Frog Jump
Begin with the feet in stride position, the hips externally rotated (toes and knees pointed out). Pull both knees up toward the shoulders. This is one Frog Jump. Push both arms down in front or press them down be-

— Forward Train (position 2)

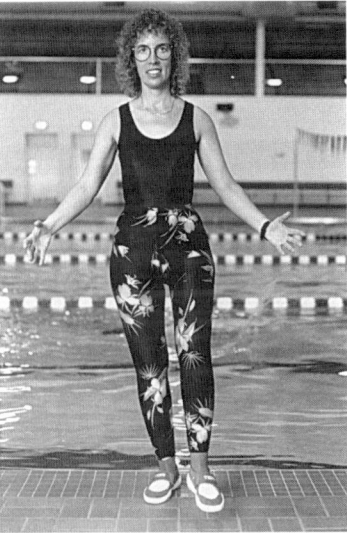

— Forward Train (position 4)

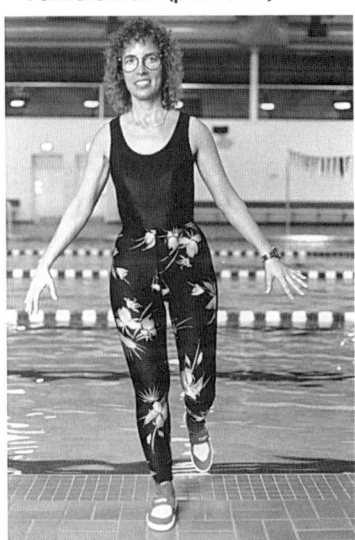

– Frog jump

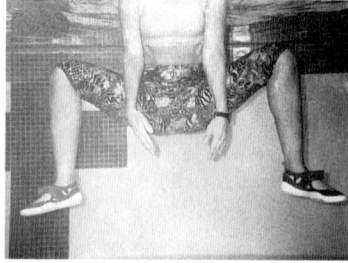

hind during the Frog Jump. This move works the iliopsoas and gluteals. Maintain proper body alignment and a posterior pelvic tilt during the Frog Jumps.

Gastrocnemius Stretch

Take a big step forward, with the left foot in front of the body and the right foot behind. Be sure the toes of the right foot point forward or even slightly inward. The heels must be down on both feet. Lean forward slowly and hold, as the calf muscle of the back leg stretches.

– Gastrocnemius Stretch

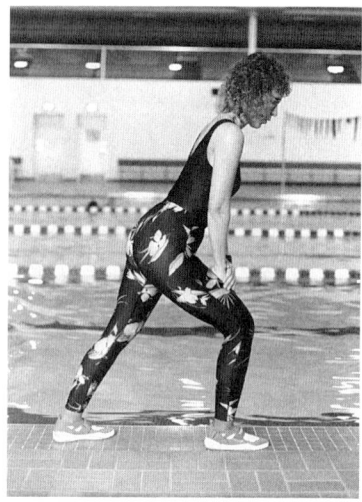

If the buoyancy of the water makes it difficult to feel this stretch, think about pulling the toes of the back foot up. Reverse for Gastrocnemius Stretch left.

Gluteal Stretch

Pull the right knee toward the chest and hold it, with the hands under the knee (behind the thigh). Stand up straight on the left foot, which should be pointed straight ahead, with the knee slightly bent. Bring the knee up, as close to the chest as possible, and hold. Reverse for left Gluteal Stretch.

– Gluteal Stretch

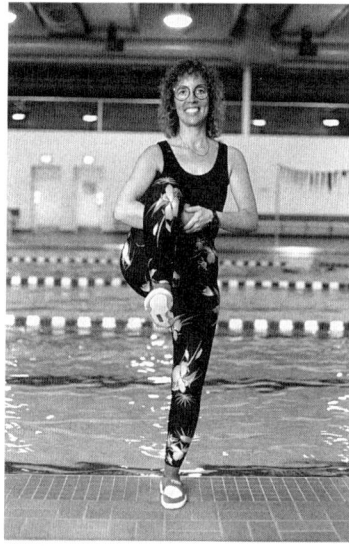

Golfing

Use both arms to mimic a golfswing. Repeat on both the left and right sides of the body.

Hamstring Stretch

Stand, facing the pool edge. Put the bottom of the right foot against the pool side, or put the right heel into the pool gutter. Stand up straight. The left foot on the pool bottom should be pointed straight ahead, with the knee slightly bent. While looking straight ahead, bend forward at the waist, and then straighten the right leg until a stretch is felt in the back of the right thigh. Reverse for the left leg. An alternative Hamstring Stretch is to begin in the Gluteal Stretch position, with the knee tucked up, close to the chest. While keeping the knee close to the chest, straighten (extend) the leg until an easy stretch is felt in the hamstrings.

– Hamstring Stretch

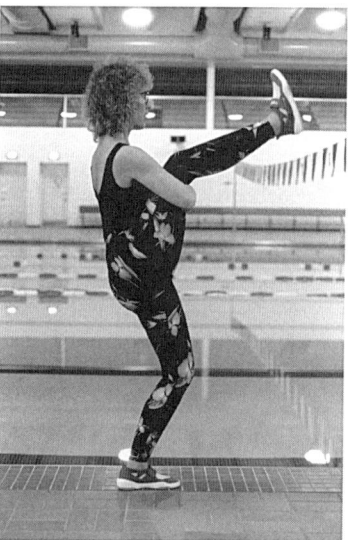

Heel Diamond

Buoyancy is needed. In a supine position, place the insteps of the feet together. Keeping them together, flex the knees and hips a in lateral motion (pulling the heels toward the body), and return to a normal, semistraight position. This move works adductors and abductors.

Heel Hit Across

Bounce once on the left foot, while reaching the left hand back to touch the right heel as it pulls up in front of the body and to the right of the right hip (knee flexion with internal hip rotation). Bounce once on the right foot, while reaching the right hand back to touch the left heel as it pulls up in front of the body and to the left of the left hip. Heel Hit Across works the quadriceps and hamstrings. **This move can compromise the knee joint.** It is important to keep the torso tall and the spine straight during Heel Hits.

— Heel Hit Across

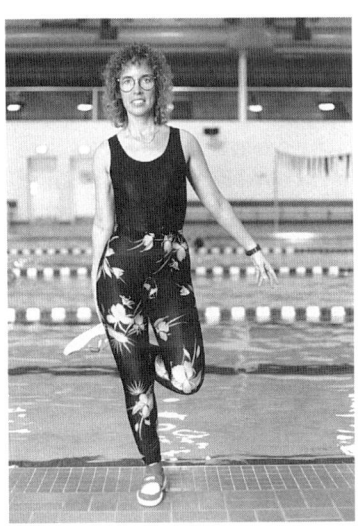

— Heel Hit Behind

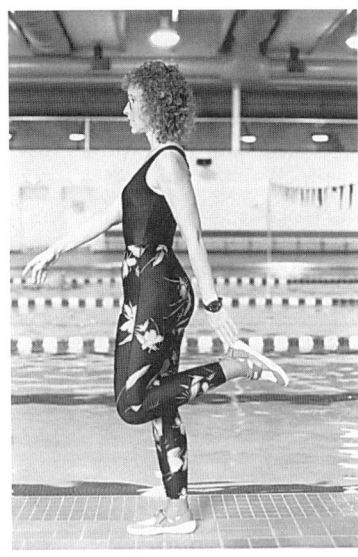

— Heel Hit Front

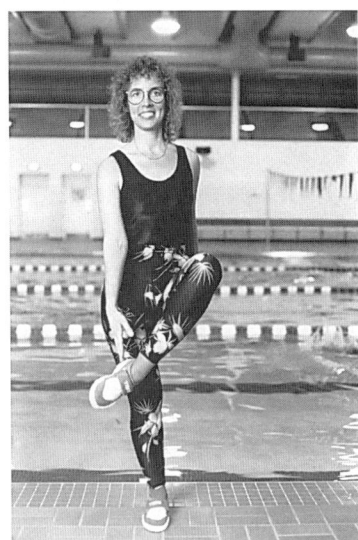

Heel Hit Behind

Bounce once on the left foot, while reaching the left hand back to touch the right heel as it pulls up behind the left leg. Bounce once on the right foot, while reaching the right hand back to touch the left heel as it pulls up behind the right leg. Heel Hits Behind work the hamstrings and quadriceps. It is important to maintain proper body alignment with a posterior pelvic tilt to avoid compromising the lower back. It is important to keep the torso tall and the spine straight during Heel Hits.

Heel Hit Front

Bounce once on the left foot, while reaching the left hand down to touch the right heel as it pulls up in front of the left thigh. Bounce once on the right foot, while reaching the right hand down to touch the left heel as it pulls up in front of the right thigh. Heel Hit Front works the adductors and abductors. It is important to keep the torso tall and the spine straight during Heel Hits.

Heel Jack

Begin with the feet in stride position. Bounce once on the left foot, while tilting slightly back to the left and touching the right heel forward to the right diagonal on the pool bottom. This is the first count. Bounce once with both feet together for the second count. Bounce once on the right foot, while tilting slightly back to the right and touching the left heel forward to the left diagonal on the pool bottom. This is the third count. Bounce once with both feet together for the fourth count. This is one set of

Heel Jack

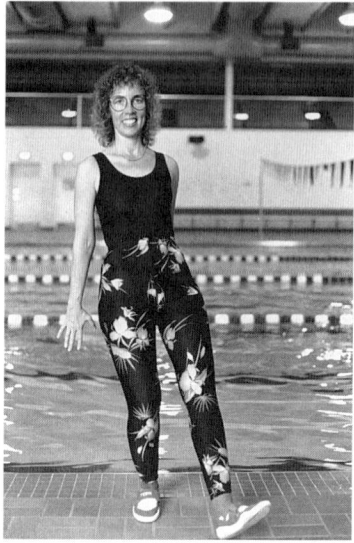

slow Heel Jacks. The arms can press down behind as the heel touches forward and out. Heel Jacks work the abdominals, obliques, and tibialis anterior. Heel Jacks can be done quickly by leaving out the second and fourth counts. During the fast Heel Jacks, punch the left arm through the water, down toward the right foot while the right heel touches. Punch the right arm through the water, down toward the left foot while the left heel touches.

Heel Jack in Three

Begin with the feet in stride position. Bounce once on the left foot, while tilting slightly back to the left and touching the right heel forward to the right diagonal to the pool bottom. This is the first count. Bounce once with both feet together for the second count. Bounce once on the right foot, while tilting slightly back to the right and touching the left heel forward to the left diagonal to the pool bottom. This is the third count. Bounce with both feet together once for the fourth count. Bounce once on the left foot, while tilting slightly back to the left and touching the right heel forward to the right diagonal. This is the fifth count. Bounce both feet together once for the sixth count. Bounce once on the left foot, while tilting slightly back to the left and touching the right heel forward to the right diagonal. This is the seventh count. Bounce both feet together once for the eighth count. Cue as "right, bounce, left, bounce, right, bounce, right, bounce." Repeat the Heel Jack in Three to the left (counts 9 through 16), cueing as "left, bounce, right, bounce, left, bounce, left, bounce." The Heel Jack in Three can be done quickly by leaving out all of the even-numbered counts (all of the bounces done with the feet together).

Heel Tilt

Begin with the feet together. Touch the right heel forward, while tilting the body back slightly and bending the left knee. (The weight is on the left foot.) This is the first count. Step the right foot next to the left to return to the beginning position for the second count. Touch the left heel forward, while tilting the body back slightly and bending the right

Heel Tilt

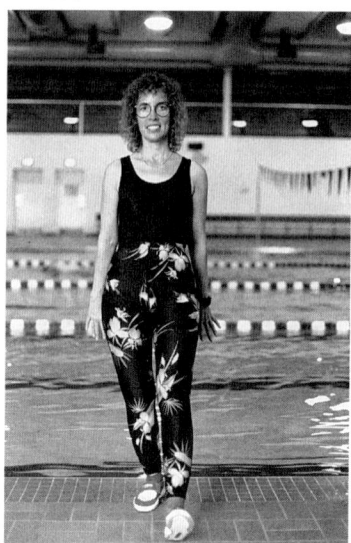

knee. (The weight is on the right foot.) This is the third count. Step the left foot next to the right to return to the beginning position for the fourth count. This is one set of Heel Tilts. Press both arms down and back as the heels touch forward, and return to slight abduction at the sides of the body as the feet step together. To increase the abdominal work, press both arms forward (as in Safe Arms) as the heels touch forward. The Heel Tilt works abdominals and tibialis anterior. Fast Heel Tilts are done by leaving out counts 2 and 4, and touching the left heel out as the right heel returns. During fast Heel Tilts, punch the left arm forward through the water as the right heel touches forward, and punch the right arms forward as the left heel touches.

Heel Turns

Begin with the feet in stride position. To do Heel Turns right: Touch the heel of the right foot to the pool bottom, with the toes pointed to the right (external hip rotation). This is the first count. Touch the toes of the right foot to the pool bottom, with the heel pointed to the right (internal hip rotation). This is the second count. Touch the heel of the right foot to the pool bottom, with the toes pointed to the right (external hip rotation). This is the third count. Bounce both feet together for the fourth count. This is one-half set of Heel Turns. To do Heel Turns left: Touch the heel of the left foot to the pool bottom, with the toes pointed to the left (external hip rotation). This is the first count. Touch the toes of the left foot to the pool bottom, with the heel pointed to the left (internal hip rotation). This is the second count. Touch the heel of the left foot to the pool bottom, with the toes pointed to the left (external hip rotation). This is the third count. Bounce both feet together for the fourth count. This is one full set of Heel Turns.

Flag Arms work well with Heel Turns (with the right forearm coming up and the left forearm going down as the right heel touches, and the right forearm going down and the left forearm going up as the right toe touches for Heel Turns right; the left arm going up and the right arm going down as the

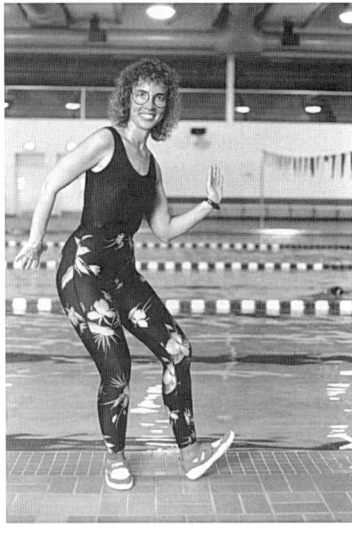

— Heel Turns (position 1)

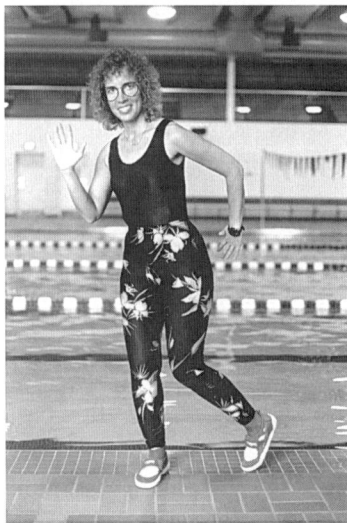

— Heel Turns (position 2)

left heel touches, and the left arm going down and the right arm going up as the left toe touches for Heel Turns left). Heel Turns work the hip rotators, adductors, abductors, gastrocnemius, and tibialis anterior. They can be varied by using Heel Turn Doubles and Singles. Heel Turns right would be two heel touches and two toe touches, followed by the Heel Turns right described above. Heel Turns left would be two heel touches and two toe touches, followed by the Heel Turns left described above. They would be cued as "heel, heel, toe, toe, heel, toe, heel, bounce" or "out, out, in, in, out, in, out, bounce."

Hip Flexor Stretch

See Iliopsoas Stretch.

Hoedown

Begin in stride position, with hips externally rotated (toes and knees pointed out). Bounce once on the right foot, while pulling the left foot up behind the knee of the right leg. Bounce once on the left foot, while pulling the right foot up behind the

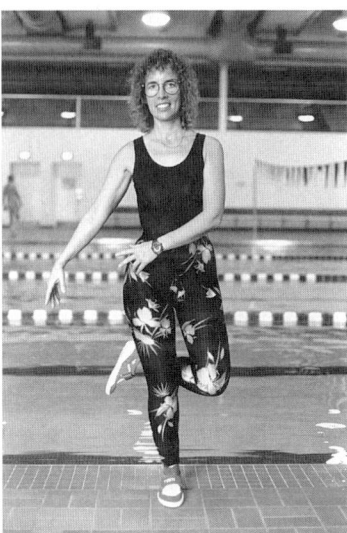

— Hoedown

left knee. This is one set of Hoedowns. Hoedown works the hamstrings and quadriceps. Swing both arms laterally to the right as the left foot pulls behind the right knee and to the left as the right foot moves. This move can be varied by doing two Hoedowns with the left foot before changing to the right foot; this is called Hoedown Doubles. Another variation, Hoedown in Three, includes one set of Hoedowns (left and right), two Hoedowns left, one set of Hoedowns (right and left), and then two Hoedowns right.

Hop

Begin with the feet in stride position, the body weight over the right foot, and the left heel lifted back (knee flexion). Jump forward on the right leg four times for the first four counts of this move. Reverse and hop forward four times on the left foot for the last four counts of the move. Hops can move laterally to the right or left or backward also. Increasing the distance covered during one hop increases the intensity of the move. Hops work the gastrocnemius, quadriceps, and hamstrings but are primarily used to increase aerobic effort.

Hopscotch

Begin by bouncing once in stride position. This is the first count. For the second count, bounce once on the right foot, while pulling the left heel up behind the right thigh. Bounce once in

– Hopscotch

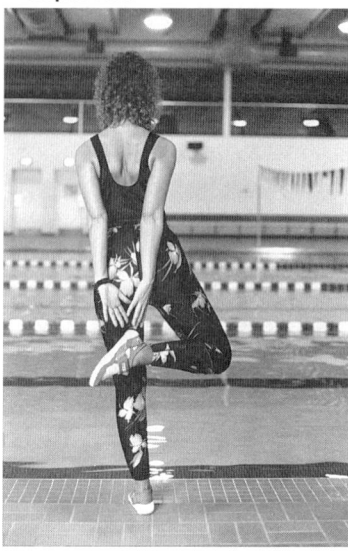

stride position with both feet down for the third count. For the fourth count, bounce on the left foot, while pulling the right heel up behind the left thigh. This is one set of Hopscotch. This move works the quadriceps and hamstrings. Arms begin extended laterally. The right arm presses down through the water toward the left heel as it pulls up behind the right thigh. Arms return to the beginning position for the third count. For the fourth count, the left arm presses down through the water toward the right heel.

Iliopsoas (Hip Flexor) Stretch

Stand, facing the pool edge, holding the pool edge with the left hand for support. Reach behind the body with the right hand, and grasp the lower-right leg, near the ankle. Push the right hip forward by contracting the right gluteals. The knee

– Iliopsoas (Hip Flexor) Stretch (version 1)

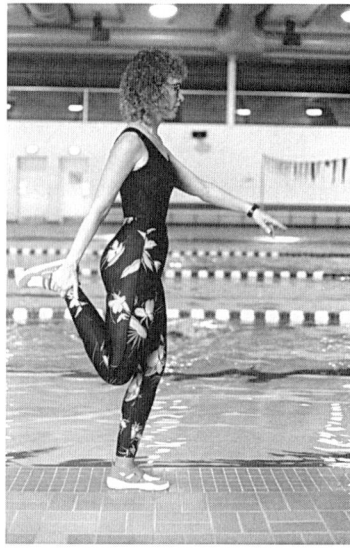

– Iliopsoas (Hip Flexor) Stretch (version 2)

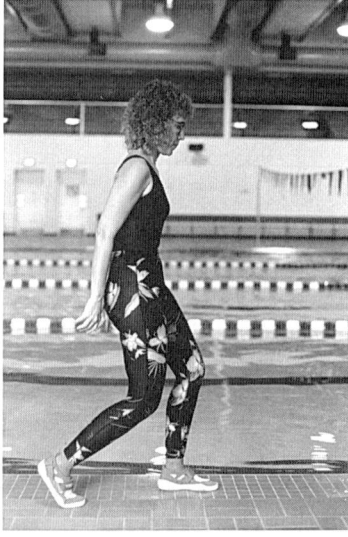

will point back about one inch. By pointing the toes up, this is also an anterior tibialis stretch. Another variation to stretch the iliopsoas is to stand in a gastrocnemius stretch position and move into a pelvic tilt. The heel of the back foot will lift off the pool bottom as the knee pushes forward during the pelvic tilt.

Jazzkick

Begin in stride position. With the hip extended, flex (bend) the right knee, pulling the heel back toward the buttocks. This is the first count. Extend (straighten) the right knee, and slightly flex (bend) the hip. This is the second count. Repeat with the left leg. This move works the quadriceps and hamstrings. It can be varied by kicking to the diagonal (with the hips externally rotated) or kicking several times with one leg before switching to the other. Jog Arms work with Jazzkick. Using both arms in an Armswing Forward Flex and Short Backstroke move also works well.

Jazzkick Diagonals

Begin with Jazzkicks forward, alternating the right and left feet. Externally rotate the hips while continuing the Jazzkicks, kicking to the right diagonal with the right foot and to the left diagonal with the left foot.

Jig

Begin with the weight on the left foot, and the right heel ex-

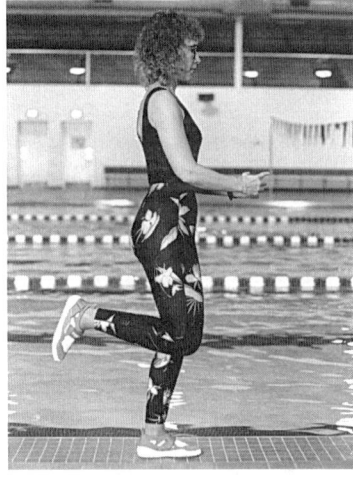
— Jazzkick (position 1)

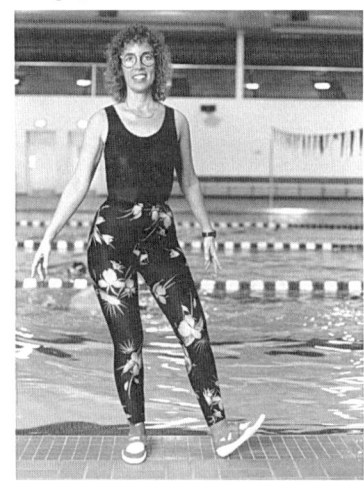
— Jig (position 1)

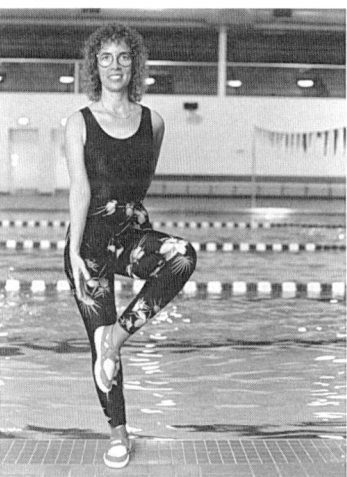
— Jig (position 2)

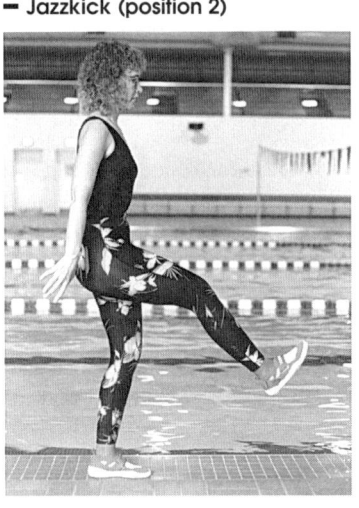
— Jazzkick (position 2)

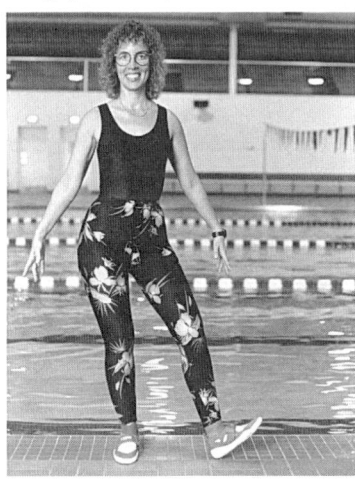
— Jig (position 3)

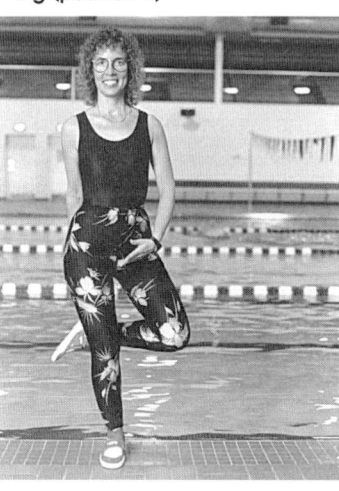
— Jig (position 4)

tended to the right and touching the pool bottom. Point the toes on the right foot to the right. Pull the right heel up in front of the left knee for the first count. Return to the beginning position for the second count. Pull the right heel up behind the left knee for the third count. Move to stride position (feet about shoulder width apart) for the fourth count. Repeat with the left leg alternating legs, or do sets of four with each leg. This move works the quadriceps and hamstrings. Adduct the left arm down through the water, in front of and behind the body toward the right heel as it comes up in front of and behind the left knee. The right arm adducts down through the water behind and then in front of the body (opposite the left arm).

Jog Arms

Hold the elbows in at the waist and the forearms down at sides (arm and elbow extension). Bring the right forearm up and forward (elbow flexion) while taking a step with the left foot. Return the right arm to the beginning position (elbow extension). Bring the left forearm up and forward (elbow flexion) while taking a step with the right foot. Jog Arms work the biceps and triceps.

Jog Doubles

Begin with the feet in stride position. Step forward on the right foot while lifting the left foot off the pool bottom for the first count. Bounce once on the right foot while keeping the left foot off the pool bottom for the second count. Step forward on the left foot while lifting the right foot off the pool bottom for the third count. Bounce once on the left foot while keeping the right foot off the pool bottom for the fourth count. This is one set of Jog Doubles. Jog Doubles can be done in place or moving forward and backward. They work the gastrocnemius.

Jog Tilt

Lean the entire body slightly forward, keeping it straight (eliminate any spinal flexion that causes a bend at the waist), and jog forward. Lean the entire body slightly backward, keeping it straight, and jog backward. The degree of tilt in the body should be extremely small. This move works iliopsoas, gluteals, and abdominals. Jog Arms or Tricep Extensions and Backstroke arms work well with the Jog Tilt.

Jump Bounce

Begin in a closed stride position. Jump forward as far as possible, making a big jump for the first count. Do a small bounce in place for the second count. Together, this is one Jump Bounce forward. Jump backward (again, a big jump covering as much distance as possible) for the first count of a Jump Bounce back. Do a small bounce in place for the second count. Jump Bounces can be done singly, with one moving forward and one moving backward, or in series with four or eight each way. Safe Arms, pushing back in the Jump Bounce forward and forward in

— Jog Tilt (position 1)

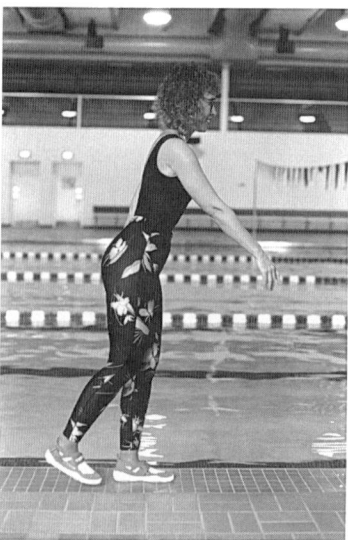

— Jog Tilt (position 2)

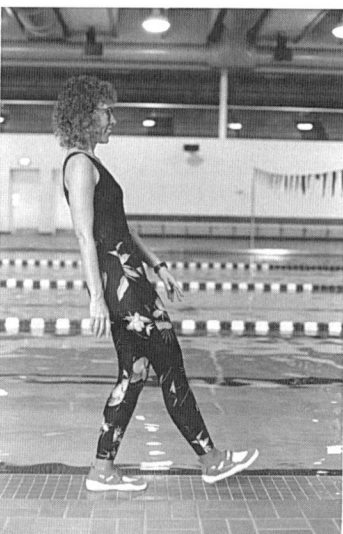

the Jump Bounce backward, work well with this move. If done slowly, increase intensity by tucking the knees to the chest during the big jump (count 1). The Jump Bounce works iliopsoas, gluteals, and gastrocnemius but is usually used for increasing aerobic training.

Jumping Jack

Begin with the feet in stride position. Jump up and push both feet out to the sides into a wide stride position. Jump up again and bring both feet together. This is one Jumping Jack. Arms can be pressed down behind, in front, or with elbows flexed or out of the water, pushing up or flying out and up. Jumping Jacks can be done "in three" by jumping out, in, out, out and then in, out, in, in. They can also be done moving forward and backward or right and left to vary the intensity. Jumping Jacks work the adductors and abductors.

Jumping Jack Crossing

Begin with the feet in stride position. Jump up and push both feet out to the sides into a wide stride position. Jump up again and bring both feet together, with the right foot crossed over (in front and to the left of) the left foot. Jump "out" again, and then jump "in," with the left foot crossed over (in front and to the right of) the right foot. This is one set of Jumping Jack Crossing. Press the arms down, with one arm in front of the body and one behind. The left arm should press in front of the body when the right foot crosses over the left, and the right arm should press in front of the body when the left foot crosses over the right. This move works adductors, abductors, deltoids, and latissimus dorsi.

— Jumping Jack Crossing (position 1)

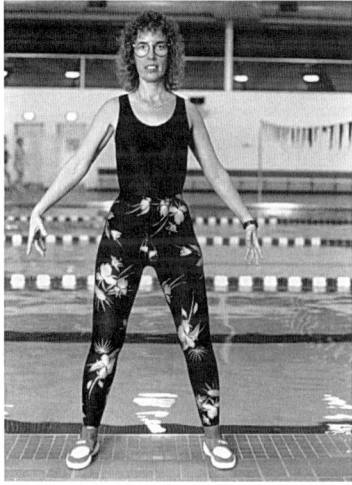

— Jumping Jack Crossing (position 2)

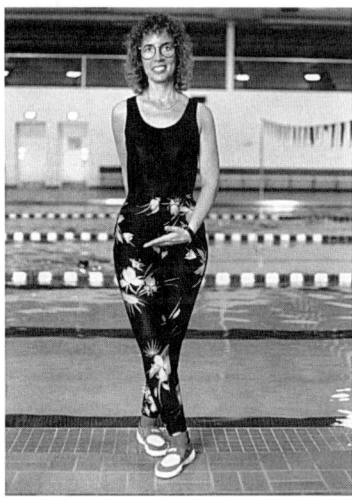

Jumping Jack Doubles

Begin with the feet in stride position. Jump up and push both feet out to the sides into a wide stride position for the first count. Bounce once with both feet in the wide stride position for the second count. Jump up and bring both feet together for the third count. Bounce once with both feet together for the fourth count. This is one set of Jumping Jack Doubles. The Jumping Jack Doubles can be varied by moving forward and backward or right and left or by pulling both knees up (in the position they're in) between each count. This move works adductors and abductors. (See Jumping Jack for arm variations.)

Jumping Jack Jump

This move is sometimes called Split Jumps. Begin with the feet together. Jump high, moving both feet out to sides and

— Jumping Jack Jump

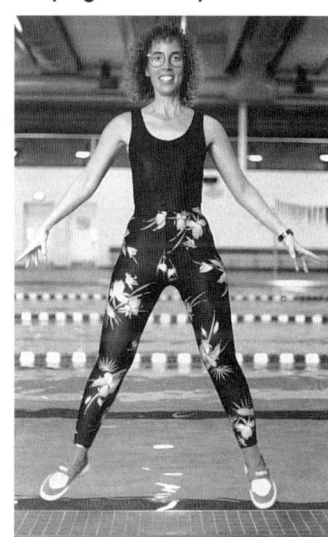

then back together; land with the feet together (beginning position). This is one Jumping Jack Jump. Any arm movements that help to maintain proper body alignment can be used. Arm movements that follow the legs out and in (a reverse press down) work well. Jumps works adductors and abductors and should be used only with well-conditioned students.

Karate Punch

Begin with the elbows in, toward the waist, flexed at about a 90-degree angle, forearms forward. Make fists. Punch the right arm across to the left until it is extended. While pulling the right elbow back to the beginning position, punch the left arm forward until it is extended. Continue punching alternate arms to a count of 1-2, 1-2. Reverse by punching the left arm across to the right and the right arm forward. Feet, knees, and hips should pivot to the left when the right arm is punching to the left and pivot to the right when the left arm is punching to the right. When punching forward, the feet should be in the forward stride position. Bounce from one position to the next, or simply pivot easily on the balls of the feet. This move works the pectorals, deltoids, biceps, triceps, trapezius, and rhomboids.

Kick

Begin with the feet in stride position. Lift the right leg (hip flexion) forward, and then return it to the beginning position (hip extension). Repeat the two movements with the left leg. Kicks can be done quickly, lifting one leg while lowering the other, or they can be done slowly, bouncing both feet together before doing the next kick. Maintain proper body alignment during Kicks, keeping the shoulders slightly back and the torso tall. Students will want to lean forward to kick higher. This should be discouraged. This move works the iliopsoas and gluteals.

Kick Corner

This move is sometimes called Kick Diagonal. Begin with the feet in stride position, with hips slightly externally rotated. Lift the right leg to the right diagonal, and return it to the beginning position. Repeat with the left leg. As with forward Kicks, Kick Corners can be done slowly or quickly. The same precautions apply. Kick Corners work the iliopsoas and gluteals.

Kick Point and Flex

Begin with the feet in stride position. Kick four or eight times, with the toes pointed forward (plantar flexed). Then kick forward the same amount of times with the toes pointed up toward the body (dorsi flexed). The kicks can be done slowly or quickly (as described in Kick) or forward or diagonally. This move works the gastrocnemius, anterior tibialis, iliopsoas, and gluteals.

Kickswing

Begin with the feet in stride position. Kick the right foot forward (hip flexion) as high as possible for the first count. Swing the right leg back into slight hip hyperextension (just

– Karate Punch (position 1)

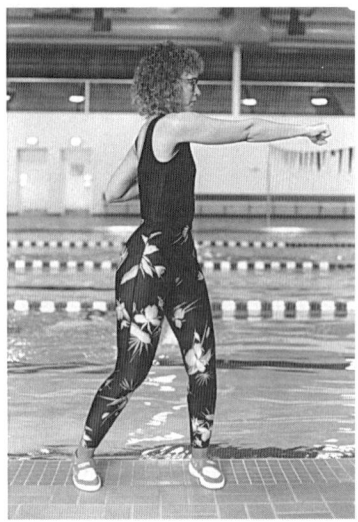

– Karate Punch (position 2)

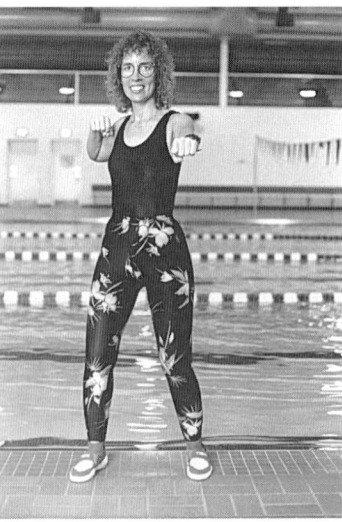

A Catalog of Movements

Kick and Point

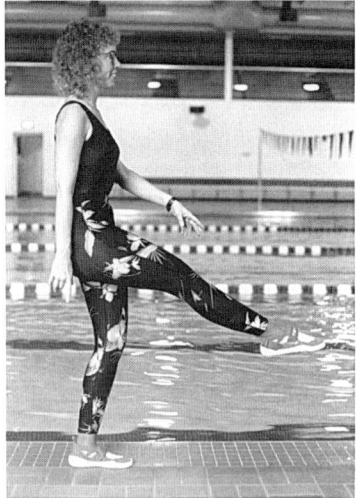

Kick and Flex

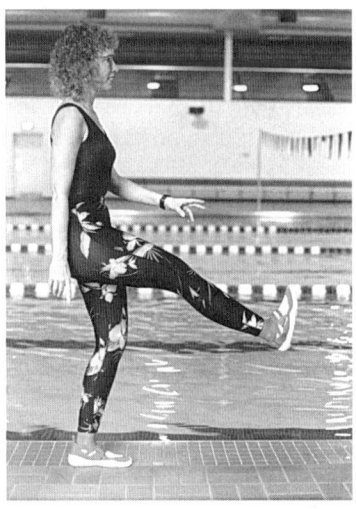

past returning to beginning position) while bouncing once on the left leg for the second count. This is one Kickswing right. Repeat counts 1 and 2 three more times. Switch and do Kickswing left four times. To protect the lower back, contract the abdominals and hold the body in a pelvic tilt during the swing portion of the move. For the Kickswing right, swing the right arm back and the left arm forward as the right leg kicks forward. Swing the right arm forward and the left arm back as the left leg kicks back. Reverse for the Kickswing left. The Kickswing works the iliopsoas and gluteals.

Kneelift

Begin with the feet in stride position. Lift the right leg (hip flexion) to approximately a 90-degree angle while bending the right knee (knee flexion) to the same angle. Repeat with the left leg. Kneelifts can be done quickly, lifting one leg while lowering the other (very much like a jog with high-lifting knees) or slowly, bouncing both feet together before doing the next Kneelift. Kneelifts can alternate right and left, doing single movements or repeating the movement two, four, or eight times on each leg. Kneelifts can be moving to the right and left to increase the intensity. Kneelifts work the iliopsoas and gluteals.

Kneelift Cross

Begin with the feet in stride position, with the right hip slightly internally rotated (toes and knees pointed in). Pull the right knee up toward the left shoulder, without allowing the shoulders to move forward. Return the right leg to the beginning position; repeat one, three, or seven more times. Repeat with the left leg. Touch the left

Kneelift Cross

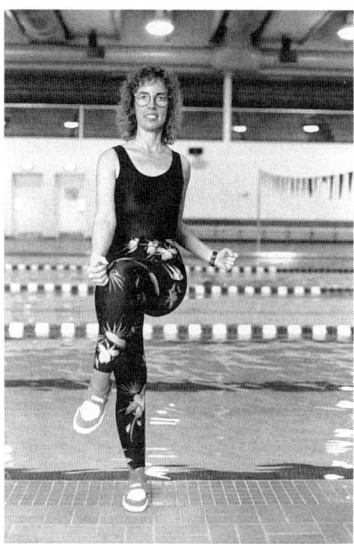

wrist to the inside (internal aspect) of the right knee and reverse. Trying to touch the left elbow to the right knee can result in simultaneous flexion and rotation of the spine, which may cause injury. Touching the wrist to the elbow allows the spine to stay erect (extended) while the spinal rotation occurs. Kneelift Crosses work the iliopsoas, gluteals, abductors, and adductors.

Kneelift Out

Begin with the feet in stride position, with both hips externally rotated (knees and toes pointed out). Pull the right knee up to the right diagonal, while keeping the torso tall (not tilting to the left), and bring it back down. Repeat with the left leg. Push both arms down in front or behind. Kneelifts Out (also called Open Kneelifts) can be

Kneelift Out

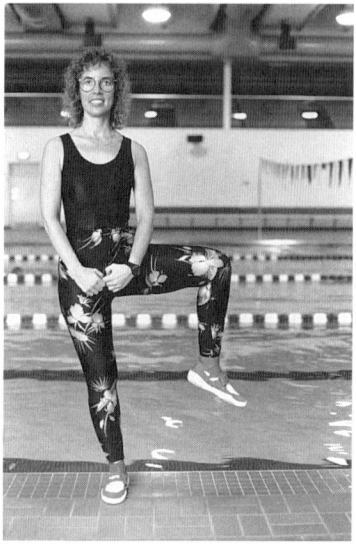

done slowly or quickly or in groups of two, four, or eight (as described in Kneelifts). This move works the iliopsoas and gluteals.

Kneeswing Combo

This is a combination of the Kneeswing Up and Back and the Kneeswing Crossing. Do one set of Kneeswing Up and Back (swing the right knee up, back, and up, and then set the right foot down; swing the left knee up, back, and up, and then set the left foot down). Follow that with one set of Kneeswing Crossing (right knee crosses, opens, and crosses, and then set the right foot down; left knee crosses, opens, and crosses, and then set the left foot down). This is one set of Kneeswing Combo. Kneeswings can be also be combined by doing Kneeswing Up and Back four times with the right leg and then four times with the left, followed by Kneeswing Crossing four times with the right leg and then four times with the left. They can also be combined doing two Kneeswings Up and Back and two Kneeswing Crossings with the right leg and then repeating with the left leg.

Kneeswing Crossing

Begin with the right knee flexed to a 90-degree angle (knee bent) and the right hip flexed to a 90-degree angle so the knee is pointing forward and the lower leg is straight down. The weight is on the left foot. Cross the right knee to the left (internally rotate the hip), while maintaining hip and knee flexion. This is the first count. Swing the knee out to the right side (externally rotate the hip), while maintaining hip and knee flexion. This is the second count. Push both arms to the right as the knee crosses to the left, and push to the left as the knee swings out to the right. Kneeswing Crossings can be done in groups of two, four, or eight with the right leg before repeating with the left leg. Kneeswing Crossings work the hip abductors and adductors.

Kneeswing Diagonal

This a Kneeswing Up and Back with the hip slightly rotated externally so that the knee is pointed to the diagonal.

Kneeswing Up and Back

Begin with the right knee flexed to a 90-degree angle (knee bent) and the hip extended so the knee is pointing straight down. The weight is on the left foot. Swing the right knee forward, keeping it flexed at a 90-degree angle. This is the first count. Swing the right knee back

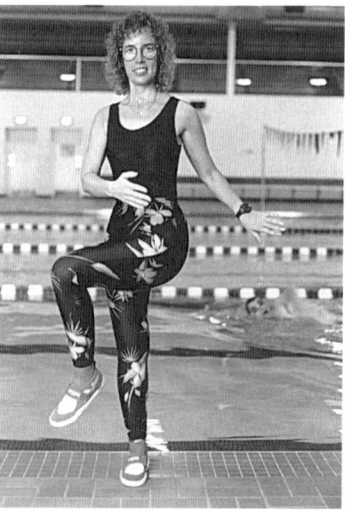

— Kneeswing Crossing (position 1)

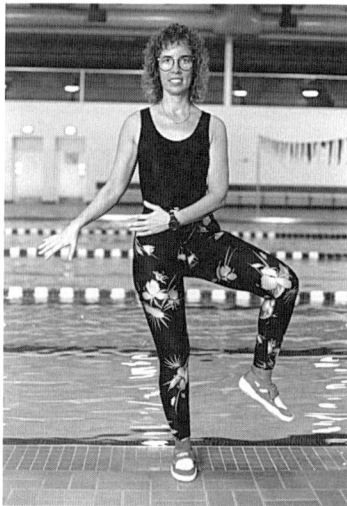

— Kneeswing Crossing (position 2)

— Kneeswing Up and Back (position 1)

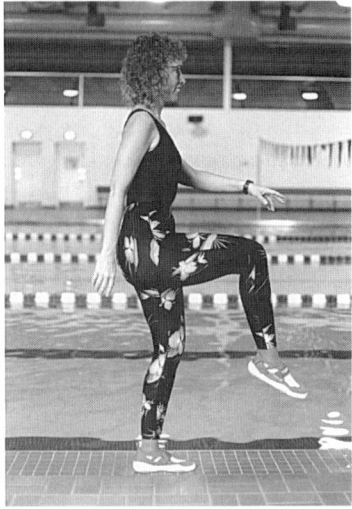

— Kneeswing Up and Back (position 2)

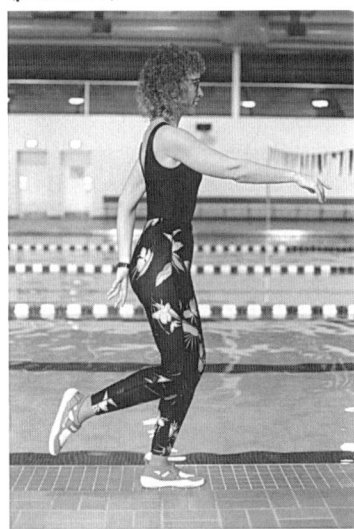

(while maintaining the knee flexion) to a slight hip hyperextension. This is the second count. Swing the left arm forward and backward with the right knee. Kneeswings with the right leg can be repeated one, three, or seven times more before changing to the left. Move forward and backward to increase the intensity. This move works the iliopsoas and gluteals.

Lateral Push

Extend the right arm laterally to the right, palm down (pronated). The left arm begins adducted across the body, so that the left hand is about parallel with the right elbow; the palm of the left hand faces down (pronated) also. Hold both arms just below the water surface. To accomplish the Lateral Push, press both arms down slightly and to the left, just below the water surface. Reverse to move in the opposite direction. Arms push to the left when the body is moving right. This is an excellent move to use when moving laterally through the water. The Lateral Push works

— Lateral Push

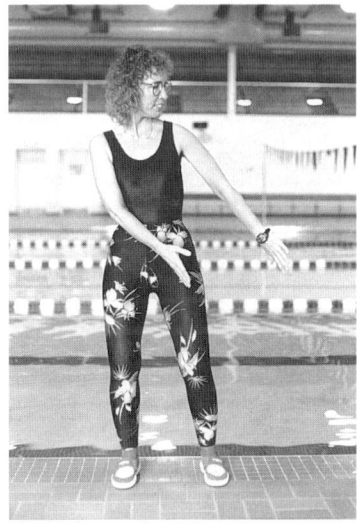

the deltoids, latissimus dorsi, trapezius, and pectorals.

Leap Forward

Begin with the arms forward, just below the water surface, with palms out and knuckles almost touching. Kick the right

— Leap Forward (position 1)

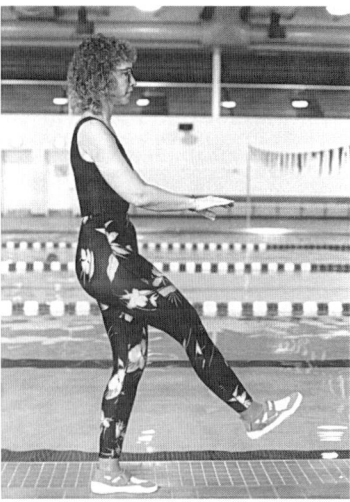

— Leap Forward (position 2)

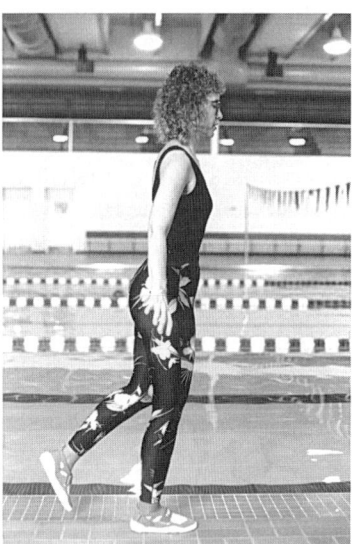

foot forward and jump forward onto it as the arms push out and back. Bring the left foot next to the right, while bringing the arms forward again. Repeat the leap with the right foot leading three more times, and then repeat it four times with the left foot leading. Jog or bounce backward to return to the beginning position. If the pool does not allow enough space to do four forward leaps with the right foot and then the left foot, leap two forward with the right foot and two forward with the left or leap four forward with the right foot leading, turn a half-turn left, and return with the left foot leading. This move works the iliopsoas, pectorals, trapezius, and gluteals.

Leap Side

Begin with the weight on the left foot, both arms extended to the right side and the right leg slightly lifted out to the side (abducted). Leap with the right leg to the right as far as possible while still facing forward and with both arms pushing down and to the left. This is the first count. Bring the left foot (adduct) next to the right, and bounce with both feet together. The arms should return to the beginning position. This is the second count. Repeat counts 1 and 2 three more times while moving to the right. To reverse the leap, begin with the left leg jumping out to the left and move left. Extend both arms to the left, and push down and to the

— Leap Side (position 1)

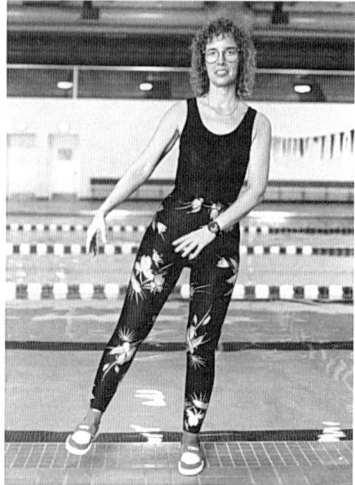

— Leap Side (position 2)

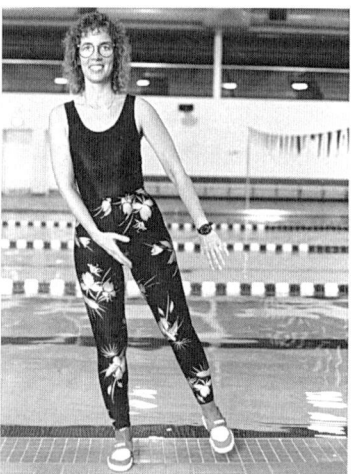

right during the jump for the first count. Leap Side works adductors and abductors. The toes of both feet should continually face forward, not to the sides, to ensure this. Leading the step with the heel will help to ensure proper forward alignment of the hips. Leap Side can be modified to work obliques by tightening the hips with the legs in the leap position, concentrating on moving from the waist, and keeping the upper torso stable.

Lift Hips

Begin with the back to the pool edge, the elbows up on the pool edge, the hips flexed at 90 degrees so that the knees are pointing forward, and the knees flexed at 90 degrees so that the feet are hanging down. The back must be flat to the pool wall. Slowly contract the abdominal muscles so that the knees move forward an inch or two. This will move the very lower back and hips away from the pool edge. Return the back to the beginning position without allowing the midback to move away from the pool wall. This move works the abdominals. If done incorrectly, with the knees moving up and down rather than forward and backward, it will work the iliopsoas muscles. If the hip joint is moving (flexing and extending), form is incorrect. If the spine is moving, form is correct, and the abdominals will be working. This move can be modified by changing the flexion in the knees and hips.

— Lift Hips

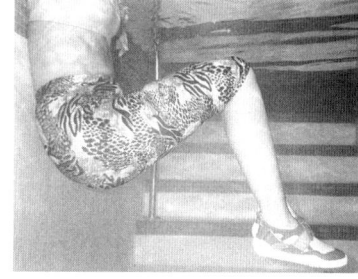

Mule Kick

Begin with the feet in stride position. Flex (bend) the right knee, while maintaining hip extension (a straight line down from the hip to the knee) in the right leg. This is the first count. Extend (straighten) the right knee, and return to beginning position for the second count. This is a Mule Kick right. Repeat with the left leg for Mule Kick left (counts 3 and 4). Mule Kicks are simple knee flexion (trying to kick the heel up to the buttocks) while keeping the knee pointed straight down (hip flexors extended). Mule Kicks can be done alternating right and then left, or four to eight can be done with the right leg before changing to the left. Mule Kicks can be done quickly (without a bounce between each kick) or slowly (with a bounce between each kick). Mule Kicks work the quadriceps and hamstrings. Optional arm movements include Elbow Press and Scissor Arms. Two other arm variations are as follows:

1. Begin with the elbows flexed at about a 90-degree angle and pulled into the waist, with forearms forward. Lift both elbows laterally as the heel kicks behind, and lower them as the foot returns. This can also be done with the arms beginning straight down at the sides of the body.
2. Begin with the arms down in front of body, with the palms on the thighs; make fists. Lift both arms forward as the heel kicks behind, and lower them as the foot returns.

Neck Stretch

Tilt the head to the right side, moving the right ear to the right shoulder. Reverse for Neck Stretch left.

— Mule Kick

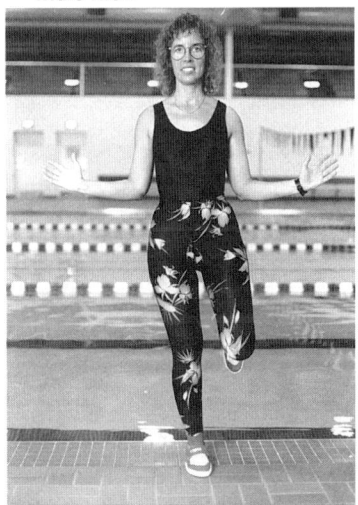

— Neck Stretch

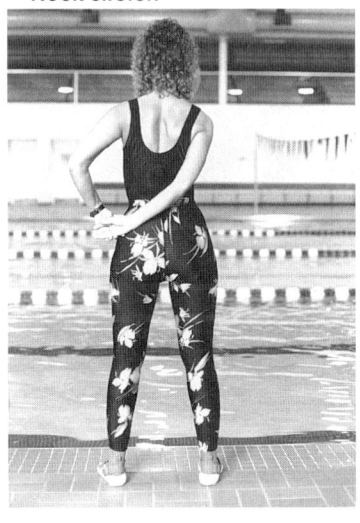

Oblique Stretch

Stand with the feet shoulder width apart, the toes pointed slightly out and the knees slightly bent. Put the left hand on the left hip, and extend the right arm up and over the head without moving the toes or knees. This should stretch the obliques. If further stretch is required, slowly bend sideways toward the hand on the hip.

— Oblique Stretch

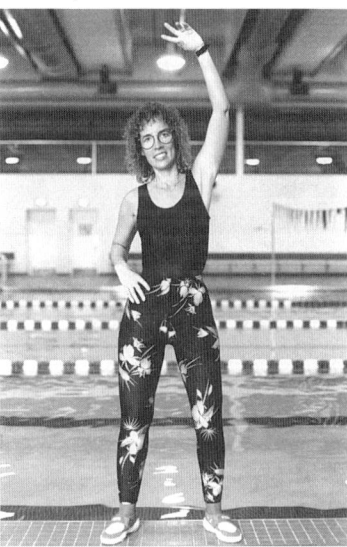

Over and Present

Begin with the arms extended laterally (out to the sides), just beneath the water surface, palms forward. With the elbow extended so the arm is straight, bring the right hand toward the left until they are almost touching. Turn the palm out (externally rotate), and push the extended right arm back to the beginning position. This can

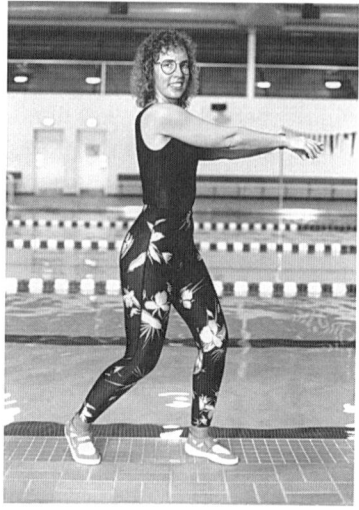
— Over and Present (position 1)

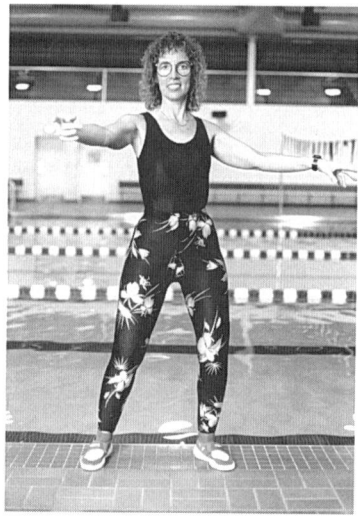
— Over and Present (position 2)

be repeated with the right arm several times before switching to the left, or it can be done alternating right and left. This works the pectorals, anterior serratus, trapezius, rhomboids, and lattisimus dorsi. To maintain integrity of the knee joint, pivot each foot to follow the knee. To work the obliques, stand with the feet shoulder width apart, and move only from the waist up. The knees should be slightly flexed, and both knees and toes should point slightly out.

Paddlekick

This move is done in a floating position, with the back to the pool edge and the elbows on the pool edge. Hold a milk jug in each hand or a kickboard under each arm. With the hips and knees flexed (bent) at a 90-degree angle (so the knees don't point forward and the feet hang down), alternately extend each knee, keeping both knees on the same plane. This move works the quadriceps and hamstrings.

Pectoral Stretch

Interlace the fingers behind the head, with the elbows pointed out to the sides. Squeeze the shoulder blades together. See also Bicep, Anterior Deltoid, and Pectoral Stretch.

Pelvic Tilt

Begin by standing in a comfortable upright position. Create an anterior pelvic tilt by using one or more of these imagery techniques:

— Pull the navel back to the spine.
— Press the stomach down toward the pool bottom.
— Tuck the buttocks under.
— Take the arch out of the lower back.

Doing any of these is one pelvic tilt. The pelvic tilt can be used during many exercise moves to protect the lower back from strain. A series of 8 to 24 standing pelvic tilts can be used during the toning portion of the workout. The pelvic tilt works the abdominal muscles.

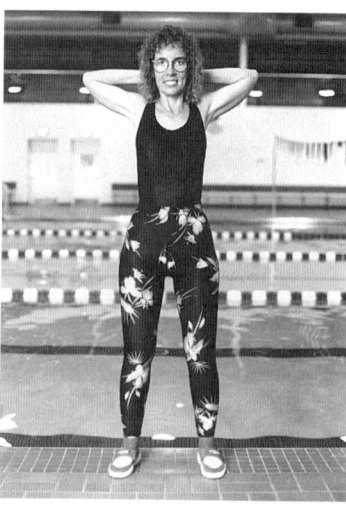
— Pectoral Stretch

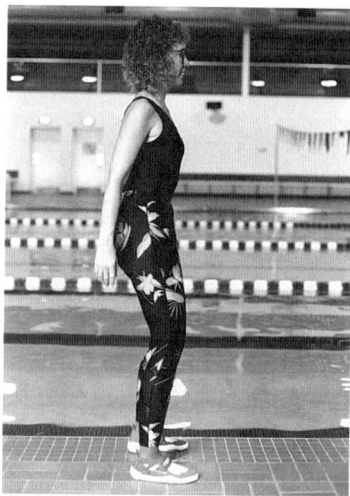
— Pelvic Tilt

Press Down Behind

Begin with the arms laterally extended (lifted to the sides), just beneath the water surface, with palms down (pronated). Push both arms down through the water until they almost meet behind the body. This portion of the move focuses on the latissimus dorsi and trapezius. To reverse, simply keep the palms down and lift the arms with force through the water to the beginning position. This portion of the move focuses on the deltoids. When used for toning, pause momentarily between the initial and reverse portions of the move.

— Press Down Behind

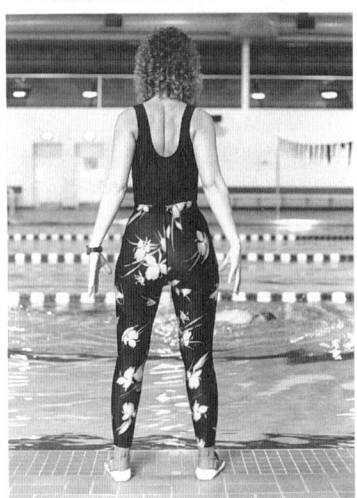

Press Down Front

Begin with the arms extended laterally (lifted out to the sides), just beneath the water surface, with palms down (pronated). Push both arms down through the water until they almost meet in front of the body. This portion of the move focuses on the pectorals and serratus anterior. To reverse, simply keep the palms down and lift the arms with force through the water to the beginning position. This portion of the move focuses on the deltoids. When used for toning, pause momentarily between the initial and reverse portions of the move.

Press Down Singles

Begin with the arms extended laterally (lifted out to the sides), just beneath the water surface, with palms down (pronated). At the same time, press the right arm down (as described in Press Down Front) and the left arm down (as described in Press Down Behind). Reverse the move (also as described). To continue, press the left arm down in front and the right arm down behind, and lift them both to the beginning position. This is one set of Press Down Singles. The deltoids, pectorals, serratus anterior, latissimus dorsi, and trapezius are all involved in this move.

Press Down with Elbows Flexed

Begin with the elbows extended laterally (lifted out to the sides), the forearms forward (90 to 120 degree elbow flexion), and the palms down. The arms should begin just below the water surface. Push both arms down through the water until the forearms almost meet in front of the body. This portion of the move works the pectorals and serratus anterior. To reverse,

— Press Down with Elbows Flexed

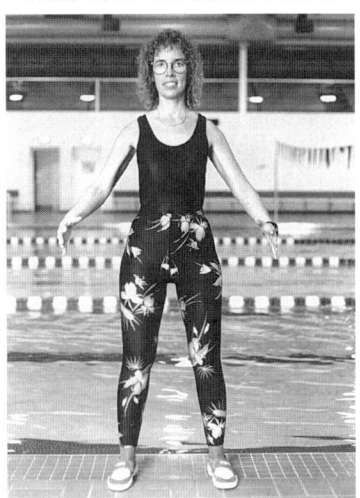

lift the arms with force back to the beginning position. The reverse portion of the move works the deltoids and trapezius.

Quadricep Stretch

Stand, facing the pool edge. Hold the pool edge with the left hand for support. Reach behind the body with the right hand,

— Quadricep Stretch

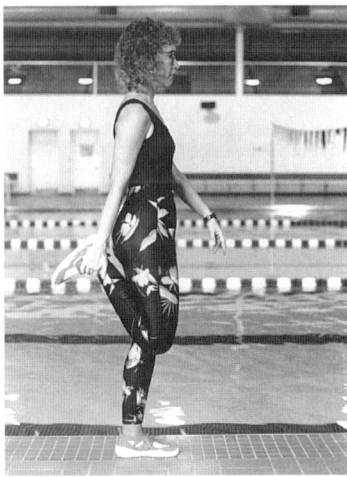

and grasp the lower-right leg near the ankle. Pull the lower-right leg and heel gently toward the right buttocks. The knee and toes should point directly to the pool bottom, straight down. Reverse for the left Quadricep Stretch.

Reach Pull-In

Begin with both arms extended to the left at shoulder level, just beneath the water surface. The feet, knees, hips, and shoulders pivot to the left to allow the palms to begin in a parallel position. This is the "Reach" position of this move. While pivoting the feet, knees, and hips forward, pull both elbows back until the shoulder blades are squeezed together. This is the "Pull-In" portion of the move. Continue to the left before switching to the right, or alternate by doing one left and then one right. It can be done bouncing into the pivot and back to the forward position or simply pivoting lightly with no bounce. Reach Pull-In involves the pectorals, deltoids, trapezius, and rhomboids.

Reverse Crossing Jog

Begin with the feet in stride position. Reverse Crossing Jog moves laterally to the right with four or eight steps before moving laterally to the left with four or eight steps. To do the move to the right: Step the right foot laterally to the right, shifting the weight to the right foot while lifting the left leg up slightly, off the pool bottom. This is the first count. Step the left foot behind the right foot, shifting the weight to the left foot while lifting the right foot up slightly for the second count. Repeat counts 1 and 2 three to seven times while moving to the right. To do the move to the left: Step the left foot laterally to the left, shifting the weight to the left foot while lifting the right foot up slightly, off the pool bottom. This is the first count. Step the right foot behind the left foot, shifting the weight to the right foot while lifting the left foot up slightly. This is the second count. Repeat counts 1 and 2 three to seven times while moving to the left. In both Reverse Cross-

– Reach Pull-In (position 1)

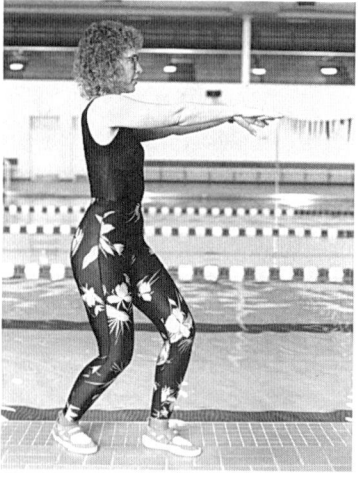

– Reach Pull-In (position 2)

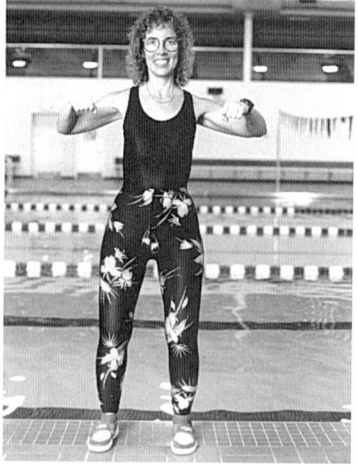

– Reverse Crossing Jog (position 1)

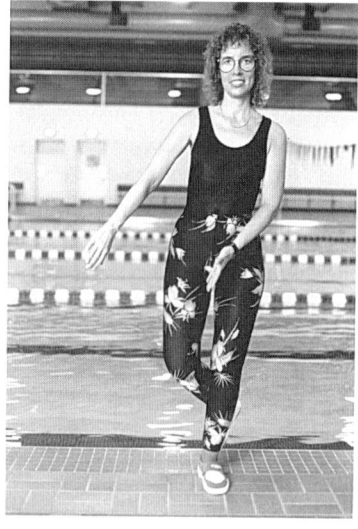

– Reverse Crossing Jog (position 2)

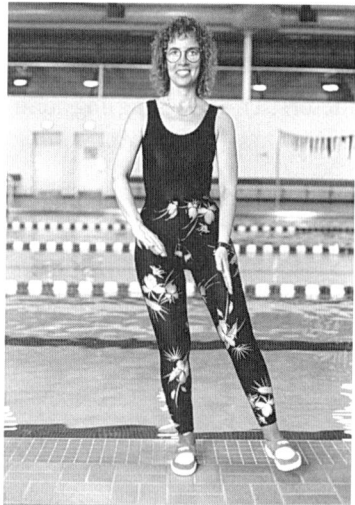

ing Jog left and right, the arms can stay on the hips or push laterally to the right (when moving left) or left (when moving right). Keep the torso facing forward to achieve the excellent oblique, adductor, and abductor work the Reverse Crossing Jog provides. This jog can also be done with the leading foot crossing behind instead of in front as described above. While moving left, the right foot would step behind the left foot for the first count of each two-count segment. While moving right, the left foot would step behind the right foot during the first count of each two-count segment. This is called Crossing Jog Behind; it also works the adductors and abductors. The Crossing Jog done in front and behind can be combined to create a grapevine move. A two-count segment of Crossing Jog in front moving left would be followed by a two-count segment behind moving left; repeat twice before reversing to the right. This can be called a Crossing Jog Combo or Grapevine. The cues would be "cross, step, back, step, cross, step, back, step."

Rhomboid Stretch

Place the palms on center of the upper back and press elbows together.

Rock in Three

Begin with the weight on the left foot, and lift the right foot slightly out to the right side (abducted). This is the first

— Rhomboid Stretch

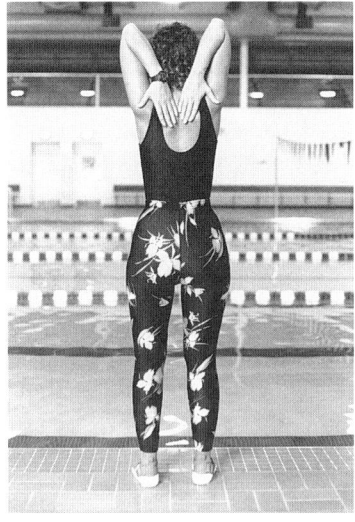

count. For the second count, step the right foot down, and lift the left foot slightly out to the left side (adducted). Step the left foot down and lift the right foot out to the right side (beginning position) for the third count. For the fourth count, pivot slightly to the right on the left foot, and kick the right leg to the right. Step the right foot down and lift the left foot out to the left side for the fifth count. Step the left foot down and lift the right foot out to the right side (beginning position) for the sixth count. Step the right foot down and lift the left foot out to the left side for the seventh count. For the eighth count, pivot slightly to the left on the right foot, and kick the left leg to the left. This is one set of Rock in Three. This move works the adductors, abductors, iliopsoas, and gluteals.

Rock Side to Side

Begin with the weight on the left foot, and lift the right foot slightly out to the right side (abducted). Step the right foot down, and lift the left foot slightly out to the left side (adducted). This is one set of Rock Side to Side. Arm movements can include Press Downs alternately or Lateral Pushes to the left (as the right leg rocks out) and right (as the left leg rocks out). The Rock Side to Side works the adductors and abductors. Lead the rocking with the heel to help keep the toes of both feet pointing forward continually and the hips in forward alignment. The Rock Side to Side can be modified to work the obliques by tightening the hip joints (with the legs in a rocking position) and concentrating on moving from the waist and keeping the upper body stable.

— Rock Side to Side

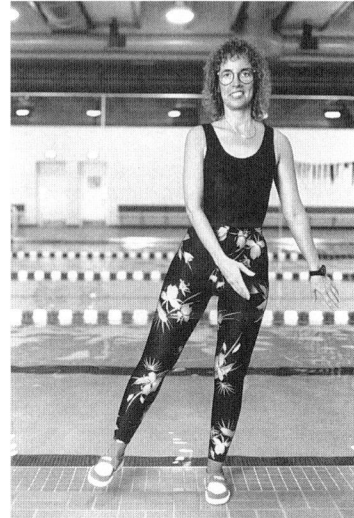

Rocking Horse

Begin with the weight on the left foot, and lift the right foot slightly in front of the body (hip flexion). Step the right foot forward. Lean the body forward over the right foot, keeping the body straight. Avoid any spinal flexion that might cause the body to bend at the waist. Lift the left foot up off the pool bottom, and kick slightly back as the weight shifts to the right foot. This is the first count of Rocking Horse. Step the left foot back to the beginning position, and lean the body slightly back over the left foot, keeping the body straight. Avoid any spinal hyperextension that might cause the body to bend backward at the waist. Lift the right foot up off the pool bottom, and kick slightly forward as the weight shifts to the left foot. This is the second count of Rocking Horse. Repeat counts 1 and 2 three more times. Then switch to Rocking Horse left, with the left foot rocking forward and the right foot rocking backward. The Rocking Horse works the iliopsoas, gluteals, and abdominals. Safe Arms, pushing back as the body leans (rocks) forward and pushing forward as the body rocks backward, works well with this move (see Safe Arms).

This move can be varied by doing it to the right and left diagonals rather than forward. This is called Rocking Horse Diagonals. Lift the right leg toward the right diagonal and turn the body in that direction before stepping on the right foot for the first count. Lift the left leg toward the left diagonal and turn the body in that direction before stepping on the left foot for the second count.

— Rocking Horse (position 1)

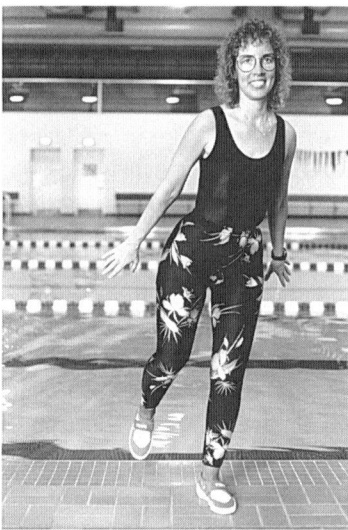

— Rocking Horse (position 2)

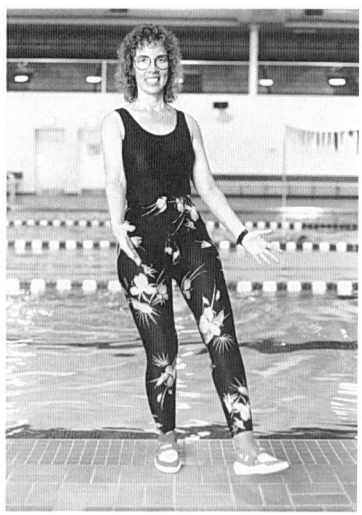

Rocking Horse Doubles

Rock forward on the right foot (as described in Rocking Horse) for the first count. Bounce once on the right foot (keeping it in first-count position) for the second count. Rock back on the left foot (as described in Rocking Horse) for the third count. Bounce once on the left foot (keeping it in the third-count position) for the fourth count. This is one set of Rocking Horse Doubles right. Repeat counts 1 through 4 three more times before switching to Rocking Horse Doubles left (with the left foot rocking forward and bouncing and then the right foot rocking back and bouncing). The Rocking Horse Doubles work the iliopsoas, gluteals, and abdominals. Safe Arms works well with this move. This move can also be varied by rocking to the diagonals.

Rocking Horse in Three

Rock forward on the right foot (as described in Rocking Horse) for the first count. Rock back on the left foot (as described in Rocking Horse) for the second count. Rock forward on the right foot to return to the first-count position. Kick the left foot forward as the body returns to an upright position for the fourth count. (This much of the move is called Rocking Horse in Three right.) Rock forward on the left foot for the fifth count, backward on the right for the sixth count, and forward on the left for the seventh count. Kick the right foot forward as the body returns to an upright position for the eighth count. (This portion of the move is called Rocking Horse in Three left.) The combination of everything done so far is one set of Rocking Horse in Three. This move works the iliopsoas, gluteals, and abdominals. Safe Arms works well with this move.

This move can be combined with Rocking Horse Doubles for a move called Rocking Horse Three and Doubles. Do a Rocking Horse in Three right, a Rocking Horse Doubles left, a Rocking Horse in Three left, and a Rocking Horse Doubles right. This is one set of Rocking Horse Three and Doubles. Students can learn well with these cues on the beats: "up, back, up, kick, up, up, back, back" (repeat these words twice for one full set of Rocking Horse Three and Doubles) **or** "right, left, right, kick, left, left, right, right; left, right, left, kick, right, right, left, left." These moves can also be varied by using Rocking Horse Diagonals.

Rocking Horse Seven and Up

Rock forward on the right foot (as described in Rocking Horse) for the first count. Rock back on the left foot (as described in Rocking Horse) for the second count. Rock forward on the right foot for the third count, backward on the left foot for the fourth count, forward on the right foot for the fifth count, backward on the left foot for the sixth count, and forward on the right foot for the seventh count. Kick the left foot forward for the eighth count. This portion of the move is called Rocking Horse Seven and Up right. Rock forward on the right foot, backward on the left, forward on the right, backward on the left, forward on the right, backward on the left, forward on the right (counts 1–7); then kick the right foot forward for count 8. This is Rocking Horse Seven and Up left. This entire move is one set of Rocking Horse Seven and Up. This move works the iliopsoas, gluteals, and abdominals. Safe Arms works well with this move.

The Rocking Horse Seven and Up can be combined with Rocking Horse Doubles for variety; it's called Rocking Horse Seven and Doubles. Do one set of Rocking Horse Seven and Up right for the first eight counts, two sets of Rocking Horse Doubles left for the second eight counts, one set of Rocking Horse Seven and Up left for the third eight counts, and two sets of Rocking Horse Doubles right for the fourth eight counts. This is one set of Rocking Horse Seven and Doubles. These can also be varied by using Rocking Horse Diagonals.

Russian Kick

This move must be done in shallow water to be accomplished successfully. With the hips and knees flexed (bent) as much as possible (almost sitting in the pool), alternately extend each knee without changing the degree of hip flexion. The arms can be held in a folded position in front of chest, like Russian dancers do, or they can punch alternately in opposition to the

— Russian Kick

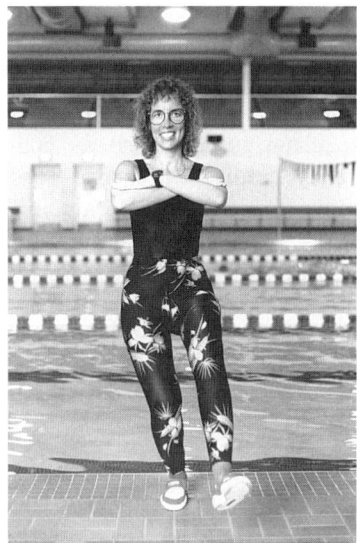

kicks. Russian Kicks work quadriceps, hamstrings, and gluteals.

Safe Arms

Begin with the arms extended out to the sides, just beneath the water surface, with the palms forward. With the elbows

— Safe Arms

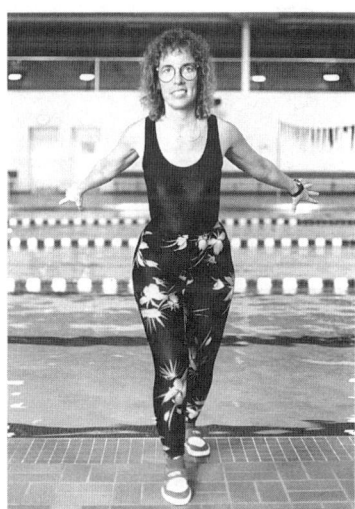

extended so the arms are straight, bring the hands together in front of the body. Turn the palms back, and with straight arms, bring the hands together (or as close as possible) behind the body. This move works the pectorals, anterior serratus, trapezius, rhomboids, and lattisimus dorsi. Rocking Horses and Forward and Back Lunges work well with Safe Arms.

Scissor Arms

Begin with the arms extended laterally, palms down. With the elbows extended so the arms are straight, push the arms straight down in front of the body until the palms meet. With the shoulders back and palms still down, pull the arms up with force to the beginning position. This move can be varied by crossing the hands in the lowered position in front of the body, increasing the range of motion involved in the movement. The serratus anterior, pectorals, lattisimus dorsi, deltoids, and trapezius are all involved in this move. Scissor Arms can be used in Jumping Jacks and most lateral movements, such as Side Step and Side Kick.

Scissors

Begin standing, with the feet together. Bounce into a cross-country ski position, with the right foot at least 12 inches in front of the left. Bounce into the reverse position, with the left foot in front of the right. When the right foot is forward, swing or punch the left arm forward and then reverse. This move can be varied by pointing the toes of the forward foot up (dorsi flexed) while tilting the body slightly back. It can also be varied by pointing the toes of the back foot down while tilting the body slightly forward. Scissors can be done moving forward, backward, or in a circle to increase the intensity. Scissors work the iliopsoas and gluteals. Tilting backward with the toes of the front foot dorsi flexed focuses work on the iliopsoas and also involves the tibialis anterior and abdominals. Tilting forward with the toes of the back foot down focuses work on the gluteals and involves the gastrocnemius.

Scissors Jump

Begin standing, with the feet together. This move is sometimes called Vertical Jump. Jump into a cross-country ski position, with the right foot in front of the left. While still suspended in the water, bring both

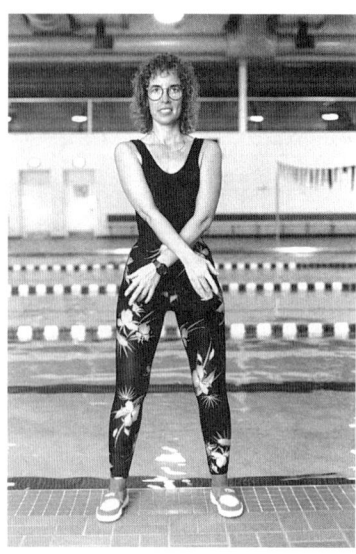
— Scissor Arms

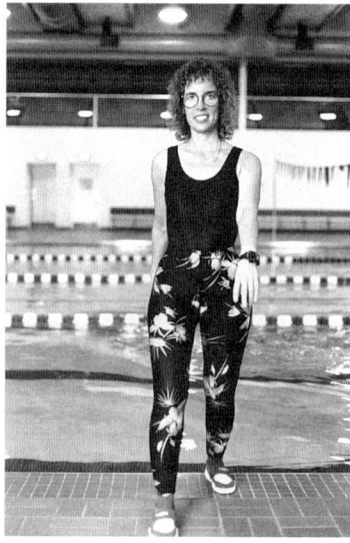
— Scissors

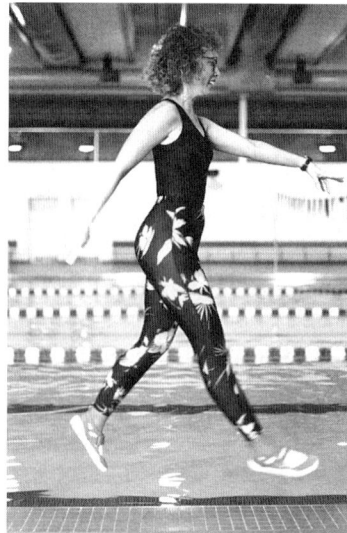
— Scissors Jump

feet together, and land with them next to each other. Jump into a cross-country ski position, with the left foot in front of the right. While still suspended in the water, bring both feet together, and land with them next to each other. Scissors Jumps work the iliopsoas, gluteals, and gastrocnemius. The left arm should swing forward as the right leg goes forward and vice versa. Scissors Jumps should be used in high-intensity classes for well-conditioned students only.

Scissors Turn

Begin standing, with the feet together. Bounce into a cross-country ski position, with the right foot about 12 inches in front of the left. This is count 1. For the second count, pivot (or bounce) a half turn to the left, keeping the feet in the same place but changing their position so that the body faces the back of the pool. Bounce twice with the feet together for counts 3 and 4. Repeat counts 1 through 4 to return facing the front. The Scissors Turn works the iliopsoas, gluteals, gastrocnemius, and obliques. It can be done with quarter turns rather than half turns. Bounce into the cross-country ski position (as stated above) for count one. For count 2, pivot or bounce a quarter turn to the left. Bounce twice with the feet together for counts 3 and 4. To face each wall with this move, repeat counts 1 through 4 four times.

Scissors with Bounce

Begin standing, with the feet together. Bounce into a cross-country ski position, with the right foot about 12 inches in front of the left. Bounce, bringing both feet together again. Bounce into a cross-country ski position, with the left foot about 12 inches in front of the right. Bounce, bringing both feet together again. The arm movements and variations written for Scissors also apply to Scissors with Bounce. The Scissors with Bounce can also be varied by twisting the body so the toes of the right foot point to the right diagonal when the right foot is forward and the toes of the left foot point to the left diagonal when the left foot is forward. This move works the iliopsoas and gluteals.

Scrunch

Buoyant bells, balls, or jugs are needed (see Chapter 8). Begin in a supine position (lying on back); flex the knees and hips. Round the shoulders forward, and "scrunch" them to the knees. Do not extend to a straight leg position. The Scrunch works the abdominal muscles.

Shoulder Shrug

Standing in stride position (with feet shoulder width apart), arms relaxed at the sides, squeeze the shoulders together in front of the body. Then squeeze the shoulders together behind the body. Shoulder Shrugs work the pectorals, deltoids, trapezius, and rhomboids. They can be done with moves like Jumping Jacks or alone for joint lubrication during the warm-up.

Side Circle

Begin standing at the pool edge, holding the pool edge to stabilize the body. The weight is on the left foot, with the right leg straight down and the right foot next to the left foot. Extend the right leg back (hip hyperextension), and circle it out to the side, around to the front, and back to the beginning position. Repeat seven more times and then reverse. During the reverse, the right leg will move forward (hip flexion), circle out to the side, and around to the back before returning to the beginning position. Repeat the Side Circles back and forward with the left leg. As the leg circles, the body should remain in good alignment. If the upper body moves around, the leg circles should be smaller. The Side Circles work adductors, abductors, iliopsoas, and gluteals. This is a toning move and should not be used during the aerobic portion of the workout.

Side Lift

The Side Lift is a toning move. It is a Side Kick done without the bounce (see Side Kick).

Side Lift Flex

This is a Side Kick with the knee slightly flexed. It is used during the toning portion of the

Side Lift Flex

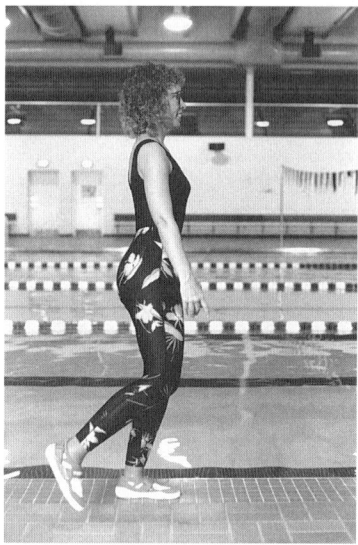

Side Press

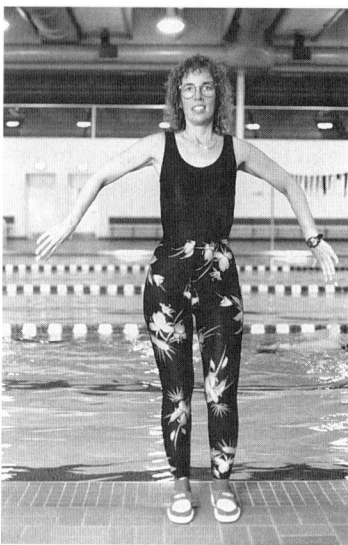

workout. Hold onto the pool edge for stability. With the knee pointing straight down (hip extension) and flexed to about a 120-degree angle, do 8 to 16 Side Kicks with no bounce. The upper body should be upright and stable. Shorten the range of motion in the leg if the upper body moves. The knee flexion will increase the water's drag on the leg and thus enhance the toning benefits. The knee joint should be consciously tightened to avoid torque. The Side Lift Flex works the abductors and adductors.

Side Press

The Side Press is a variation of the Tricep Extension (see Tricep Extension). For Side Press Out, begin with the hands on the hips and the elbows out to the side. Turn the palms away from the body (pronate), and press the forearms out to the sides (extend elbows). For Side Press In, return to the beginning position from the extended Side Press Out. The Press In concentrates on biceps, while the Press Out concentrates on triceps.

Side Step

Begin with the feet together and the arms at the sides. For the first count, step the right foot out to the right (keep the toes pointed forward and allow the knees to bend), and lift both arms out to the sides (a reverse Press Down). Shift the body weight to the right foot, and move the left foot next to the right foot's new position as arms lower for the second count. The body will be in the beginning position but two to three feet to the right of the actual starting place. Repeat counts 1 and 2 three more times, moving to the right. Then Side Step four times to the left; step the left foot out to the left, and move the right foot next to the left foot's new position. The arms can be kept straight, or the elbows can be flexed up to a 90 degree angle. Straight or slightly flexed arms will provide the highest intensity. Complete flexion will provide the the lowest intensity. The Side Step works the abductors, adductors, deltoids, and lattisimus dorsi.

Side Touch

See Touch Side.

Side Train

Begin with the feet together. For the first count, step the right foot out to the right side, and shift the body weight to that leg by lifting the left foot up from the beginning position. For the second count, step the left foot back to the beginning position, and shift the body weight to that leg by lifting the right foot up. Step the right foot back to the beginning position for the third count, and shift the body weight to that leg by lifting the left foot up from the beginning position. For the fourth count, step the left foot back to the beginning position. This is one Side Train right. Repeat counts 1 through 4 three or seven more times. Reverse to do four or eight Side Trains left. Lateral Pushes to the left (as the right foot steps right during the Side Train right) and right (as the left foot steps left during the Side Train left) can be used.

A Catalog of Movements

— Side Train (position 1)

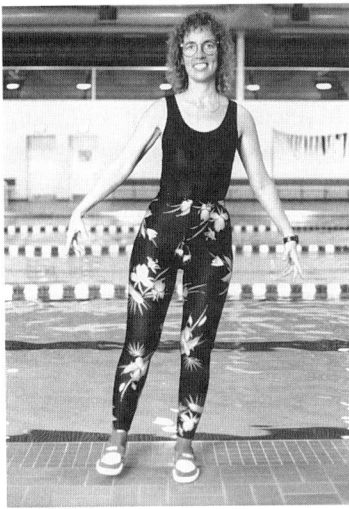

— Side Train (position 2)

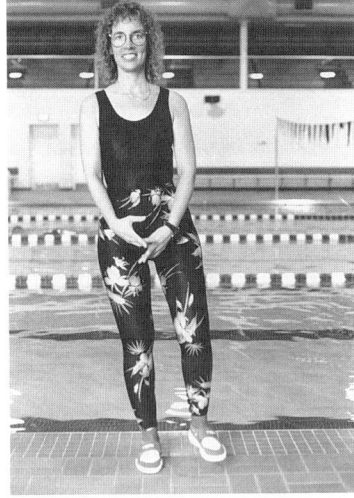

— Side Train (position 3)

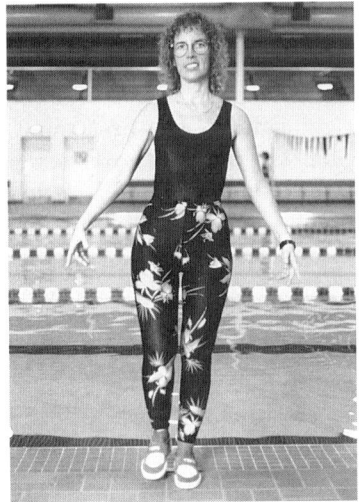

— Side Train (position 4)

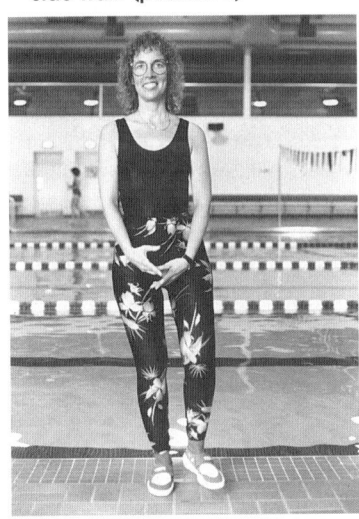

Repeat the move to the left for a Sidebend left. The Sidebend works the obliques. Be careful to bend to the *side* only, not forward or backward during the Sidebend. This is a much smaller move than participants expect it to be. Emphasize the small range of motion that will be experienced.

Sidekick

Begin in stride position. Lift the right leg out to the side (abduct) while bouncing once on the left leg for the first count. Return the right leg to the beginning position (adduct), and bounce on both feet for the second count. Abduct the left leg while bouncing once on the right leg for the third count; adduct the left leg to the beginning position, and bounce on both feet for the fourth count. This is one set of Sidekicks. Properly

— Sidekick

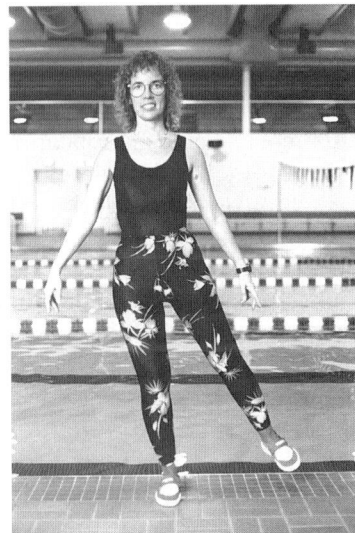

A reverse Press Down, with the elbows flexed or the arms straight, can also be used (with the lift coming during the step to the right during the Side Train right and during the step to the left during the Side Train left). The Side Train works abductors and adductors.

Sidebend

Begin with the feet in stride position, knees slightly flexed, hips tucked under, and abdominals contracted. While bending sideways at the waist, tilt the upper torso toward the right (lateral spinal flexion right). This a Sidebend right.

position the leg, with the toes pointing forward and the heel pointing slightly out to the right, before kicking out to the right. The Sidekick can be varied by doing two, four, or eight with the right leg before switching to the left leg. Press Down Behind and Press Down Front arm moves both work well with the Sidekick. The Sidekick works the adductors and abductors.

Sidekick Forward and Backward

Begin in stride position. Lift the right leg out to the side (abduct), and bounce once on the left leg for the first count. Return the right leg (adduct) to just in front of the left ankle while bouncing once on the left leg for the second count. Abduct the right leg while bouncing once on the left leg for the third count. Adduct the right leg to just behind the left ankle while bouncing once on the left leg for the fourth count. This is one Sidekick Forward and Backward. If used during the toning portion of the workout, this move should be repeated four or eight times before switching to the left leg. If used during the aerobics portion, it should be done only once on the right leg before switching to the left leg. Also incorporate hand movements if used during the aerobics portion. Press Down the left arm in front of the body (and the right arm behind) when the right leg is adducted in front of the left

Sidekick Forward

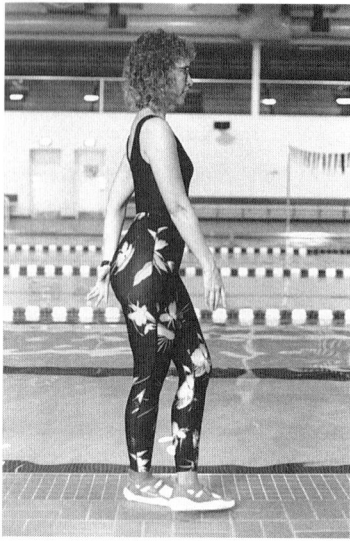

Sidekick Backward

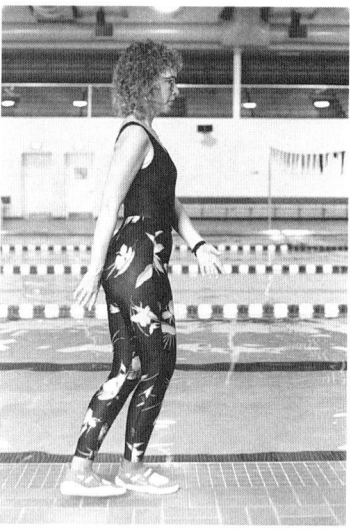

ankle, and Press Down the right arm in front of the body (and the left arm behind) when the left leg is adducted behind the right ankle. Sidekick Forward and Backward works the adductors and abductors.

Ski Bounce

Begin with the feet in stride position. Bounce, moving both feet together to the right and then to the left, as if schussing down a ski hill. This move works the quadriceps and hamstrings if done with concentration on flexing and extending the knees. It works obliques if done with concentration on the movement coming from the waist and keeping the upper torso stable. Tricep Extensions back work well with the Ski Bounce.

Slide

The Slide is a bouncing side-step, moving laterally to the right and then to the left. Begin in stride position for the Slide right: Step the right foot to the right side for the first count. Step the left leg next to the right, while lifting the right foot up off the pool bottom for the second count. Repeat counts 1 and 2 three to seven times moving to the right. For the Slide left: Step the left foot to the left for the first count. Step the right leg next to the left, while lifting the left leg up off the pool bottom for the second count. Repeat counts 1 and 2 three to seven times moving to the left. This is one full set of Slides. Press Down arm moves work well with the Slide. The Slide works the adductors and abductors.

Spider Crawl

Begin facing the pool edge, with the feet on the pool wall and the hands holding the gutter. Crawl or shuffle down the pool wall in one direction; then switch direction. The feet should remain in contact with the pool wall, and the hands should remain palms down on the edge of pool. The more frequently direction is changed, the higher the intensity of the move.

Stroke

Begin with the left hand on the left hip and the right hand extended laterally to the left, palm facing forward. Move the right hand just below the water surface, pushing to the right; push until the body has to pivot right as the right arm reaches slightly behind it on the right side. Repeat with the left arm beginning on the right, the palm catching the water and pushing it to the left. For a faster pace, shorten the range of motion. This move works the pectorals, deltoids, rhomboids, and trapezius.

– Stroke

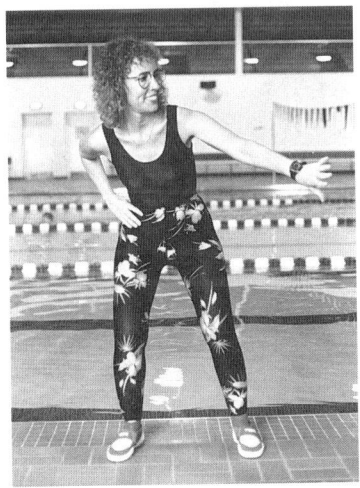

Swing Twist

Begin with feet in stride position. Bounce both feet to turn the toes to the right for the first count (feet pivot but stay in place on pool bottom). This is a Swing Twist right. Bounce both feet (in place) to turn the toes to the left for the second count. This is a Swing Twist left. The entire move to both sides is one set of Swing Twists. During the Swing Twist right, push both arms to the left, and during the Swing Twist left, push the arms to the right. This move can be varied by moving forward and backward, right and left, or in a circle. The Swing Twist works the obliques.

– Swing Twist

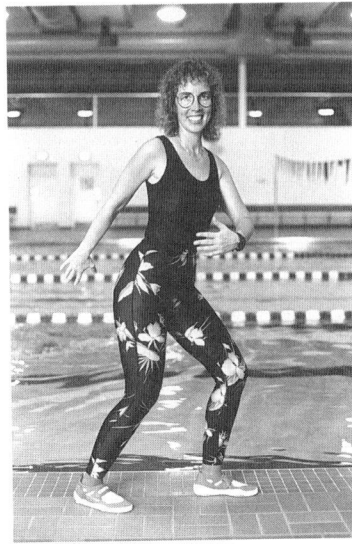

Swing Twist Doubles

Begin with the feet in stride position. Bounce both feet to turn the toes to the right for the first count (feet pivot but stay in place on pool bottom). Bounce once in that position for the second count. Bounce both feet (in place) to turn the toes to the left for the third count. Bounce once in that position for the fourth count. This is one set of Swing Twist Doubles. This move can be varied like the Swing Twist. It works the obliques.

Swing Twist in Three

Begin with one set of Swing Twists for counts 1 and 2. On counts 3 and 4, do Swing Twist Doubles right. On counts 5 and 6, do Swing Twists left and right. On counts 7 and 8, do Swing Twist Doubles left. The toes turn right, left, right, right, left, right, left, left. This move can be varied like the Swing Twist. It works the obliques.

Swing Twist with Back Toes Down (see photo at the top of the next page)

Begin doing a Swing Twist (as described in Swing Twist). During the Swing Twist right, point the toes of the back foot (left) down (plantar flex) toward the pool bottom. During the Swing Twist left, point the toes of the back foot (right) down toward the pool bottom. Pointing the back toes down during the Swing Twist adds gluteal work to the move, which ordinarily works the obliques. The "Toes Down" adaption can be used during Swing Twist, Swing Twist Doubles, and Swing Twist in Three.

— Swing Twist with Back Toes Down

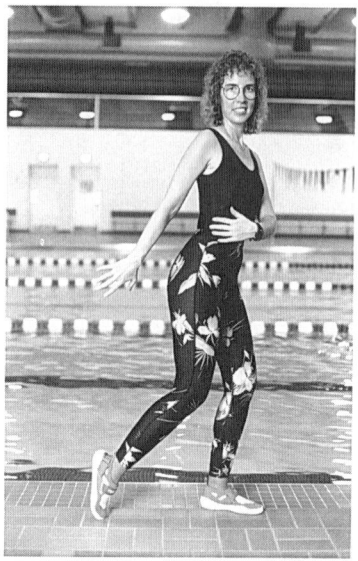

Swing Twist with Front Toes Up

Begin doing a Swing Twist (as described in Swing Twist). During the Swing Twist right, point the toes of the front foot (right) up toward the body (dorsi flex). During the Swing Twist left, point the toes of the front foot (left) up toward the body. The Swing Twist with Front Toes Up works the obliques and tibialis anterior. The "Toes Up" adaption can be used during Swing Twist, Swing Twist Doubles, and Swing Twist in Three.

Swish

Begin in stride position, with the toes pointed slightly out (slight external hip rotation) and the arms extended laterally (abducted), just beneath the water surface. (The elbows are straight, and the arms are straight out to the sides.) Rotate the spine (twist) to the right, so that the right hand moves back about 6 to 12 inches and the left hand moves forward about 6 to 12 inches. Return to the beginning position. Then twist to the left, so the arms move 6 to 12 inches in the opposite direction. The body should not move from the hips down. Students will think this is an arm movement; it is not. The arms stay in place in relation to the torso. The movement comes from the waist, which causes the arms to move. Students who are unable to accomplish this move without moving the lower body should pivot to the right during the Swish right and vice versa. This will protect the knee joints. The Swish works the obliques.

Touch Back

Begin with the feet in stride position. Move the toes of the right foot backward on the pool bottom for the first count. Return to the beginning position for the second count. Move the

— Swing Twist with Front Toes Up

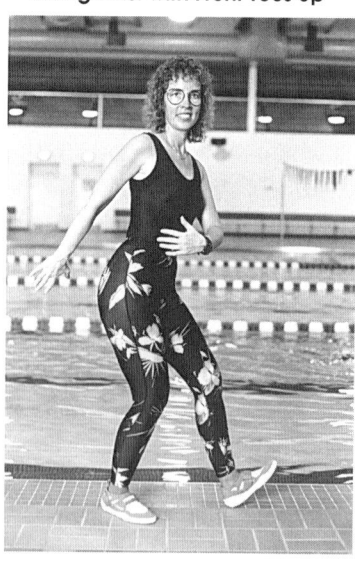

— Swish

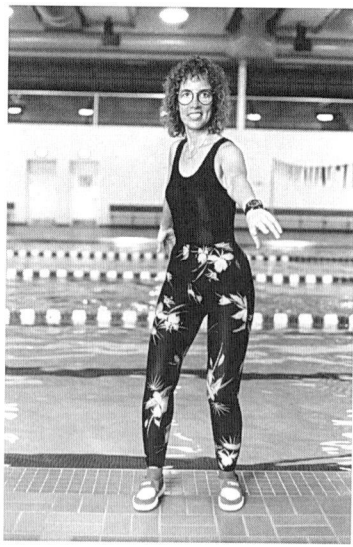

— Touch Back

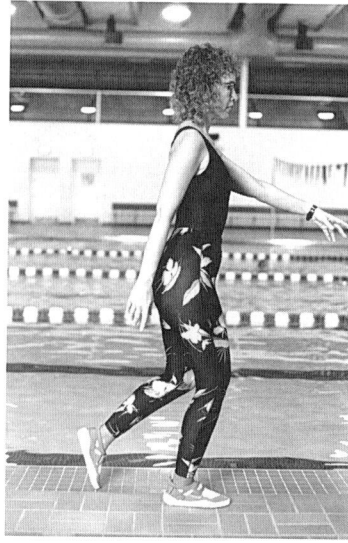

toes of the left foot backward on the pool bottom for the third count. Return the left foot to the beginning position for the fourth count. Swing the right arm forward and the left arm backward as the toes of the right foot touch back. Touch Backs can be done in series of four or eight with the right leg before changing to the left leg. They can also be done alternately (as described above) or in threes: right, left, right, right and left, right, left, left. Touch Backs work the gluteals and iliopsoas. They are sometimes called Back Touches.

Touch Forward

Begin with the feet in stride position. For the first count, move the toes of the right foot forward on the pool bottom. This will cause slight hip flexion. Swing the left arm forward and the right arm backward as the toes touch forward. Return to the beginning position for the second count. Repeat counts 1 and 2 using the left foot for counts 3 and 4. Touch Forwards can be done four or eight times with the right foot before changing to the left foot or alternately (as described above). Touch Forwards work the gluteals and iliopsoas. They are sometimes called Forward Touches.

Touch Side

Begin with the feet together. Move the toes of the right foot to the right side along the pool bottom for the first count. Return to the beginning position for the second count. Move the toes of the left foot to the left side along the pool bottom for the third count. Return to the beginning position for the fourth count. This is one set of Touch Sides. Touch Sides can be done slowly with the feet bouncing together between each touch (as described above) or quickly in a rocking-type movement, with the right foot returning to beginning position as the left foot is touching to the left and vice versa. Armswing Sides work well with Touch Sides. This move can be done in a series or four or eight with the right foot before changing to the left foot. Touch Sides work the adductors and abductors. They are sometimes called Side Touches.

Touch-Up

Do a Touch Side with the right foot while bouncing once on the left foot for the first count (see Touch Side). Do a Kneelift Cross with the right foot while bouncing once on the left foot for the second count (see Kneelift Cross). Repeat counts 1 and 2 three times before changing to the left foot. Do a Touch Side with the left foot while bouncing once on the left foot for the first count. Do a Kneelift Cross with the left leg while bouncing once on the right foot for the second count. Repeat counts 1 and 2 three more times with the left foot. This is one full set of Touch-Ups. Since it is not recommended to bounce more than eight times successively

— Touch-Up (position 1)

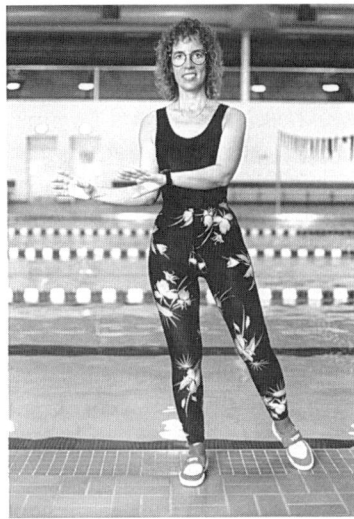

— Touch-Up (position 2)

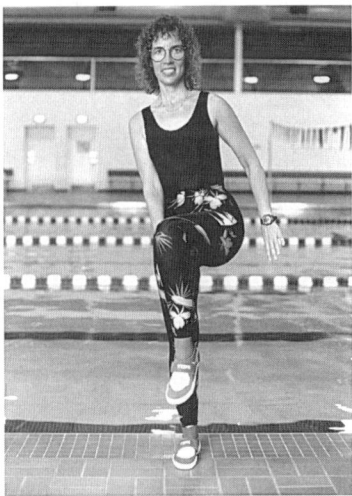

on one foot, do not do more than four Touch-Ups on one foot before changing to the other, unless weight is equally displaced between both legs during the Touch Side. Tricep Extensions pressing back as the knee comes up work well with Touch-Ups. Touch-Ups work the iliopsoas, gluteals, and abductors.

Trapezius Stretch

With the fingers interlaced in front of the body, arms at shoulder height, turn the palms outward as arms extend forward until a stretch is felt in the upper back. The trapezius can be stretched further by doing Neck Stretches to each side; then relax the chin and drop it down on the chest (see Neck Stretch). An alternative Trapezius Stretch can be done by placing both hands on either side of the neck. Tilt the head forward and down.

— Trapezius Stretch

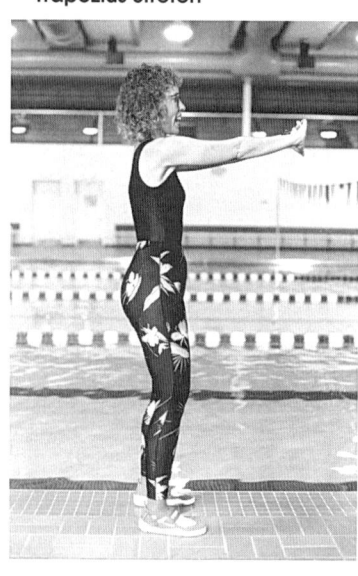

— Tricep Extension Back

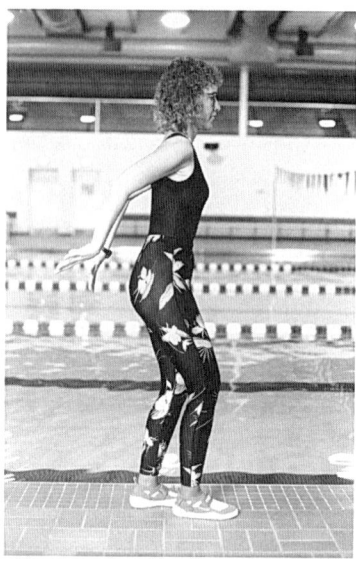

— Tricep Extension Out

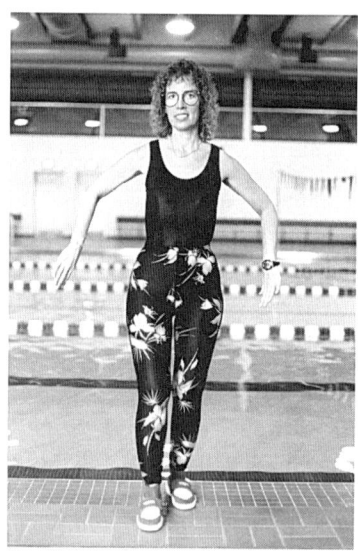

— Tricep Extension Forward

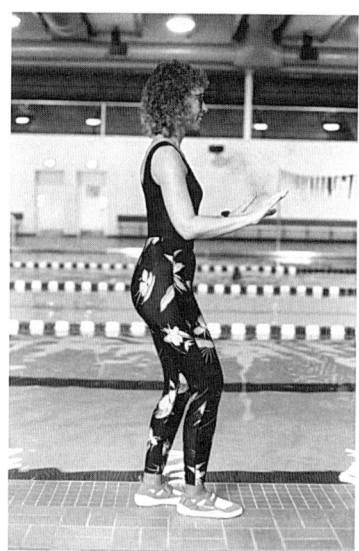

Tricep Extension

This move is the reverse of the Bicep Curl but with the palms facing the other way (pronated) (see Bicep Curl). Tricep Extensions back begin with the elbows flexed at about a 90-degree angle. The forearms are down next to waist, and the elbows are about three to six inches back from the body. The arms (shoulders) are slightly hyperextended. In this position, press the forearms back through the water (elbow extension). Tricep Extensions out begin in the same position but with the palms facing out (away from the body). Press the forearms out through the water. Tricep Extensions forward begin with the elbows next to the waist and completely flexed. Extend the elbow or press the palms down to the outer thighs. These moves all work the triceps and biceps.

Tricep Stretch

With the arms overhead, hold the elbow of the right arm with the left hand. Gently pull the right elbow to the left behind the head, stretching the tricep. To increase the stretch, bend the elbow of the right arm. This also stretches the latissimus dorsi. Reverse for the left arm.

Tricep Stretch

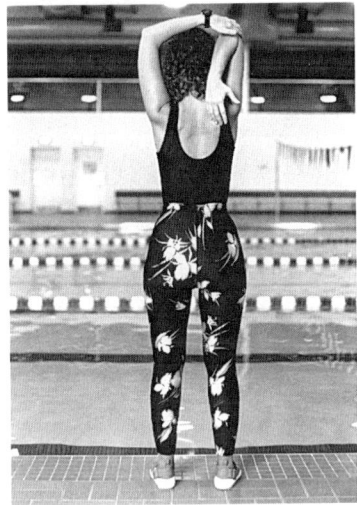

Tuck Jump

Begin with the feet in stride position and the arms extended laterally, just below the water surface. Pull both knees up to the chest while pressing the arms down through the water and under the knees. The abdominal muscles should be contracted. Tuck Jumps work iliopsoas and gluteals.

Twist

Begin with the feet in wide stride position, knees slightly flexed, hips tucked under, abdominals tightened, and ribs lifted. While keeping the toes, knees, and hips pointed forward, twist the upper torso toward the right (spinal rotation right). This is the first count. Return to the beginning position for the second count. Twist the torso to the left for the third count, and return to the beginning position for the fourth count. This is one set of Twist. It can be varied to protect the knee joints by pivoting the feet, knees, and hips in the same direction as the twist. The Twist works obliques.

Two-Step

The Two-Step is simply two Side Steps right followed by two Side Steps left (see Side Step).

Waist Curl

The Waist Curl is a Bicep Curl in which the elbows stay close to the waist (see Bicep Curl). It can be done forward, with the forearms forward moving up and down; in, with the forearms across the body moving up and down; and out, with the forearms out to the sides moving up and down. The palm always faces up (supinated). Waist Curls work the biceps and triceps.

Waterpull

Begin with both arms extended laterally to the left; then pull the elbows in toward the waist, palms facing forward. This is the beginning position. Push both arms through the water to the right and then to the left. The range of motion will be short because of the flexed position of the elbows. Lowering the arms deeper into the water and then bringing them back to the surface will increase the interest and intensity of this move. This move works the biceps and triceps but can be modified to work the pectorals, deltoids, rhomboids, and trapezius by extending the elbows. It is often done without any foot movement for upper-body toning, but Rock Side to Side can work well with it.

Tuck Jump

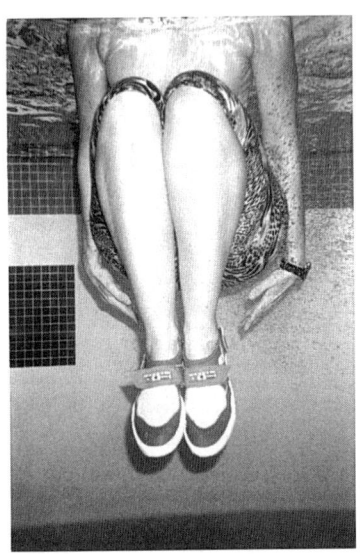

Waterpull

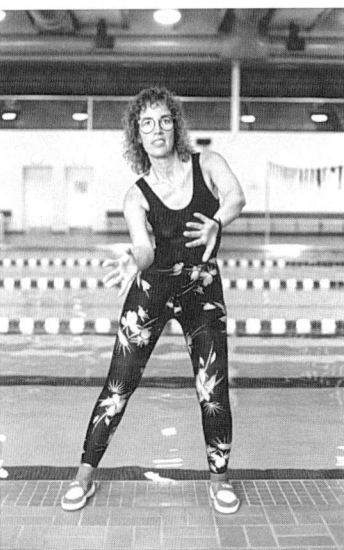

Wind-Up and Present

Begin with the arms extended laterally, palms down. With the elbow extended so the arm is straight, press the right arm down in front of the body; continue moving it left and up until it is parallel with the left arm. This is the "Wind-Up" portion of the move. Turn the right palm out and push across, just below the water surface, to the beginning position. This is the "Present" portion of the move. Continue with several, using the right arm and then switching to the left, or alternate using the right and left arms. The pectorals, deltoids, trapezius, and rhomboids are all involved in Wind-Up and Present. To involve the obliques, keep the lower body stationary with the feet in a wide stance, pointed slightly outward. If working the obliques is not desired, keep the knee joints safe by pivoting the feet and knees in the same direction.

— Wind-Up and Present (position 1)

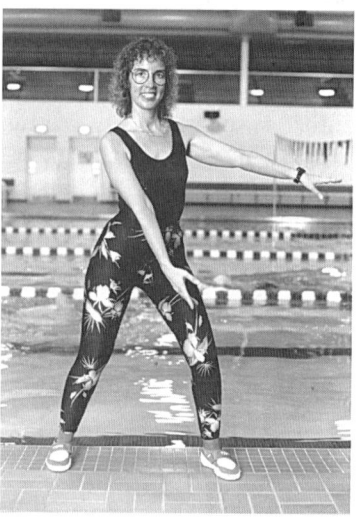

— Wind-Up and Present (position 2)

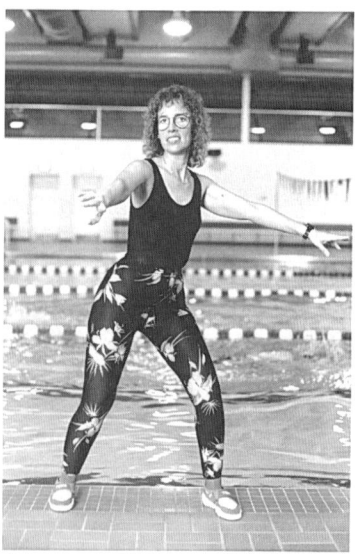

Successful Combinations

Hopscotch Combo

Do one set of Hopscotch left and right for the first four counts. Do two Hopscotches left for counts 4 through 8. Do one set of Hopscotch right and left for counts 9 through 12. Do two Hopscotches right for counts 13 through 16. The Hopscotch combo is cued as "bounce, left, bounce, right, bounce, left, bounce, left, bounce, right, bounce left, bounce, right, bounce, right."

Jumping Jack and Tuck

Jump apart for the first count; jump together for the second count. Tuck Jump, with both knees moving to the chest, for the third count. Land with both feet together for the fourth count. This is one Jumping Jack and Tuck. Jumping Jack and Tuck can move backward by using Safe Arms moving forward. Jumping Jack and Tuck can move forward by using Safe Arms moving backward.

Jumping Jack in Three

Jump apart for the first count; jump together for the second count. Jump apart for both the third and forth counts. Jump together for the fifth count. Jump apart for the sixth count. Jump together for both the seventh and eighth counts. This is one set of Jumping Jack in Three. The instructor may cue it as "out, in, out, out, in, out, in, in." If the music tempo is slow enough, lift the knees on the extra bounce during the fourth and eighth counts. The fourth-count double Kneelift would resemble a Frog Jump, and the eighth-count double Kneelift would resemble a Tuck Jump.

Kick Combo

Kick the right foot forward for the first count; bounce and bring the feet together for the second count. Diagonal kick with the right foot for the third count; bounce and bring the feet together for the fourth count. Sidekick with the right leg for the fifth count; bounce and bring the feet together for the sixth count. Back Kick with the right leg for the seventh count; bounce and bring the feet together for the eighth count. This is one half of a Kick Combo.

Finish it by repeating with the left leg. Kick Combo Doubles is another variation in which every kick is repeated twice before moving on to the next.

Knee Combo

Begin with a Kneelift Cross for the first count. Bounce and bring the feet together for the second count. Kneelift forward for the third count, bounce and bring feet together for the fourth count, Kneelift out for the fifth count, bounce and bring the feet together for the sixth count, Mule Kick for the seventh count, and bounce and bring the feet together for the eighth count. This is one half of Knee Combo. Repeat with the left leg to complete the combo. Knee Combo Doubles can be done by simply repeating each Kneelift twice before moving to the next step.

Knee Knee Knee Kick

This move can be done slowly with a bounce between each step but is described here as a fast Knee Knee Knee Kick. Begin with a Kneelift right for the first count and a Kneelift left for the second count. Do a Kneelift right for the third count and without touching the right leg down, kick the right leg forward from the Kneelift for the fourth count. Kneelift left for the fifth count, and Kneelift right for the sixth count. For the seventh count, Kneelift left, and without touching the left leg down, kick the left leg forward for the eighth count. This is one set of Knee Knee Knee Kick. This move can be varied by externally rotating the hips slightly so that the knees point to the diagonal.

Kneelift Kick

Kneelift with the right leg for the first count, bounce and bring the feet together for the second count, kick the right leg forward for the third count, bounce and bring the feet together for the fourth count, Kneelift with the left leg for the fifth count, bounce and bring the feet together for the sixth count, kick forward with the left leg for the seventh count, and bounce and bring the feet together for the eighth count. The Kneelift Kick can be varied by internally rotating the hips slightly to create a Crossing Kneelift Kick and by externally rotating the hips slightly to create a Diagonal Kneelift Kick.

Kneeswing Combo

This is a combination of the Kneeswing up and back and the Kneeswing Crossing. Do one set of Kneeswing up and back (swing right knee up, back, up, then set right foot down; swing left knee up, back, up, then set left foot down). Follow that with one set of Kneeswing Crossing (right knee crosses, opens, crosses, then set right foot down; left knee crosses, opens, crosses, then set left foot down). This is one set of Kneeswing Combo. The Kneeswings can also be combined by doing Kneeswing up and back four times with the right leg and then four times with the left leg, followed by Kneeswing Crossing four times with the right leg and then four times with the left leg. They can also be combined doing two Kneeswings up and back and two Kneeswing Crossings with the right leg and then the left leg.

Kneeswing Kickswing

Do one Kneeswing up and back with the right leg for the first two counts. Do one Kickswing up and back with the right leg for the third and fourth counts. Repeat counts 1 through 4 to finish Kneeswing Kickswing right. Do one Kneeswing up and back with the left leg for the first two counts. Do one Kickswing up and back with the left leg for the third and fourth counts. Repeat counts 1 through 4 with the left leg to finish the full Kneeswing Kickswing Combo.

Run and Kick

Turn to the right, and jog six steps, moving forward to the right (jogging right, left, right, left, right, left) for the first 6 counts. Step and pivot on the left foot to face the left wall for the seventh count. Kick the right foot forward for the eighth count. Jog six forward to the left wall (jogging right, left, right, left, right, left). Step and pivot on the left foot to face the right wall for the seventh count. Kick the right leg forward for the eighth count. This is one set of Run and Kick.

Running Tires

Jog with the feet apart, mimicking the tire running football players use as drills. The knees should come up, the upper torso should stay in a vertical position, and the jogging should be fairly rapid.

Scissors Turn Kick Bounce

Do a Scissors Turn to face the back of the pool for the first two counts. Kick the right leg forward for the third count; bounce and bring the feet together for the fourth count. Do a Scissors Turn to face the front of the pool for counts 5 and 6. Kick the right leg forward for count 7, and bounce and bring the feet together for the count 8.

Scoot

Do a reverse Crossing Jog for three counts, moving to the right (step right with the right foot, step behind with the left foot, step right with the right foot). Do an open Kneelift left for the fourth count. Do a reverse Crossing Jog going left for counts 5, 6, and 7 (step left with left foot, behind with the right foot, and left with the left foot). Do an open Kneelift right with the right knee for count 8. Jog backward for three counts (right, left, and right) for counts 9, 10, and 11. Kneelift left for the twelfth count. Rocking Horse in Three with the left leg forward for counts 13 to 16. This is one set of Scoot.

Slide Square

Slide to the right, with the right foot leading for the first four counts. Turn one-quarter turn left; Slide with the left foot leading for counts 5 through 8 (four more counts). Turn one-quarter turn right; Slide with the right foot leading for counts 9 through 12. Turn one-quarter turn left; Slide with the left foot leading for counts 13 through 16. When making the square, face the outside when sliding right with the right foot leading and face inside when sliding left with the left foot leading.

Tennis Strokes

Swing the right arm back and then horizontally across the body, mimicking a tennis forehand stroke. A single- or double-handed backstroke can also be used.

Touch Combo

Touch Forward with the right foot while bouncing once on the left foot for the first count. Touch Side with the right foot while bouncing on the left foot once for the second count. Touch Back with the right foot while bouncing once with the left foot for the third count. Bounce and bring both feet together for the fourth count. Touch Forward with the left foot for the fifth count while bouncing once on the right foot. Touch Side with the left foot while bouncing once on the right foot for the sixth count. Touch Back with the left foot while bouncing once on the right foot for the seventh count. Bounce and bring both feet together for the eighth count. This is one set of Touch Combo.

Touch Lift Cross Kick

Side Touch with the right foot while bouncing once on the left foot for the first count. Kneelift with the right foot while bouncing once on the left foot for the second count. Bounce and bring both feet together for the third count. Diagonal Kick with the left foot while bouncing once on the right foot for the fourth count. Side Touch with the left leg while bouncing once on the right foot for the fifth count. Kneelift with the left foot while bouncing once on the right foot for the sixth count. Bounce and bring both feet together for the seventh count. Diagonal Kick with the right leg while bouncing once on the left foot for the eighth count. This is one full set of Touch Lift Cross Kick.

Touch Lift Cross Rock

Side Touch with the right foot while bouncing once on the left foot for the first count. Kneelift with the right foot while bouncing once on the left foot for the second count. Bounce and bring both feet together for the third count. Diagonal Kick with the left foot while bouncing once on the right foot for the fourth count. Rock forward to the left diagonal on the left leg while kicking the right foot back to the right diagonal for the fifth count. Rock back to the right diagonal on the right foot while kicking the left foot forward to the left diagonal for the sixth count. Rock forward to the left diagonal on the left foot while kicking the right foot back to the right diagonal for the seventh count. Rock back to the right diagonal on the right leg while kicking the left foot forward to the left diagonal for the eighth count. This is one-half set of Touch Lift Cross Rock. Side Touch left with the left foot while bouncing once on the right foot for the ninth count. Kneelift with the left foot while bouncing once on the right foot for the tenth count. Bounce both feet together once for the eleventh count. Diagonal Kick with the right foot while bouncing once on the left foot for the twelfth count. Rock forward to the right diagonal on the right leg while kicking the left foot back to the back left diagonal for the thirteenth count. Rock back to the back left diagonal on the left foot while kicking the right foot toward the right diagonal for the fourteenth count. Rock forward to the right diagonal on the right foot while kicking the left foot back to the back left diagonal for the fifteenth count. Rock back to the back left diagonal on the left leg while kicking the right foot toward the right diagonal for the sixteenth count. Repeat the eight-count sequence, reversing lefts and rights, to do one full set of a Touch Lift Cross Rock.

KEY WORDS

Muscle balance
Skeletal framework
Muscle groups

Opposing muscles
Muscle pairs

Safety
Contraindicated

SUMMARY

— Muscle imbalances reflect differences in the relative strengths and flexibilities of the various muscles surrounding a joint or body part.
— The human body is designed to be balanced in all ways.
— The most important factor in successful aquatic exercise programming is a basic understanding of why each movement is being used.
— Participants should remember to work opposing muscles of a pair at least equally.
— Safety is another reason for knowing why a move is used.

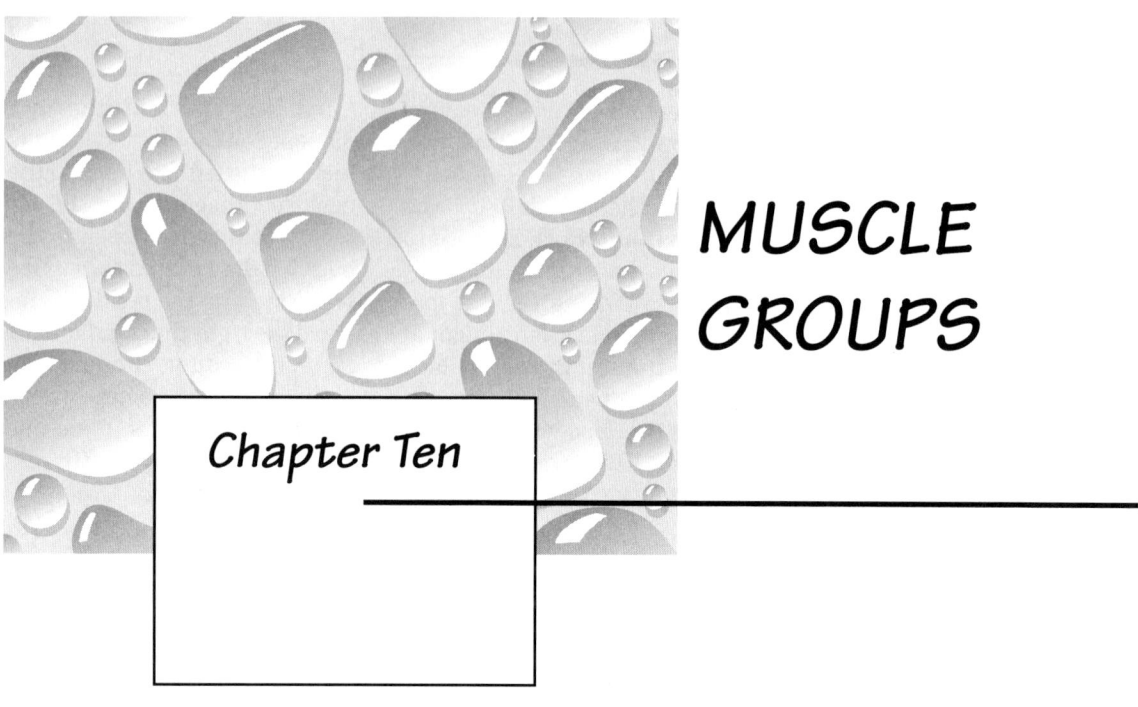

MUSCLE GROUPS

Chapter Ten

ALIGNMENT AND MUSCLE BALANCE

Good postural **alignment** allows the human body to move safely. From a front view, the shoulders should evenly align over the hip joints, and the pelvis should rest over the hip joints in a balanced position. From the side, the spine should have an anterior curve in the cervical and lumbar areas and a posterior curve in the thoracic area. The ear, shoulder, hip, and ankle joints should fall in line. When deviation from good postural alignment exists in one area, there is always a reactive deviation in another area.

Aquatic exercisers should not only practice proper postural alignment, but the exercises used should promote **muscle balance.** Muscles should be strong enough to contract fully when needed and to relax fully when contraction is not needed. Muscles that are **hypertoned** are unable to relax fully.

All the muscles surrounding each joint should be toned equally so there is good balance and give and take among them. Each muscle should be of appropriate resting length, so that bones and other body parts hang in proper neutral positions.

Muscles that are subjected to repeated overload adapt by becoming stronger and wider. Unless they are specifically overloaded with a stretch, they also become permanently tighter and shorter. When one muscle is consistently strengthened and the opposing muscle ignored, the strengthened muscle becomes permanently shortened and the opposing or antagonistic muscle remains lengthened, weak, and inefficient.

Muscle groups at a joint often work in pairs to first flex and then extend a part of the body. A good example of a **flexor/extensor pair** is the hamstring/quadricep muscle group. The hamstrings flex (bend) the knee, and the quadriceps straighten (extend) it.

Muscle balance is achieved when both muscles in a pair are developed to the same degree. Imbalance, resulting from overdevelopment or underdevelopment of one member of the pair, can cause poor posture, pain, tendon tightness, and eventual misalignment of the body's framework.

MOVEMENTS FOR MAJOR MUSCLE GROUPS

The rest of this chapter outlines the major muscle groups. Each section ends with a list of toning, aerobic, arm, and stretch movements. (See descriptions of most in Chapter 9.)

When designing a workout, be sure to include at least two moves for each major muscle group in every hour-long program.

1. *Pectoralis/Trapezius/Rhomboids*
   The **pectorals** are the chest muscles. The **trapezius** is a diamond-shaped muscle in the upper back and neck. The **rhomboids** are small-back muscles located beneath the trapezius.

   The exercises listed below work the trapezius, rhomboids, and pectorals. When arm movements go in front of or across the front of the body, they work the pectorals. When they move toward the sides and back, they work the trapezius and rhomboids.

DIAGRAM 10-1 Pectorals

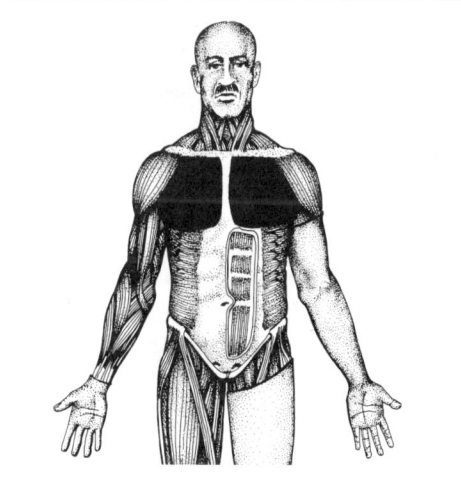

DIAGRAM 10-2 Trapexius

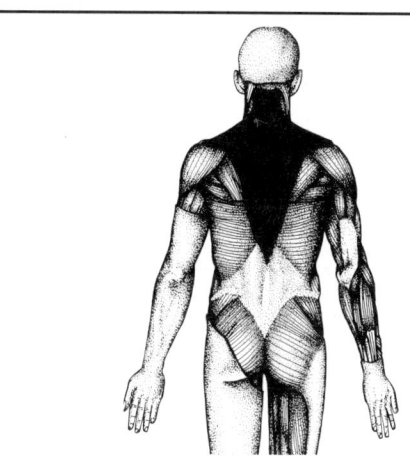

– elbow press single
– elbow press with forearm down
– safe arms
– over and present
– scissor arms
– backstroke
– wind-up and present
– bow and arrow
– reach pull in
– stroke
– waterpull
– shoulder shrug
– backstroke side

2. *Hamstrings/Quadriceps*
   The **hamstrings** are located in the back of each thigh. The **quadriceps** are located in the front of each thigh.

   The exercises listed below work the quadriceps and hamstrings: the hamstrings, as the knee is bent, and the quadriceps, as the knee is straightened.

– jazzkick
– flick kick
– jig
– hoedown
– hopscotch

DIAGRAM 10-3 Quadriceps/Hamstrings

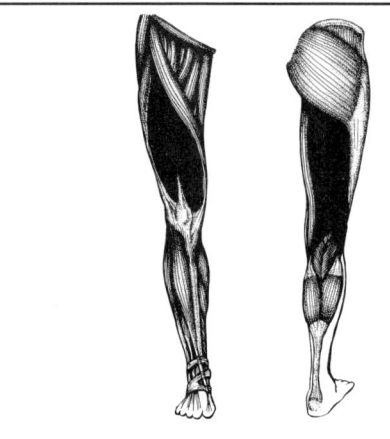

- heel hits behind
- heel hits across
- mule kick
- ski bounce
- paddlekick
- forward lunge
- Russian kick

3. *Biceps/Triceps*

The **biceps** are located on the front of each upper arm. The **triceps** are located on the back of each upper arm.

DIAGRAM 10-4 Biceps/Triceps

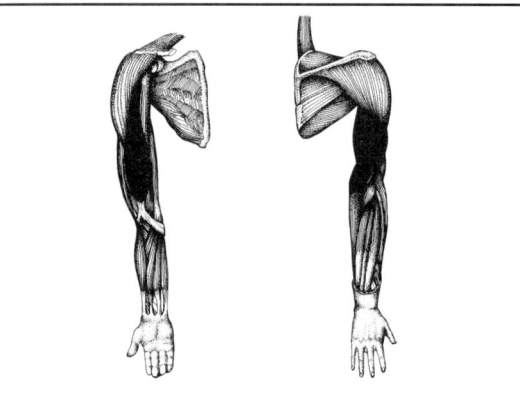

The exercises listed below will work the biceps and triceps. As the elbow bends, the biceps will contract. As the elbow straightens, the triceps contract.

- waist curl
- tricep extensions back (also forward, out)
- side press out, in
- jog arms
- lateral push
- backstroke

4. *Iliopsoas/Gluteals*

The **iliopsoas** (hip flexors) are located on the front of the hip. The **gluteus maximus** (called the **gluteals**) are located on the buttocks.

The exercises listed below work the iliopsoas when the hip flexes or the leg moves forward. As the leg comes back and lowers through the water, the gluteals contract.

- tuck jump
- frog jump
- kick
- kick corner
- kneelift
- back kick (swing)

DIAGRAM 10-5 Iliopsoas/Gluteus Maximus

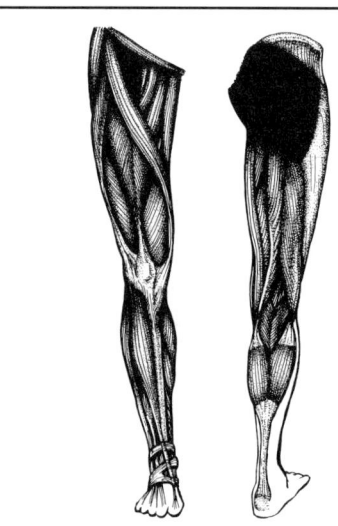

- scissors
- knee swing
- back lunge
- leap forward
- forward train
- forward walking/jogging movements
- flutter kick
- scissor jump

5. *Adductors/Abductors*

The **adductors** are located on each inner thigh. The **abductors** are located on the outside of each thigh.

The exercises listed below work the hip adductors and abductors. As the limb moves laterally, the abductors contract. As the limb returns to anatomical position, the adductors contract.

- crossing jog
- side kick
- side circles
- jumping jacks
- cross kick
- heel hits front
- fling
- fling kick
- knee swing crossing

- wringer
- leap side
- rock side
- side train
- side step

6. *Obliques*

The **obliques** are located under and to the side of the rectus abdominus muscle. They are midriff muscles.

The exercises listed below work the obliques.

- waterpull
- twist
- karate punch
- press down and behind with sidebend
- over and present
- side scissors
- rock side
- leap side
- scissor turn
- swing twist
- ski bounce

DIAGRAM 10–6 Adductors/Abductors

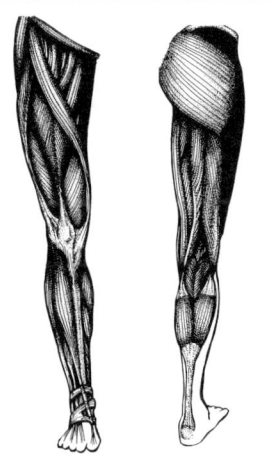

DIAGRAM 10–7 Obliques

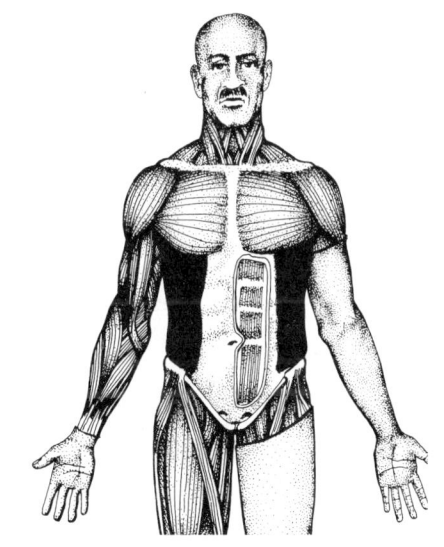

DIAGRAM 10-8 Rectus Abdominus

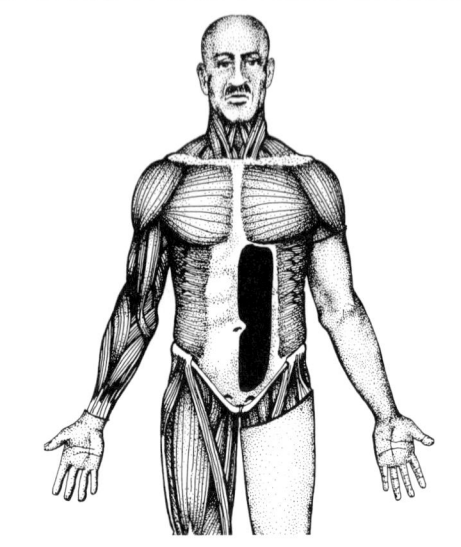

DIAGRAM 10-9 Deltoids

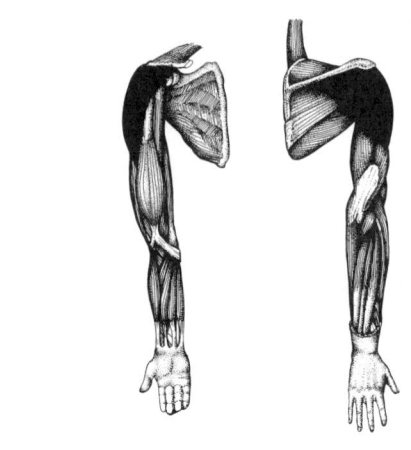

7. *Abdominals / Erector Spinae*

The **erector spinae** is a large back muscle. The **abdominals** *(rectus abdominus)* is a large muscle located from the ribs to the pelvis.

There is a misconception that exercises that flex the hip are abdominal exercises. The rectus abdominus does not cross the hip joint and therefore is not the primary mover in hip flexion.

The exercises listed below will work the abdominals and back muscles.

- knees tucked crunch
- lift hips
- heel jack
- heel tilt
- pelvic tilt
- curl down
- jog tilt

8. *Deltoids (Medial) / Latissimus Dorsi*

The **medial deltoid** is a cap on the shoulder. The **latissimus dorsi** is a large back muscle in the middle on each side of the back.

The exercises listed below will work the medial deltoid and latissimus dorsi. As the arms lift (abduct), the deltoid contracts. As they lower (adduct), the latissimus dorsi contracts.

- press down behind
- press down front
- press down alternate
- press down (one front, one back)
- press down with elbows bent

DIAGRAM 10-10 Latissimus Dorsi

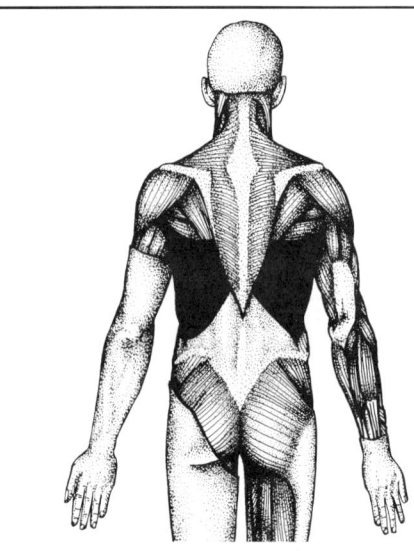

9. *Anterior and Posterior Deltoids*

The **anterior deltoids** are located on the front of each shoulder. The **posterior deltoids** are located on the back of each shoulder.

The exercises listed below will work the anterior deltoids as the arm moves forward and the posterior deltoids as the arm moves backward.

- armswing, forward and backward
- with both elbows bent or straight arms
- swing forward and backward, alternating arms forward and backward

10. *Gastrocnemius/Tibialis Anterior*

The **gastrocnemius** is located in the calf of each lower leg. The **tibialis anterior** is located in the front of each lower leg.

The exercises listed below will work the gastrocnemius as the toe points down (plantarflexes) and the tibialis anterior as the toe points up toward the shin (dorsiflexes).

- bounce
- most jogs
- heel jack

DIAGRAM 10–11 Gastrocneumius

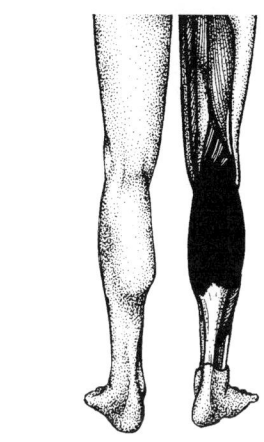

- heel tilt
- scissor with front toe up
- swing twist with toe up
- kick and point, kick and flex

KEY WORDS

Alignment
Muscle balance
Hypertoned
Flexor/extensor pair
Pectorals
Trapezius
Rhomboids
Hamstrings

Quadriceps
Biceps
Triceps
Iliopsoas
Gluteals
Adductors
Abductors
Obliques

Abdominals
Erector spinae
Medial deltoids
Latissimus dorsi
Anterior deltoids
Posterior deltoids
Gastrocnemius
Tibialis anterior

SUMMARY

- Good postural alignment allows the human body to move safely.
- Aquatic exercisers should not only practice proper postural alignment, but the exercises they use should promote muscle balance.
- Each muscle should be of appropriate resting length, so that the bones and other body parts hang in proper neutral positions.
- Muscle groups often work in pairs to first flex and then extend a part of the body at a joint.

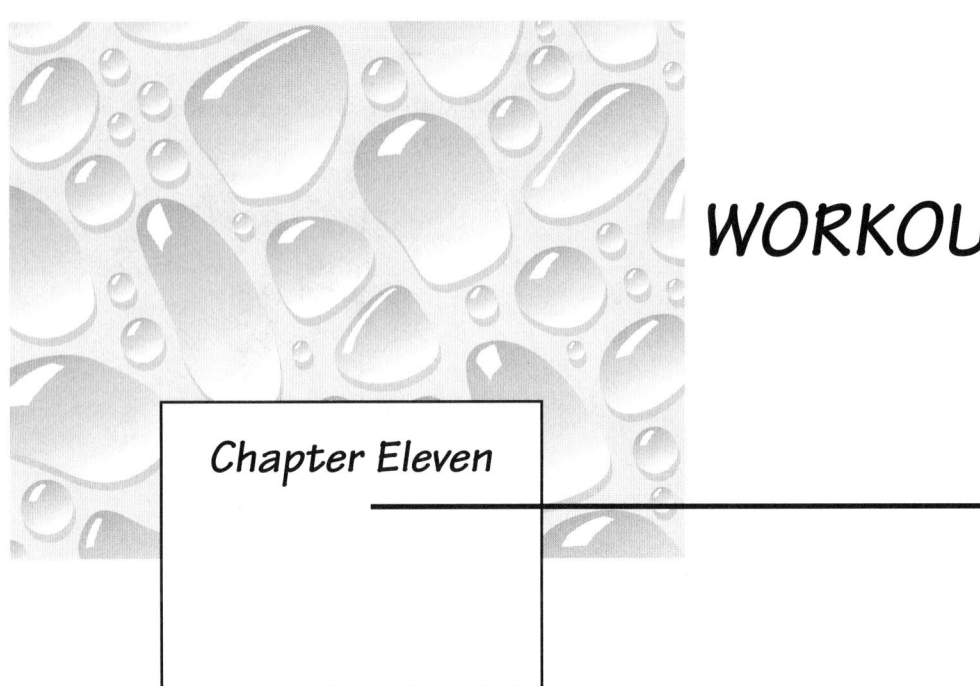

WORKOUTS

Chapter Eleven

SAMPLE CLASS PROGRAMS

Strength Training

— **Thermal Warm-Up**

Do the following for 1 minute each:
A. Jog or walk, forward and back (usually, 8 or 16 jogs forward and 8 or 16 jogs backward, depending on pool size)
B. Continue jogging or walking, bending the knee and pulling the heel back to the buttock
C. Continue jogging or walking, using high kneelifts
D. Change to walking or jogging sideways (8 or 16 to the right, 8 or 16 to the left)
E. Jumping jacks with arms beneath the water surface

— **Prestretch**

Hold the following stretches for 10 to 15 seconds each:
A. Quadricep right, quadricep left
B. Hamstring right, hamstring left
C. Calf right, calf left
D. Hip flexor right, hip flexor left
E. Pectorals
F. Trapezius

— **Weight Training**

1. Do the following for 90 seconds each with force:
   A. Bicep curls up
   B. Tricep extensions down
   C. Pectoral presses (elbow press forward) with elbows bent
   D. Trapezius/rhomboid pulls (elbow press back) with elbows bent
   E. Latissimus dorsi presses (press down behind)
   F. Deltoid lifts

2. Do the following with the right leg for 90 seconds each with force; then repeat with the left leg:
   A. Knee flexion (mule kick)
   B. Hip flexion (kick forward)

C. Hip abduction (side lift)
D. Knee extension (flick kick)
E. Hip extension (back kick)
F. Hip adduction (cross kick)
G. Hip circumduction (circles)

— **Cooldown**

Walk for 2 to 3 minutes.

— **Poststretch**

Do the following stretches for 20 to 30 seconds each:
A. Quadricep stretch, right and left
B. Gluteal stretch, right and left
C. Abductor stretch, right and left
D. Hamstring stretch, right and left
E. Iliopsoas stretch, right and left
F. Adductor stretch, right and left
G. Bicep stretch
H. Tricep stretch, right and left
I. Pectoral stretch
J. Trapezius stretch
K. Deltoid (medial) stretch, right and left

Water Walking

Wearing shoes is recommended.

— **Thermal Warm-Up**

Do the following for 45 seconds each:
A. Walk with small steps, 12 forward and 12 backward, using walking arms (the right arm swings forward as the left leg steps forward), elbows bent.
B. Repeat A with shoulder rolls.
C. Walk forward in a circle, rolling from heel to toe
D. Walk backward in a circle, rolling from toe to heel.
E. Walk forward around the circle on the toes.
F. Walk backward around the circle on the heels.
G. Do toe circles for 20 seconds with the right foot and 20 seconds with the left foot.

— **Prestretch**

A. Calf stretch, right and left (15 seconds each)
B. Walk forward around the circle; push both arms forward for trapezius/rhomboid stretch (20 seconds)
C. Walk backward around the circle, using a shoulder blade pinch to stretch the pectorals (20 seconds)
D. Walk forward to the right corner; walk back using mule kicks (20 seconds)
E. Repeat D to the left corner and back (20 seconds)
F. Quadricep stretch, right and left (15 seconds each)
G. Hip flexor stretch, right and left (15 seconds each)
H. Hamstring stretch, right and left (15 seconds each)
I. Calf stretch, right and left (15 seconds each)
J. Walk forward and backward using sidebends (30 seconds)

— **Cardiovascular Warm-Up**

1. Do the following in circle formation for 45 seconds each:
   A. Moving forward, take exaggerated, long strides, keeping the knees bent. Add jogging arms, with the hands cupped.
   B. Keep the knees bent and move double time with smaller steps. Change the arms to punching.
   C. Repeat A and B.
2. Face the center of the circle, and do the following for 45 seconds each:
   A. Walk sideways using lateral push arms. Move 8 to the right and 8 to the left repeatedly until the time allotment is finished.
   B. Walk sideways using deltoid lift arms. Move 8 to the right and 8 to the left repeatedly until the time allotment is finished.
   C. Walk in and out of the circle using breaststroke and backstroke arms.

D. Add high knees to 2C and continue.
E. Straighten the legs to a goose step, moving in and out of the circle.
F. Repeat B, C, D, and E.

– **Aerobics**

Do the following exercises for 60 seconds each:

Group 1—In scatter formation:
A. Walk forward on the toes (bent elbow, walking arms); walk back on the heels.
B. Walk sideways using sidekicks. Move 8 to the right and 8 to the left repeatedly until the time allotment is finished.
C. Walk forward and back using mule kicks.

Group 2—In scatter formation:
A. Walk in a square with the knees and toes pointed somewhat out.
B. Repeat A, moving backward.
C. Walk forward and backward, using side bends.
D. Walk, leaning forward while moving forward and leaning backward while moving backward.

Group 3—In circle formation:
A. Walk forward into the circle, using high knees.
B. Continue with high knees, but cross the right foot over the left and lower the right as the step is taken (strut).
C. Walk backward around the circle, crossing the right foot behind the left and the left behind the right.

Group 4—In circle formation:
A. Walk around the circle, using high knees.
B. Continue walking around the circle, but change to a goose step.
C. Continue walking around the circle, but change to a flick kick.
D. Repeat A through C, moving backward around the circle.

Group 5—In circle formation:
A. Walk around the circle, contracting and releasing the abdominals.
B. Walk backward, using diagonal kicks.
C. Move forward, using sidekicks and stepping across.
D. Turn around and go back (again, facing forward), using sidekicks and stepping behind.

– **Cooldown**

Do the following in scatter formation for 1 minute each:
A. Walk 4 low and 4 high (2 sets forward and 2 sets back).
B. Walk 4 fast and 8 slow, forward and back.
C. Walk sideways, 2 slow and 4 fast (2 sets right, 2 sets left).
D. Over and present.
E. Walk forward and back, using shoulder rolls.

– **Upper-Body Toning**

Do the following for 45 seconds each (3-1/2 minutes total):
A. Elbow press
B. Elbow press back
C. Bicep curls
D. Tricep extensions
E. Push across

– **Edge-of-Pool Toning**

Do the following for 1 minute each:
A. Side lifts—Do 10 with force on the lift out and 10 with force on the return. Repeat.
B. Knee flexion (mule kick)—Do 10 with force on pulling the heel back and 10 with force on straightening the leg.
C. Knee swings
D. Turn the other side to the pool edge and repeat with the other leg.

- **Stretch**

    Hold each for 30 seconds (5 minutes total):
    A. Quadricep stretch, right and left
    B. Calf stretch, right and left
    C. Hamstring stretch, right and left
    D. Pectoral stretch
    E. Iliopsoas stretch, right and left
    F. Back stretch, push forward
    G. Adductor stretch, right and left

Aerobics

Do the following workout 3 times on nonconsecutive days:

- **Thermal Warm-Up**

    Do the following for 1 minute each (4 minutes total):
    A. Hoedowns
    B. Jazz kicks
    C. Sidekicks
    D. Cross kicks

- **Stretch**

    Do the following for 15 seconds each (3 minutes total):
    A. Quadricep stretch, right and left
    B. Calf stretch, right and left
    C. Hamstring stretch, right and left
    D. Pectoral stretch
    E. Iliopsoas stretch, right and left
    F. Back stretch
    G. Adductor stretch, right and left

- **Cardiovascular Warm-Up**

    Do the following for five minutes total:
    A. Hopscotches, 1 minute
    B. Sidekicks (repeat 4 left, 4 right), 1 minute
    C. Forward kicks, slow and fast, 2 minutes
    D. Kneelifts fast, 1 minute

- **Aerobics**

    Do each of the following for 60 seconds:

    Group 1
    – Jumping jacks
    – Jumping jacks crossing
    – Forward kicks fast
    – Forward kicks slow

    Group 2
    – Sidekicks
    – Mule kicks fast
    – Mule kicks doubles
    – Flick kicks (repeat 8 left, 8 right)
    – Jazzkicks

    Group 3
    – Diagonal kicks fast
    – Diagonal kicks slow
    – Diagonal kicks slow (repeat 4 left, 4 right)
    – Jog forward slow and backward fast
    – Jumping jacks, slow and fast

    Group 4
    – Scissors
    – Scissors with front toes up
    – Scissors with back toes down
    – Jog tilt (8 leaning forward, 8 leaning backward)
    – Kneelifts

- **Cooldown**

    Do the following for 1 minute each (3 minutes total):
    A. Jog in place, fast and slow
    B. Rock from side to side
    C. Mule kicks

- **Upper-Body Toning**

    Do the following for 45 seconds each (3-1/2 minutes total):

    A. Elbow press
    B. Elbow press back
    C. Bicep curls
    D. Tricep extensions
    E. Push across

- **Edge-of-Pool Toning**

    Do the following for 1 minute each:

A. Side lifts—Do 10 with force on the lift out and 10 with force on the return in. Repeat.
B. Knee flexion (mule kick)—Do 10 with force on pulling the heel back and 10 with force on straightening the leg.
C. Knee swings
D. Turn the other side to the pool edge and repeat with the other leg.

– **Stretch**

Hold each for 30 seconds (5 minutes total):
A. Quadricep stretch, right and left
B. Calf stretch, right and left
C. Hamstring stretch, right and left
D. Pectoral stretch
E. Iliopsoas stretch, right and left
F. Back stretch, push forward
G. Adductor stretch, right and left

Toning

– **Thermal Warm-Up**

A. Walk fast in a big circle, moving clockwise, for 30 seconds.
B. Move back around the circle for 30 seconds.
C. Walk fast with high knees, moving counterclockwise, for 30 seconds.
D. Back up for 30 seconds.
E. Walk sideways, moving right 8 to 10 steps and then left 8 to 10 steps, for 1 minute
F. Walk with sidebends around the circle for 30 seconds.
G. Back up with sidebends for 30 seconds.
H. Walk around the circle counterclockwise, kicking the heel toward the buttocks, for 30 seconds.
I. Back up, kicking the heel toward the buttocks, for 30 seconds.
J. Walk around the circle on the heels for 30 seconds.
K. Back up around the circle on the heels for 30 seconds.

– **Prestretch**

Hold each of the following for 15 to 20 seconds:
A. Calf stretch, right and left
B. Iliopsoas stretch, right and left
C. Hamstring stretch, right and left
D. Quadricep stretch, right and left
E. Adductor stretch, right and left
F. Pectoral stretch
G. Back stretch

– **Toning**

At the pool edge, do each of the following for 24 reps or 1 minute. Do those exercises that are repeated on the right and left sides for 1 minute on each side.
A. Bicep curls, right and left
B. Mule kicks, right and left
C. Tricep extensions, right and left
D. Flick kicks, right and left
E. Swing the arms, forward and backward (with emphasis on arm extension or pull back)
F. Kickswing, right and left (with emphasis on hip extension)
G. Deltoid lift (both arms together)
H. Side lifts, right and left (hip abduction)
I. Press down (both arms together)
J. Cross kicks, right and left
K. Elbow press forward
L. Abdominal crunches
M. Elbow press back
N. Kick swing, right and left (with emphasis on hip flexion or kick)
O. Swing the arms together, forward and backward (with emphasis on swing forward or shoulder flexion)
P. Punch across (alternating arms)

– **Cooldown and Poststretch**

A. Do A and B from Warm-Up
B. Bicep stretch, 15 to 20 seconds
C. Trapezius stretch, 15 to 20 seconds
D. Do C and D from Warm-Up

E. Quadricep stretch, right and left
F. Hip flexor stretch, right and left
G. Do E from Warm-Up with tricep stretch, right and left, and neck stretch, right and left
H. Do F and G from Warm-Up
I. Abductor stretch, right and left
J. Adductor stretch, right and left
K. Do H and I from Warm-Up
L. Hamstring stretch, right and left
M. Calf stretch, right and left
N. Back stretch

Flexibility

— Warm-Up

Do the following in circle formation:
A. Walk fast, moving clockwise, for 30 seconds.
B. Back up for 30 seconds.
C. Walk fast with high knees, moving counterclockwise, for 30 seconds.
D. Back up for 30 seconds.
E. Walk sideways, moving 8 to 10 steps to the right and 8 to 10 steps to the left, for 1 minute.
F. Walk forward with sidebends around the circle for 30 seconds.
G. Back up with sidebends.
H. Walk, kicking the heels toward the buttocks, moving counterclockwise, for 30 seconds.
I. Back up, kicking the heels toward the buttocks, for 30 seconds.

— Arms

Use the following arm movements with A through I above:
A. Tricep extensions
B. Bicep curls
C. Punching the opposite arm forward
D. Backstrokes
E. Deltoid lifts
F & G. Press downs
H & I. Swing the corresponding arm forward and up and the opposite arm down and backward.

— Flexibility

Upper Body—Jog or walk while doing the following stretches to keep body temperature at a comfortable level. If the body becomes chilled and muscles tighten, stop stretching and go through the Warm-Up phase more vigorously until body temperature is warm enough for comfortable, relaxed stretching.

Hold each of the following for 20 to 30 seconds:

A. Push both arms up, lifting from the ribs
B. Trapezius stretch
C. Pectoral stretch
D. Tricep stretch, right and left
E. Bicep stretch
F. Neck stretch, right and left
G. Walk with shoulder rolls

Lower Body—Hold each of the following stretches for 30 seconds:

A. Do C and D from the Warm-Up
B. Iliopsoas stretch, right and left
C. Gluteal stretch, right and left
D. Do E from the Warm-Up
E. Adductor stretch, right and left
F. Abductor stretch, right and left
G. Do F and G from the Warm-Up
H. Oblique stretch, right and left
I. Do H and I from the Warm-Up
J. Quadricep stretch, right and left
K. Hamstring stretch, right and left
L. Walk forward on the toes and backward on the heels for 1 minute
M. Calf stretch, right and left
N. Tibialis anterior stretch, right and left
O. Back stretch
P. Abdominal stretch

— Cooldown

Walk slowly around the pool for 3 minutes.

Aqua Circuit Training

— Thermal Warm-Up

Do each of the following for 1 minute:
A. Jumping jacks and sidekicks
B. Kneelifts moving forward, crosskicks back
C. Heelhits, front and back
D. Kneeswing combo in place, up and back (4 right, 4 left), cross (4 right, 4 left)

— Prestretch

Do each of the following for 10 to 15 seconds:
A. Quadricep stretch, right and left
B. Iliopsoas stretch, right and left
C. Hamstring stretch, right and left
D. Scissors with pectoral stretch
E. Calf stretch, right and left
F. Back stretch

— Cardiovascular Warm-Up

Do each of the following for 1 minute:
A. Kicks, slow and fast
B. Jumping jacks crossing
C. Slides (16 right, 16 left)
D. Ski bounces
E. Swing twists in 3

— Aerobics

For each of the following, spend 1 minute doing each station movement and 2 minutes doing each aerobic segment:

- *First station*—Elbow press, forward and backward
- *Aerobics*—Jog forward, heelhits back (any mix); add jazzkick
- *Second station*—Mule kicks, right leg
- *Aerobics*—Swing twist singles and doubles (any mix); vary with the toes of the back foot down and the toes of the front foot up; move forward and backward and side to side
- *Third station*—Bicep curls, tricep extensions
- *Aerobics*—Side steps and scissors (any mix)
- *Fourth station*—Mule kicks, left leg
- *Aerobics*—Bounce square; add scissors moving forward, jumping jacks back
- *Fifth station*—Kickswings, right leg
- *Aerobics*—Sidekicks, 4 right and 4 left
- *Sixth station*—Deltoid lifts, press down
- *Aerobics*—Jump bounce, 4 forward and 4 back; add kicks, slow and fast
- *Seventh station*—Kickswings, left leg
- *Aerobics*—Slide; add kicks forward, ski bounces back
- *Eighth station*—Side leglifts, right leg
- *Aerobics*—Mule kicks, slow and fast; add jumping jacks and jumping jacks crossing
- *Ninth station*—Side leglifts, left leg
- *Aerobics*—Back kicks, slow and fast; add back kicks forward, kneelifts back
- *Tenth station*—Abdominal crunches
- *Aerobics*—Kicks and fling kicks; add flings and heelhits front
- *Eleventh station*—Crosskicks, right leg
- *Aerobics*—Rockinghorse 7 and up; add tuck jumps
- *Twelfth station*—Crosskicks, left leg
- *Aerobics*—Kneelifts forward, heel hits back, slow and fast; add rocking side to side
- *Thirteenth station*—Flick kicks, right leg
- *Aerobics*—Jumping jacks square, 4 each direction (right, back, left, forward); add crossing kneelifts, 4 right and 4 left
- *Fourteenth station*—Flick kicks, left leg
- *Aerobics*—Scissors and ski bounces

— Cooldown and Flexibility

Do the following and hold the stretches for 20 to 30 seconds each:

A. Swing twists with flag arms
B. Walk 8 forward, kick, walk 8 backward; repeat 3 times
C. Bounce 8 times
D. Adductor stretch, right and left
E. Side step with tricep stretch
F. Side step with neck stretch
G. Side step with shoulder stretch

H. Swing twist 16 times
I. Iliopsoas stretch, right and left
J. Kneeswing combo, 4 sets
K. Hamstring stretch, right and left
L. Pectoral stretch
M. Corner jazzkick 32 times
N. Quadricep stretch, right and left
O. Back stretch
P. Heel jacks 32 times
Q. Calf stretch, right and left
R. Push both arms up

Sport Specific

— Thermal Warm-Up

Do each of the following for 1 minute:
A. Walk with long, exertive strides, forward and backward.
B. Jog forward and back, with high knees. Use bicep curls and tricep extensions.
C. Sidestep 8 to 10 steps to the right and 8 to 10 steps to the left. Use deltoid lift and press down arms.
D. Jog in place, with heels kicking up and back (like mule kicks). Use elbow press forward and backward.

— Prestretch

Hold each of the following for 10 to 15 seconds:
A. Calf stretch, right and left
B. Iliopsoas stretch, right and left
C. Hamstring stretch, right and left
D. Back stretch

— Cardiovascular Warm-Up

Do the following combination movements/stretches:
A. Do 16 sidesteps to the right while doing a tricep stretch right.
B. Do 16 sidesteps to the left while doing a tricep stretch left.
C. Repeat A and B.
D. Do 32 jumping jacks while doing a pectoral stretch.
E. Do 32 jumping jacks while doing a deltoid lift and press down.
F. Do 8 jumping jacks moving forward and 8 moving back; repeat this sequence (8 up, 8 back) 4 times.
G. Do 32 scissors.

— Aerobics

Balance and Coordination
A. Do 32 ski bounces while doing tricep extensions.
B. Do 16 ski bounces moving forward and 16 moving backward; repeat this sequence (16 up, 16 back) 4 times.
C. Do 32 ski bounces in place with the right foot only.
D. Repeat C with the left leg.
E. Bounce 4 times moving sideways to the right and 4 times moving sideways to the left; add the lateral press arm movement. Repeat this sequence (4 right, 4 left) 4 times.
F. Repeat E using only the right foot.
G. Repeat E using only the left foot.
H. Bounce 16 times in a square, so that the first bounce makes the right corner of the square (bounce right, back, left, forward to make the square). Bounce another 16, so that the first bounce makes the left corner of the square (bounce left, back, right, forward). Add the jump rope arm movement.
I. Repeat H using the right leg only.
J. Repeat H using the left leg only.

Intervals
A. Do scissors at moderate intensity for 30 seconds; swing the arms alternately forward and backward.
B. Do scissors at high intensity for 30 seconds. Use more power, lengthen the stride, use a larger range of motion with the arms, and push up off the pool bottom with more effort.
C. Repeat A and B (3 times).

Power
A. Do tuck jumps, 8 moving forward and 8 moving backward. Do the sequence (8 up, 8 back) covering a moderate amount of distance and twice covering the largest distance possible.
B. Do jump bounces, 1 forward and 1 backward; do 16 sets.
C. Do 3 small bounces and 1 big jump, covering a maximum distance on the big jump. Move 4 forward and 4 backward; repeat this sequence (4 up, 4 back) 4 times.
D. Run with long strides to form a circle; move forward around the circle for 2 minutes.

Intervals
A. Do jumping jacks at moderate intensity for 30 seconds.
B. Do jumping jacks at high intensity for 30 seconds.
C. Repeat A and B (3 more times).

Sport Stations
Spend 1 minute each at 4 different stations of your choice:
A. Baseball bats
B. Tennis racquets
C. Power mule kick drills
D. Basketball jumps
E. Run and hurdle
F. Sprinting
G. Run and long jump
H. Golf clubs

— Cooldown and Flexibility
A. Walk for 2 minutes with varied strides.
B. Sidestep 16 to the right while doing a right shoulder stretch.
C. Sidestep 16 to the left while doing a left shoulder stretch.
D. Sidestep 16 to the right while doing a right tricep stretch.
E. Sidestep 16 to the left while doing a left tricep stretch.
F. Calf stretch, right and left, 15 seconds each
G. Do 24 scissors.
H. Iliopsoas stretch, right and left, 15 seconds each
I. Hamstring stretch, right and left, 15 seconds each
J. Do 24 jumping jacks.
K. Back stretch, 15 seconds
L. Pectoral stretch, 15 seconds
M. Repeat A.

Bench Aerobics
— Thermal Warm-Up
Do each of the following for 1 minute:
A. Walk forward and backward, using tricep extensions and bicep curls.
B. Sidestep 8 right and 8 left, using deltoid lift and lateral press.
C. Jog forward 16 using mule kicks; jog backward 16 with kneelifts.
D. Jumping jacks

— Prestretch
Hold each of the following 10 to 15 seconds:
A. Calf stretch, right and left
B. Quadricep stretch, right and left
C. Iliopsoas stretch, right and left
D. Hamstring stretch, right and left
E. Pectoral stretch
F. Back stretch

— Cardiovascular Warm-Up
Do each of the following:
A. Jog out and in, 8 sets
B. Kneelifts, 32 reps
C. Sidekicks, 32 reps
D. Back kicks, 32 reps
E. Kneeswings (8 right, 8 left), 4 sets
F. Jog out and in, 8 sets

– Aerobics

Do each of the following for 1 minute:
A. Step up, up, down, down, leading with the right foot.
B. Do jumping jacks without the bench.
C. Step up, up, down, down, leading with the left foot.
D. Do jumping jacks without the bench.
E. Step up, hold, down, down, alternating the right and left feet on the "up" step (right foot steps up, left foot steps down, right foot steps down, left foot steps up, right foot steps down, left foot steps down). Hold the "up" for 2 counts.
F. Do kneelifts without the bench.
G. With the right side to the bench, step up and down, with the right foot always stepping up on the bench and the left foot always stepping down on the pool bottom.
H. Do scissors without the bench.
I. With the left side to the bench, step up and down, with the left foot always stepping up on the bench and the right foot always stepping down on the pool bottom.
J. Do scissors without the bench.
K. With legs straddling the bench, do jumping jacks. (This move should not be done if the bench is in waist-deep water.)
L. Walk around the bench in a circle, moving clockwise. (Do not step up or down on the bench.)
M. With legs straddling the bench, step down, up, up, hold, alternating the right and left feet on the "down" step (right foot steps down, left foot steps up, right foot steps up, left foot steps down, right foot steps up, left foot steps up). Hold the second "up" for 2 counts.
N. Do sidekicks without the bench.
O. Step up, kneelift, step down, step down, alternating the right and left feet on the step "up" (step up with the right foot, kneelift with the left leg, step down with the left foot, step down with the right foot; repeat this sequence with the opposite foot).
P. Do back kicks without the bench.
Q. With legs straddling the bench, step up, kick, step down, step down, alternating the on the step "up" (step up with the right foot, kick forward with the left leg, step down with the left foot, step down with the right foot; repeat this sequence with the opposite foot).
R. Do jumping jacks without the bench.

– Cooldown

Do each of the following for 1 minute:
A. Walk forward and backward, using tricep extensions and bicep curls.
B. Walk forward and backward with high kneelifts.
C. Sidestep, right and left
D. Sidekicks
E. Kneeswing 8 right and 8 left until the time allotment is up.

– Flexibility

Hold each of the following for 10 to 15 seconds:
A. Calf stretch, right and left
B. Iliopsoas stretch, right and left
C. Quadricep stretch, right and left
D. Hamstring stretch, right and left
E. Abductor stretch, right and left
F. Pectoral stretch
G. Back stretch

Deep Water: Using Flotation Vests or Belts

– Thermal Warm-Up

Do each of the following for 1 minute:

A. Jog forward at moderate intensity, using tricep extensions.
B. Jog backward at moderate intensity, using bicep curls.

C. Do jumping jacks with deltoid lifts and press downs.
D. Do scissors, with arms alternately swinging forward and backward.

— Prestretch

Do each of the following for 10 to 15 seconds:
A. Hamstring stretch, right and left
B. Quadricep stretch, right and left
C. Iliopsoas stretch, right and left
D. Pectoral stretch
E. Back stretch
F. Calf stretch, right and left (at the edge of the pool, pressing the foot of the leg to be stretched against the pool wall)

— Cardiovascular Warm-Up

Do each of the following for 1 minute:
A. Jog with high knees, staying in place.
B. Jog with high knees, moving forward by using breaststroke arms.
C. Jog with high knees, moving backward by using backstroke arms.
D. Jog with heels kicking up and back (mule kick), staying in place.
E. Repeat D, moving forward using breaststroke arms. (The abdominals must be contracted, and no hip flexion should occur.)
F. Repeat D, moving backward using backstroke arms.

— Aerobics

1. Do each of the following for 1 minute:
   A. Scissors at moderate intensity, staying in place
   B. Scissors, moving forward by using crawl arms
   C. Scissor jumps, using enough force to push the body up and out of the water
   D. Scissors, moving backward by using single arms alternating the backstroke

2. Do each of the following:
   A. Scissor and jumping jack combo (1 scissor, 1 jumping jack); repeat for 1 minute
   B. Kneelifts in 3, 4 sets in place and 4 sets moving forward; 4 sets in place and 4 sets moving backward
   C. Scissors, 16 times each: toes pointed out, toes pointed down, toes pointed up. Repeat this sequence (16 out, 16 down, 16 up) 2 times
   D. Mule kicks, 16 moving forward, kneelifts, 16 moving backward; repeat this sequence (16 forward, kneelifts, 16 backward) 4 times
   E. Scissors, 16 with long, slow strides, 16 with short, fast strides; repeat this sequence (16 long, 16 short) 2 times

3. Do each of the following for 1 minute:
   A. Jumping jacks in place
   B. Jumping jacks, moving forward using breaststroke arms (the abdominals must be contracted, and hip hyperextension should not occur)
   C. Jumping jacks (legs should close with enough force to push the body up and out of the water)
   D. Jumping jacks, moving backward using backstroke arms
   E. Jumping jacks crossing
   F. Jumping jacks, alternating with toes pointed down and up

— Cooldown

Do each of the following for 1 minute:
A. Jog forward with mule kicks
B. Jog backward with kneelifts
C. Mule kicks in place
D. Kneelifts in place
E. Heel hits in front
F. Heel hits behind

— Toning and Flexibility

1. Work at the edge of the pool, with one side to the pool wall (work the same side, right or left, for entire sequence). Repeat each movement 32 times; hold each stretch for 15 seconds.
   A. Side leglift
   B. Adductor stretch
   C. Kickswing
   D. Iliopsoas stretch
   E. Side leg circles
   F. Abductor stretch
   G. Mule kicks
   H. Hamstring stretch
2. Switch sides, turning the other side to the pool wall. Repeat A through H. Again, repeat each movement 32 times; hold each stretch for 15 seconds.
3. Continue as follows:
   A. With the back to the pool edge, do elbow presses forward and backward
   B. With the back still to the pool edge, do pectoral stretch
   C. Facing the pool edge, do deltoid lifts and press downs
   D. Back stretch
   E. Calf stretch, right and left (press the foot of the leg being stretched against the pool wall)

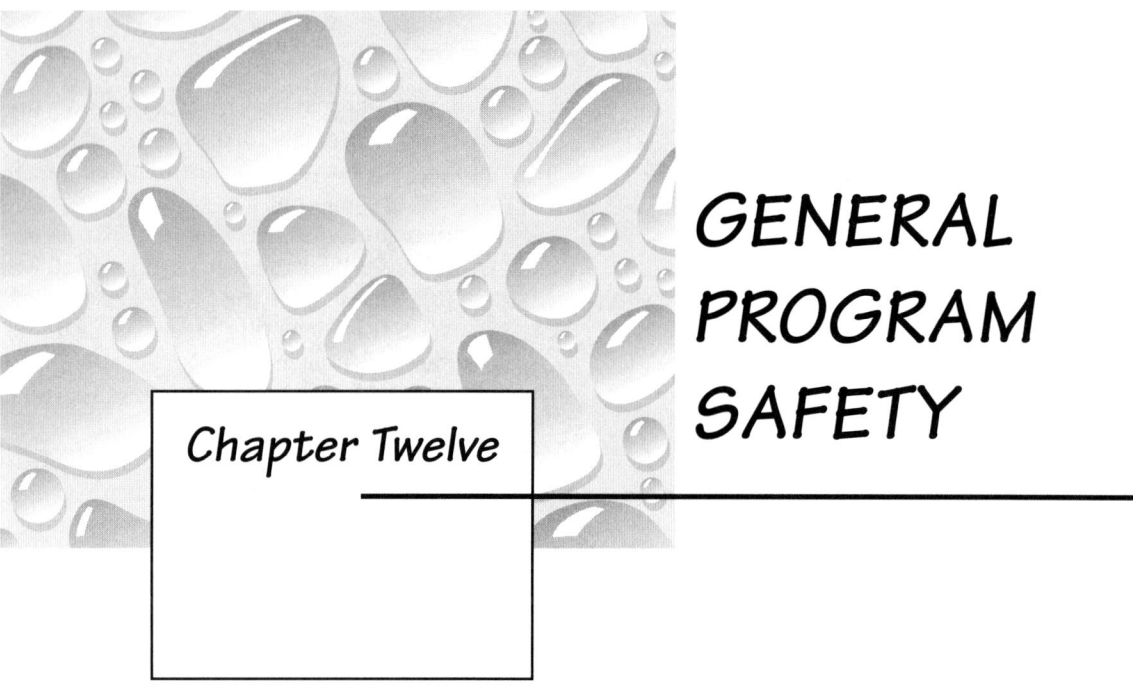

GENERAL PROGRAM SAFETY

Chapter Twelve

PROGRAMMING INFORMATION

Certification Standards

The individual who creates an aquatic exercise program should have an Aquatic Exercise Association or comparable certification. This **certification** gives individuals information on the following:

1. general exercise, including basic anatomy, kinesiology, and exercise physiology
2. physical laws applied to water exercise
3. pool, water, and air conditions, program guidelines, and leadership
4. emergency training, basic water rescue, and injury prevention
5. aquatic equipment, its use and precautions
6. nutrition and weight loss
7. legal issues

Contraindicated Exercises

Aquatic exercise programs tend to have a large variety of populations and body types. For that reason, exercises that are safe for one person may not be for another.

Some exercise is **generally contraindicated,** which means that it is harmful to the exerciser's physical well-being. This means that the exercise is contraindicated for everyone. **Relatively contraindicated** means that the exercise is contraindicated for some individuals.

To create the safest possible program, an aquatic exerciser should be aware of two specific concepts when doing programming or choreography:

1. *The purpose of each exercise*—With this knowledge, moves that may aggravate some students' conditions can be replaced with other moves that have the

same exercise purpose. For instance, a prone flutter kick primarily works the hip flexors (iliopsoas) and elevates heartrate. Since prone flutter kicks have a high risk potential, an instructor could replace them with standing forward kicks, which have a lower risk potential but still work the hip flexors (iliopsoas) and elevate heartrate. If forward kicks aggravate a student's low back, the forward kicks could be changed to kneelifts, which also work the hip flexors and elevate heartrate.

2. *High-risk areas in the average body*—The student must be aware of specific areas to protect. Always compare the ratio of benefits of an exercise to its risk. If the benefit outweighs the risk, the student should use the move. There is risk associated with every type of move. Only those that seem to be high risk or cause discomfort should be eliminated.

High-Risk Areas

High-risk areas include knees, shoulders, neck, low back, ankles, and feet.

Knees. Knees can be protected by remembering that their function is simple flexion and extension. Safe moves for the knee joint will not hyperextend it, twist it, move it too quickly, or overflex it.

Movements should be slow and controlled when the knee joint is involved. Ballistic or percussive movements in the knee can cause injury. Extremely fast flexion and extension can cause damage to the joint capsule, tendons, and ligaments. Students sometimes use excessively fast movements during the toning portion at the end of class to feel the muscles working. Using force rather than speed during toning ensures a better and safer workout.

Shoulders. Shoulder impingement has become a concern of low-impact aerobic students. It also should be a concern of aquatic exercise instructors and students. Seventy percent of the U.S. population has degenerative shoulder problems.

Shoulder impingement can occur in aquatic exercise when students spend a sustained period of time hanging from their arms on kickboards or at the edge of the pool, using the arms overhead excessively or vigorously, and moving arms in and out of the water repeatedly.

Neck. The **cervical vertebrae** and discs can be injured during aquatic exercise. The cervical area of the spine has several functions, including flexion and extension (bending and straightening), lateral flexion (sideways tilting), and rotation (turning). A safe rule for aquatic exercise instructors is to allow the cervical area of the spine to move in only one of those directions at a time. This is a conservative way of viewing each of the moves the students do.

Hyperextension of the cervical area of the spine should be eliminated from aquatic exercises. Students look up but not all the way up. Full-neck circles should be eliminated and replaced with a look down, a look somewhat up, a look to the right, then left, and a neck stretch (with the right ear to the right shoulder and then, the left ear to the left shoulder). Percussive or ballistic moves in the cervical area of the spine also can damage the vertebrae and discs.

Low Back. Eighty to ninety percent of the population in North America experiences back pain at some time in their lives. Low-back pain is the most common problem. For that reason, exercises involving the low-back muscles should be well thought out.

The lumbar and thoracic areas of the spine have several functions. They can do spinal flexion and extension (bending forward and returning), lateral flexion (sidebends), and rotation (twisting). A good rule is to allow the back to do only one of these functions at a time.

Hyperextension of the lumbar area of the spine should be eliminated from all standing or moving exercises.

Many of the exercises that compromise the low back are those thought to work the abdominals, so students work them more vigorously and enthusiastically than they do other exercises. Very few abdominal exercises actually compromise the low back. The exercises that students and instructors think work the abdominals actually are working the iliopsoas or hip flexors. Instructors should be aware that if the spine (vertebrae) is flexing, the abdominals are working. The **Aquatic Exercise Association** has an aquatic abdominal video workshop listed in the Resources Chapter of this book (Chapter 13). If the hip joint is moving, the muscles working are the iliopsoas. Double-leg lifts and flutter kicks both work the iliopsoas. A safer way to work the iliopsoas is with standing forward kicks.

All exercises involving the lumbar area of the spine should be slow and controlled. Ballistic or percussive moves can easily cause injury in the low-back area. **Sustained spinal flexion** is not encouraged in any type of exercise for the general population.

Lower Leg, Foot, and Ankle. The lower leg, foot, and ankle are susceptible to many overuse injuries. Even though these injuries are impressively lessened by working out in the water, they still can occur. Many injuries are associated with students' specific anatomy. A person with excessive **pronation** (rolling in) of the foot is more likely to have an injury on the inside or medial side of the leg or ankle. **Supinators** (students who roll out), however, are more likely to have an injury on the outside or lateral portion of the lower leg or ankle.

Side-to-side movements need to be done with control and stability. Many other ankle/foot injuries are caused by impact. The instructor can guard against this in three ways: (1) moving students to deeper water; (2) adding a flotation belt or vest; and (3) creating a program with less bouncing and more walking or traveling moves.

Impact injuries also can be lessened by learning how to land. Students who stay on the forefoot can develop severe lower-leg and foot injuries. Consciously thinking about landing first on the forefoot and rolling the heel down to the bottom of the pool and bending the knee can decrease considerably the likelihood of injury. Adding shoes that are designed for aquatic exercise or aerobics can protect the foot and ankle and protect the bottoms of the feet from having an excessive amount of skin worn away, and from slipping.

Repetitions

Excessive reps of one move that causes bouncing on the other leg can lead to an overuse injury and cause the support leg to become destabilized. It is prudent to bounce only eight times on one foot before changing to the other. Toning exercises where no bouncing on the other foot occurs can be repeated up to 30 or 40 times.

Traveling Moves

Lateral, forward, or backward movement increases the intensity of a workout. Traveling also can increase workout risk. To minimize risk, remember proper alignment before beginning a traveling move.

Tempo

The speed, or **tempo**, of the exercise or music should allow enough time to move each exercise through a full range of motion in a controlled manner. Percussive, ballistic, or jerky types of movements can cause injuries throughout the body.

Preventive Measures

Good shoes, specifically designed for the type of aquatic exercise being performed, are essential for injury prevention and assist in keeping injuries from recurring. Shoes should fit the shape of the student's foot, have adequate cushioning in the heel and forefoot to absorb shock, and be well padded in the arch. The shoes also should have good stability for forward, backward, and lateral movement, and the heel box should be firm for heel stability. Shoes also should have good flexibility to move with the foot. The flexion should be near the toes, not at the arch. The sole of the shoe should have adequate gripping power to hold on slippery pool bottoms. Comfort, fit, cushioning, stability, flexibility, and gripping are the characteristics of a good aquatic shoe.

A gradual progression, from warm-up and stretching to higher-intensity activity and gradual recovery and stretching at the end of class, also reduces the likelihood of injury recurrence. Individual pacing and progressive overload must continually be kept in mind. While variety of movement is important, tricky steps and awkward transitions should be avoided. Continuous reps of the same movement have little value during the aerobic portion of the class and can lead to overuse injuries. Staying in any one position, out of proper alignment, for too long also has the potential for harm. Students should not whip, hurl, or flail body parts but rather move slowly with control and always be aware of how they feel. Any movement that causes pain should be eliminated.

Maintaining good alignment allows muscles to work without strain and assists in preventing injury recurrence. Good alignment allows the safe transfer of body weight and enables the joints and spine to absorb shock efficiently. Participants should think about "standing tall" when exercising. **Footstrikes** should not be done with the toes only but should begin on the toes and allow the heels to contact the pool bottom while rolling through the foot. The knees and hips should bend each time jumping, bouncing, or landing occurs.

General Problems

Overexertion

Students should avoid overexertion. The symptoms of **overexertion** are breathlessness, extreme fatigue, dizziness, an extremely red face, nausea, and poor heartrate response. The heartrate response could indicate either a very high heartrate or a very poor recovery rate. A poor recovery rate would be indicated by a high heartrate even 5 or 10 minutes after the cooldown.

Overexertion can be avoided by gradually warming up, monitoring intensity during the aerobic section, and adequately cooling down.

Overuse

The majority of injuries associated with exercise are a result of overuse. Too much bouncing, incorrect body mechanics and alignment, improper footwear, and inappropriate water depth can all cause aquatic exercise injuries. Environmental conditions also can take their toll.

Overuse injuries include shinsplints, stress fractures, tendonitis, bursitis, plantarfasciitis, chondromalacia patella, lower-back pain, neuroma, and metatarsalgia. With the exception of stress fractures, these overuse injuries occur in soft tissues and are unlikely to show up on x-rays. Participants often ignore or deny the injury and attempt to continue exercising in spite of the symptoms. This can result in an increased injury and other injuries brought on by an altered gait.

Soft-tissue injuries should be recognized as they develop. Localized pain—tenderness or pain on or around a bony area or joint—is an indication of injury. Radiating pain—involving nerves and tingling sensations—is another sign of injury. Swelling or inflammation can also indicate tissue damage. Swelling may occur after the overuse injury, because it takes time for the inflammation to develop. Discoloration of the skin and movement impairment also are warning signs of injuries.

Overuse injuries can often be treated with the following three-step plan:

1. Reduce or stop the stress that is causing the injury.
2. Reduce inflammation.
3. Correct any factors that may cause an injury to recur.

Overtraining

Participants who exercise too much—that is, at too high an intensity, for too long a time, or too frequently—may experience symptoms of overtraining. This can occur with individuals who are beginning to exercise, as well as those who suddenly double their workout time. **Overtraining** occurs when the concept of progressive overload is ignored.

While a basic musculoskeletal injury may not occur, a participant should watch for these signs and symptoms of overexercising:

1. persistent muscle aches and soreness
2. energy loss
3. depression
4. insomnia
5. irritability
6. elevated resting heartrate

If a participant exhibits any of these symptoms, he or she should modify his or her workout by decreasing frequency, intensity, or duration, as appropriate.

Heat-Related Injuries

Heartrates and Heat. One of the heart's basic functions is to move the blood that feeds the muscles in our bodies. When our muscles are relaxed, or not involved in activity, the heart pumps slowly but gets the blood (and the "food" the blood carries) to the muscles and other parts of the body. When muscles are in use, or moving, the heart has to beat faster to achieve the same function. The "food" the blood is carrying is oxygen, and the more oxygen the muscles need, the more calories the body burns.

Because of that, many people think that a high heartrate is a sign of calorie usage, so they do whatever they can to achieve a high heartrate. It is true that more calories are used if the heartrate is elevated due to increased oxygen consumption. However, if the heartrate goes up for other reasons, such as fright, heat, or the "pressor effect" (caused by using arms overhead), it may not correlate to increased calorie usage and it may not be beneficial. Remember this: The level of oxygen consumption (how much oxygen the muscle is using), not the heartrate, determines the amount of calories used and, therefore, the true workout intensity.

Another of the heart's functions is to help the body maintain a safe core temperature. When heat in the body increases, the heart helps cool it down. It starts to beat faster to transport the heat out of the deep tissues to the surface for cooling. When the heart beats faster to assist the body with heat dissipation, it is not the same kind of increased heartrate that causes calorie consumption. That increase results when muscles are being used vigorously, and it leads to aerobic conditioning. The increased heartrate that results when the body needs cooling, does not provide conditioning.

To illustrate this point, consider an example: The heartrate increases when a body is lying in the hot sun. It is obvious that even though the heartrate is up, the body is not working cardiovascularly. The increase in heartrate is due simply to the heat, not conditioning.

If students' heartrates are increasing because of heat-related factors and not because of muscles' use, two things may happen. Even though they feel like they are getting a high-intensity workout, (1) they may not increase calorie burning, and (2) they may be prime candidates for heat-related injuries.

Heat Build-Up and Dissipation. There are two basic ways to increase heat in the body: The body can produce heat, or it can pick up heat. Instructors and students can use this information in reverse to decrease body heat on hot days. Bodies produce heat themselves through cellular metabolism, muscular activity, ingestion of food, some drinks and drugs, lack of body fluids, and hormonal actions. Bodies can pick up heat from the sun's rays or reflections from sand and snow; from environmental factors, such as air or water temperature and humidity; and from the amount and type of clothing worn.

Our bodies possess a **thermoregulatory mechanism** that adjusts constantly so that the heat gained is offset exactly by the amount dissipated. While the mechanism is complicated and includes circulation, sweating, neuroimpulses, and endocrine responses, we can easily understand the two major mechanisms by which the body dissipates heat to maintain normal temperature.

The first is *sweating,* which provides our mainline of defense against overheating. The sweat glands in the skin produce sweat, which evaporates, transforming the liquid into a vapor state. There is a resultant loss of heat from the skin. It is thought that 80% of heat dissipation occurs from sweating and evaporation from the head.

The second major mechanism, set in motion when the core temperature of the body increases, is *conduction/convection.* As heat is generated in the body, blood vessels dilate to increase bloodflow to the skin. This bloodflow carries the heat from the core, or deeper tissue, to the surface for cooling. Convection then occurs when cool air or water currents move over the body surface and carry the heat away.

Both themoregulatory mechanisms increase the body's heartrate. The heart must beat faster when the heat is transported via the bloodstream to the body surface for dissipation through sweating or radiation. This increased heartrate is cardiovascular stress and not a sign of increased workout intensity.

Heat and the Elderly. The elderly are more vulnerable to heat stress than younger people because their bodies do not adjust as well to heat. They perspire less. They also are more likely to have health problems requiring medications that work against the body's natural defenses to adjust to heat.

Prevention of Heat-Related Problems. Depending on the cause of heat stress, there are various ways to prevent injuries. Since the purpose of exercise is to increase cellular metabolism and muscular activity, students generally do not want to lessen body heat by decreasing the workout intensity. There are several other ways to avoid heat-related problems.

1. *Eliminate bouncing in the workout.* This can decrease some of the heat generated while still working the muscles and burning calories.
2. *Decrease the intake of food, and eliminate alcoholic or hot beverages.* Hot or heavy meals add heat to the body. Alcohol acts as a diuretic, resulting in faster water loss, which can lead to dehydration. In addition, alcohol promotes a sense of well-being, making the participant less aware of the danger signs of heat stress.
3. *Stay out of direct sunlight or wear a well-ventilated, protective hat.* This helps lessen heat build-up. Since water dissipates heat at least four times faster than air (some studies show that it removes extra body heat 25 times faster than cool air), dipping the hat in the water, wetting the hair, or wetting the face, neck and shoulders helps cool the body.
4. *Increase air movement by using fans if there is no breeze.* A breeze helps the body dissipate heat by speeding up evaporation.
5. *Increase the exercise water depth.* This assists in cooling the body if the water temperature is below 88 degrees Fahrenheit. Decreasing the water depth increases impact (biomechanical stress), thereby increasing heat build-up. However, if the water temperature is high (over 88 degrees) and the air temperature is comfortable with a slight breeze, a shallower water depth may help cool the body, since more of

the body will be exposed to the cooling air temperature and air circulation.

6. *Exercise during the coolest parts of the day.* Offer workouts until 10:30 A.M. and then again after 5:30 P.M. to protect the instructor and students from the hottest part of the day.
7. *Keep clothing to a minimum if working out in a warmer than normal environment.* Wear light-colored, natural-fiber clothing: white cotton is a good choice if it works in the water for the instructor and students. Stay away from dark-colored clothing, since it absorbs heat, and also avoid materials that do not allow heat out. Tight clothing retards heat dissipation. Students should wear a swimsuit rather than a full-sleeve unitard. They should eliminate tight-fitting vests or other equipment on hot days. Since swimcaps do not allow evaporation to occur, they should be left in the locker room.
8. *Keep wet.* Allow the skin to stay wet with sweat and/or pool water rather than drying it with a towel. This allows evaporation to cool the skin.
9. *Consider weight.* Thin people tolerate heat better than heavy ones because they have a better ratio of body surface to body weight. The core body temperature of thin people can be decreased more quickly because there is less mass. It is harder for the overweight body to dissipate excess heat because body fat is an effective insulation.
10. *Drink plenty of water.* The single most important item in preventing heat injury is fluid. The thermoregulatory system cannot function without an adequate supply of water. A person who exercises for 30 to 60 minutes should consume 8 to 10 glasses of water that day. Exercising in a warmer than normal environment obviously increases the fluid requirements.

Cold-Related Injuries

Aquatic exercisers often have to deal with many variables that make them chilled, cold, or hypothermic, including: air temperature; wind velocity or ventilation; water temperature; air humidity; length of exposure to the cold; a person's age, body size, build, and level of fitness; and water depth. Internal environmental factors that can affect a student's core temperature include medications, time of day of the class, types of food eaten, the amount of fluids ingested, and the type of clothing worn.

Exercise modifications in a cool environment may include a longer warm-up. While the average warm-up time is 5 to 10 minutes, it may take 15 minutes of warm-up for morning classes because participants have not had a chance to move around much. Evening classes may be able to get by with a 10 to 12 minutes of a warm-up in a cool environment. Exercisers should be aware that even though heartrates are in a "warmed-up" zone, the muscles may still be too cold to accommodate fast, forceful movements. The fact that the heart has warmed up does not mean that the rest of the body is ready for vigorous exercise. Instructors usually have to rely on students to let them know how the warm-up is going.

In some instances, the pool environment may be too cool to conduct a class. When students step into cool water (below 80 degrees Fahrenheit), blood vessels constrict and the blood is shunted from the muscles to the internal organs in an attempt to keep them nourished and warm. It is essential to have the blood circulating in the active muscles during exercise. The muscles are unable to function if their oxygen needs are not met. When muscles get cold, they shorten. Exercising with cold muscles can lead to injury. The safe range of water temperature and air temperature varies from person to person. Some participants will be able to exercise in extremely cool conditions, while others may exhibit symptoms of mild **hypothermia** in 78-degree Fahrenheit water.

If the water and air environment allow the instructor to warm up the students and go through an aggressive workout, students and instructors have to be cautious to protect themselves again at the end of the workout. Moisture rapidly conducts heat away from the body. After working out in the pool, students should have a towel nearby to dry themselves as thoroughly as possible. They should move immediately to the locker room to take a warm shower and put on dry clothes. In cool weather, students need to ensure that they are completely dry—including their hair—before leaving the exercise area. Since 40% of the body's heat is lost through the head in cold weather, it is important that the students attempt to keep their hair dry and wear a warm hat when leaving the exercise facility. Hypothermia can occur in weather as moderate as 50 degrees Fahrenheit if the victim is partially wet.

Sun Exposure and Skin Cancer

Exercisers in outdoor pools can be prime candidates for skin cancer. Repeated exposure to the sun's ultraviolet rays can do serious damage to the skin, sometimes causing different types of skin cancer. Aquatic exercisers are at an unusually high risk because exposure is both to direct sunlight and **ultraviolet reflections** off the surface. Additional factors that affect the likelihood of developing skin cancer and the extent of its damage are: heredity, age, skin type, length of exposure each day, and what precautions are taken to protect the skin.

Damage to skin through skin cancer is almost 100% preventable if the proper precautions are taken. Students and instructors working in direct sunlight should always wear a wide-brimmed hat to keep the face and ears out of the sun. A bandana around the neck and a lightweight, long-sleeve top and full-length pants also protect the skin.

Participants and instructors should always wear sunscreen or sunblock products on the exposed areas. These products should have a skin protection factor (SPF) of 15 or higher. A sunscreen or sunblock should be applied two to three times a day or any time after participants get wet or sweat.

The sun's rays are most intense between the hours of 10 a.m. and 3 p.m., and ultraviolet rays penetrate the air more easily at high altitudes than at sea level. Aquatic exercisers also should be aware that the sun's rays can reach down three feet into the water.

The aquatic student and instructor should be extremely familiar with their skin and any blemishes, birthmarks, and moles. Any change in their appearance should be reported immediately to a medical professional.

Participants who have experienced skin cancer should be especially careful in noting all the precautions and taking preventive measures. Skin cancer can recur frequently. Routine check-ups are essential.

KEY WORDS

Generally contraindicated
Relatively contraindicated
Shoulder impingement
Cervical vertebrae
Hyperextension
Sustained spinal flexion
Tempo

Pronation
Supinators
Aquatic Exercise Association
Certification
Footstrike
Overexertion

Overuse injury
Overtraining
Thermoregulatory mechanism
Heat stress syndromes
Hypothermia
Ultraviolet reflections

SUMMARY

- In order to create the safest possible program, an exerciser should be aware of the purpose of each exercise and the high-risk areas in the average body.
- Knees can be protected by remembering that their function is simple flexion and extension.
- Seventy percent of the U.S. population has degenerative shoulder problems.
- Without proper care, the cervical vertebrae and discs can be injured during aquatic exercise.
- Eighty to ninety percent of the population in North America experiences back pain at some time in their lives.
- While lower leg, foot, and ankle injuries are impressively lessened by working out in the water, they still can occur.
- Traveling can increase the risk of the workout.
- The speed, or tempo, of the exercise or music should allow enough time to move each exercise through a full range of motion in a controlled manner.
- The individual who creates an aquatic exercise program should have an Aquatic Exercise Association or comparable certification.
- Good shoes, specifically designed for the type of aquatic exercise being performed, are essential for injury prevention and will assist in keeping injuries from recurring.
- Students should avoid overexertion.
- The majority of injuries associated with exercise are a result of overuse.
- Participants who try to exercise too much—that is, at too high an intensity, for too long a time, or just too frequently—may experience symptoms of overtraining.
- If students' heartrates are increasing because of heat-related factors, they may not increase caloric consumption and may be prime candidates for heat-related injuries.
- The elderly are more vulnerable to heat stress than younger people because their bodies do not adjust as well to heat.
- The single most important item in preventing heat injury is fluid.
- Aquatic exercisers often have to deal with many variables that make them chilled, cold, or hypothermic.
- Exercisers in outdoor pools can be prime candidates for skin cancer.

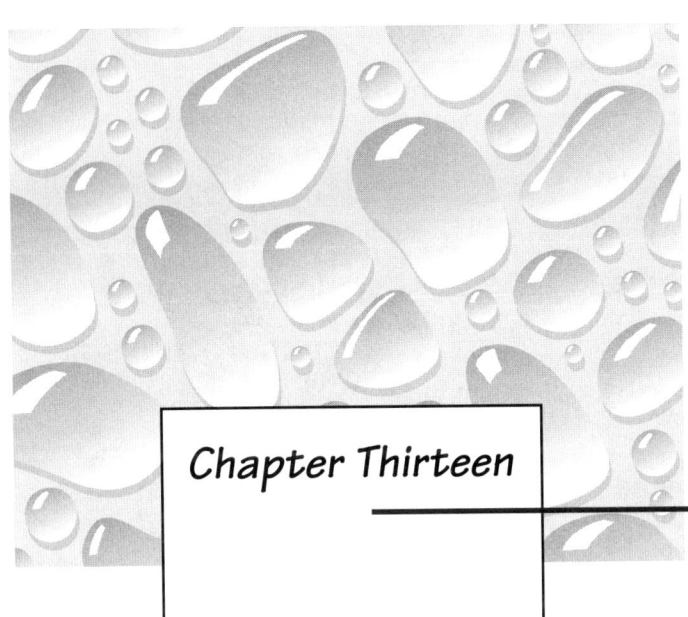

RESOURCES

Chapter Thirteen

The Resources are organized alphabetically under the following headings (see page numbers indicated):

Aqua Wear	164
Choreography	164
Consultants	165
Equipment	165
Filters, Chemicals, and Air Products	175
Health Products	177
Music Sources	177
Organizations	178
Pool Products	180
Publications*	181
Books	181
Catalogs	184
Magazines and Newsletters	185
Shoes	186
Signs and Charts	187
Skin and Hair Care Products	187
Training and Workshops	188
Video- and Audiocassettes	189

*Refer to the References for additional source information.

AQUA WEAR

"Do It in the Water" Swim Cover-Up
WW Enterprises of
 Wisconsin, Ltd.
P.O. Box 371
DePere, WI 54115
414-336-2142

An attractive, one-size-fits-all, dropped sleeve cover-up made of 50% cotton and 50% polyester. It is available in white with an aqua and black design.

Easy Access Swim Suits (Model 5505)
Danmar Products, Inc.
221 Jackson Industrial Drive
Ann Arbor, MI 48103
1-800-783-1998

The tank suit is made with two zippers on each side for easy dressing. The shoulder straps have three snaps, making adjustment quick and comfortable. A matching detachable skirt converts the suit into an ideal cover-up, even if incontinence products are being worn.

Swim Caps
Speedo Activewear
11111 Santa Monica Blvd.
Los Angeles, CA 90025
213-473-0032

There are several kinds of caps—Lycra, Latex, silicone—that protect hair and streamline the head in water. Latex is the most popular for racing. Silicone is the most durable.

"Swimmer" Tank Suit
McArthur Towels, Inc.
P.O. Box 448
Baraboo, WI 53913
1-800-356-9168/
608-356-8922

A black, nylon, long-lasting tank suit; sizes are indicated by color-coded stitching inside the suit.

Swimming Goggles
Swans Sports, USA
21 Airport Blvd. #E
South San Francisco, CA
 94080
415-589-9301

Swans' swim goggles and accessories are made of the finest materials on the market today. Swans sells goggles and accessories to meet all consumer demands.

The Wet Wrap
D. K. Douglas Company, Inc.
299 Bliss Road
Longmeadow, MA 01106
1-800-334-9070

— The Wet Wrap

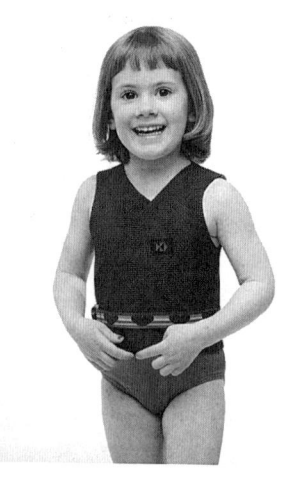

A unique wetsuit vest worn for warmth during exercise, therapy, or recreation.

CHOREOGRAPHY

AEROBIC Q-SIGNS™
Webb International
Tamilee Webb
968 Emerald Street, Suite 54
San Diego, CA 92109
619-755-4489/
FAX 619-755-3564

AEROBIC Q-SIGNS™ is a visual cueing system through which the instructor conveys direction, position, and number of steps. Use allows a consistent form of communication in all classes, regardless of location or type of participants (e.g., foreign language or hearing impaired).

Aqua Choreography Workshop
Aquatic Exercise Association
P.O. Box 497
Port Washington, WI 53074
414-284-3416

This workshop focuses on music selection, steps, combos, and movements that involve specific muscle groups. Other topics include designing a safe workout, checking cardiorespiratory potential, sample routines, and toning exercises.

Aquatic Circuit, Interval, and Sport-Specific Training Workshop
Aquatic Exercise Association
P.O. Box 497
Port Washington, WI 53074
414-284-3416

This workshop reviews the concepts behind, and benefits of, different types of classes, along with the equipment that can be used and actual moves that can be done. All three types of programs—circuit, interval, and sports—are tried in the water.

Aqua-Tunes
Aqua-X/A-X Enterprises
P.O. Box 842
San Marcos, CA 92079-0842
619-743-5760

This resource provides instructors and participants with a program packet of music and exercises for a complete one-hour class, including instructions on which music to use and which specific exercises to use with each tune. The program packet has a "crib sheet" to be used at poolside, listing each tune and the exercises choreographed to it. A second "crib sheet" is used for the second portion of the class for exercises performed at the wall and in deep water. A page of cross-references is provided, along with a detailed choreography sheet and a music reference sheet.

CONSULTANTS

Aquatic Consulting Services
Alison Osinski
3833 Lamont Street, 4C
San Diego, CA 92109
619-270-3459

This service is geared to meet a variety of aquatic consulting needs—in, on, near, or under the water: pool design, site inspections, staff screening and selection, lifeguard audits, custom signs, expert testimony, document development, equipment specification and testing, programming, training and certification programs, and water-quality analysis.

Aquatic Programming Services
Ruth Sova
P.O. Box 497
Port Washington, WI 53074
414-284-3416

Consulting services are geared to provide aquatic fitness programming and marketing assistance.

Northeast Aquatic Designs (NEADS)
Winthrop Knox
11 Midland Road
Lynnfield, MA 01940
(617) 334-2522

Produce a fun, effective, and safe pool/spa/sauna environment. NEADS is a design/consulting firm that specializes in health clubs, offering more experience than the average professional and utilizing current CAD methods.

Swimming Pool Consulting Services
Kurt E. Carmen
1666 Twin Oaks Drive
Toledo, OH 43615
419-534-3043

Professional consulting on the design, equipment specification, engineering, operation and maintenance of aquatic facilities.

EQUIPMENT

Advance Athletic Equipment, Inc.
3440 N. Pacific Highway
Medford, OR 97501
1-800-223-5816/
503-773-6870

Advance Resilient Athletic Floors cushion the body during indoor sports and aerobic dance. The floor is made of two layers of wood over coil springs, topped with carpet or hardwood, available in portable or permanent formats. The company also carries gymnastic equipment, ballet barres, glassless mirrors, and weight room and locker room flooring.

CHAPTER THIRTEEN / RESOURCES

Aerobic Workbench
P.O. Box 2575
Largo, FL 34649
813-391-7419

The Aerobic Workbench is made of fiberglass to provide strength and durability. It weighs less than 20 pounds. Two different sizes are available. The special construction allows for aquatic step or bench workouts without shifting on the pool bottom.

Ankle Buoy #975
Sprint/Rothhammer
    International, Inc.
P.O. Box 5579
Santa Maria, CA 93456
1-800-235-2156

Ankle buoys provide resistance for legs while exercising. Soft, high-density, EVA (closed cell foam) foam straps attach the weights to the ankle, toning muscles as the leg moves through the water.

Aqua Accessories
Gwen McDonald, OTR
15 Atwood Street
Wakefield, MA 01880
617-246-2508

Aqua Ark
Life Tec, Inc.
1710 S. Wolf Road
Wheeling, IL 60090
1-800-822-5911/
708-459-7500

The Aqua Ark uses properties of buoyancy, heat, and resistance to accelerate the rehabilitation of injured persons. It employs a unique flotation vest, front- and rear-tether system, patient lift. It is used in deep water for both upper- and lower-extremity rehabilitation.

Aqua Arm (Model 6850)
Danmar Products, Inc.
221 Jackson Industrial Drive
Ann Arbor, MI 48103
1-800-783-1998

Development of wrist, arm, and shoulder strength, flexibility, and range of motion is promoted through resistance training programs of all levels. The Aqua Arms are a set of yellow and blue paddles made of flotation plastic with two six-inch discs at either end. A wrist strap may be added for individuals who have problems grasping for extended periods.

— Aqua Arm (Model 6850)

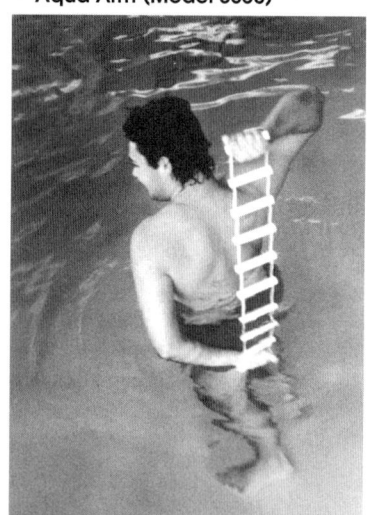

Aqua Champion
Speedo Activewear
11111 Santa Monica Blvd.
Los Angeles, CA 90025
213-473-0032

This webbed glove is designed to strengthen arm muscles and hand pull.

Aqua Jazz
Aqua Jazz, Inc.
1642 S. Parker Road, #201
Denver, CO 80231
303-751-4474

Aqua Jazz is a remarkably easy and effective year-round fitness program, featuring specially designed AquaWings and AquaBoots for a total body workout. A complete instruction manual covers a series of fun, nonrepetitive exercises that are easily adapted to individual fitness levels and needs. Even nonswimmers can enjoy Aqua Jazz.

AquaJogger
Excell Sports Science
145 E. 29th Street
P.O. Box 5612
Eugene, OR 97405
503-484-2454

A water exercise buoyancy belt, the AquaJogger holds the participant stable and upright in deep water, providing buoyancy and total freedom of movement for arms and legs.

Aqua-Rider

Hughes Toy Company
24675 Glenwood Drive
Los Gatos, CA 95030
408-353-2136

Made of polyethylene plastic, the Aqua-Rider is an almost indestructible flotation unit. It provides adjustable balance chambers, so that individual body weight can be balanced, allowing the participant to be suspended in water without effort, free to do anything. This flotation unit is so stable when adjusted that under supervision, nonswimmers and the physically disabled have become active in the water.

Aquarius Water Workout Station

Robert W. Jahn II, President
Aquarius Health and Fitness Products, Inc.
631 U.S. Highway 1, Suite 300
North Palm Beach, FL 33408
407-585-0754

Wave of the Future, the Aquarius Water-Workout Station taps into our greatest natural resource—water—to provide a safe and efficient muscle-training program. This novel approach can be used in a variety of programs: fitness, relaxation, toning, rehabilitation, cardiovascular conditioning, weight loss, and arthritic relief.

Aqua Space Weights

Swimnastics by Nancy Benson
P.O. Box 1258
Oak Brook, IL 60522-1258
708-393-4224

Aqua Space Weights are hollow, oval, hand-held plastic weights. They can be used hollow to work against buoyancy or filled with water or other materials to work against weight. They are perfect for creating additional resistance in Swimnastics workouts. Available in blue, red, and yellow.

Aquatic Harness

Churchill Fitness Agency
708 Lakeshore
701 Dorval
Quebec H9S 2C4 Canada

The harness is comprised of a web belt and two soft plastic lines that hook onto a lane ring. It fits any size.

Aquatoner

Kona Fitness, Inc.
P.O. Box 5775
Asheville, NC 28813
1-800-237-0469/
704-252-8268

The Aquatoner is a water-resistance exerciser that works the whole body, promoting strength, endurance, mobility, and physical therapy. Three streamlined paddles connect at the center; there is a central handle on one side and a foot/leg/arm attachment on the other. The surface area can be adjusted by overlapping or un-

– Aquarius Water Workout Station

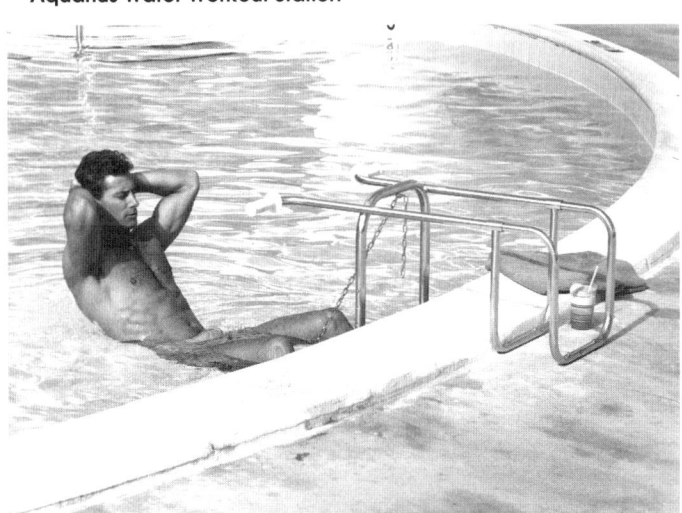

– Aquatoner

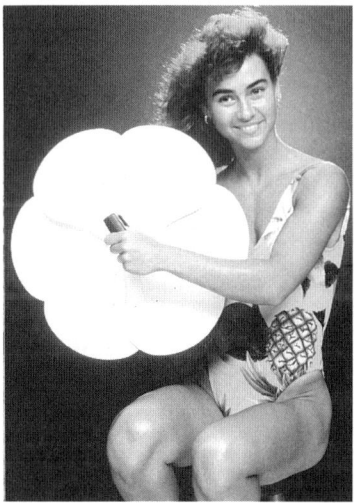

folding from 96 to 250 square inches, allowing the user to control force and velocity through a full range of motion.

Aquatoning Bar
Kona Fitness, Inc.
P.O. Box 5775
Asheville, NC 28813
1-800-237-0469/
704-252-8268

A water-resistance exerciser for the upper body, this 3-foot PVC bar has stainless steel end elbows and caps to which two Aquatoners attach, parallel to the bar. Exercises done with the bar include standing bench presses, shoulder raises, tricep and arm curls, and upper-back and latissimus dorsi workouts.

Aquatoning T-Bar
Kona Fitness, Inc.
P.O. Box 5775
Asheville, NC 28813
1-800-237-0469/
704-252-8268

This water-resistance exerciser works the upper body in movements that require the arms to be raised over the head and to exercise the upper body sitting outside of the water while still utilizing water resistance. It is a 3-foot PVC bar with stainless steel end caps that accept a handle on one end and an Aquatoner on the other end, attached perpendicular to the bar. The handle and an Aquatoner (three paddles) are included with the bar.

Aqua Tunes
1020 Berea Drive
Boulder, CO 80303
303-494-7224

This product enables swimmers to listen to music while exercising. A watersports belt, containing a molded plastic pouch and watertight clamp, attaches to a soft, webbed, nylon, adjustable belt. Patented earphone speakers also are included.

AquaWave and Wavetek
Aquatic Amusement
 Associates, Ltd.
P.O. Box 648
1 Aquatic Circle
Cohoes, NY 12047
518-783-0038

Wave equipment is custom-made for use in specifically sized indoor and/or outdoor zero-inch depth entry pools. It is extremely useful for special populations, such as senior citizens and the handicapped, and also for training purposes.

B-Wise Swim Fitness Bar
B-Wise Enterprise Inc.
3640 Villanova Court
Bethlehem, PA 18017
215-865-3508

The Swim Fitness Bar is a buoyant polystyrene barbell created for aquatic exercise. It has a small-diameter padded bar for good grip. It can be used in shallow water for underwater arm, trunk, and waist exercises. Water walking, running, and toning exercises can be done in the deep water.

Bar Float #677
Sprint/Rothhammer
 International, Inc.
P.O. Box 5579
Santa Maria, CA 93456
1-800-235-2156

Used to develop arm strength, the Bar Float can be used like a kickboard or pushed and pulled through the water for resistance.

Belt Float #670
Sprint/Rothhammer
 International, Inc.
P.O. Box 5579
Santa Maria, CA 93456
1-800-235-2156

This device is used to keep the user afloat while exercising, particularly in deep water.

Bema Schwimmflugel
Bema USA, Inc.
2015 Weaver Park Drive
Clearwater, FL 34625
813-446-2362

The original "swim wings," this product helps the participant in water exercise by providing buoyancy for arms and ankles. It can be used as a water tool for swimming and water exercise and is available in five sizes for the entire family.

Bioenergetics, Inc.
Glenn McWaters
290 Montgomery Highway
Pelham, AL 35124
1-800-433-2627

Body Buoys
Dan Chester
P.O. Box 178
Cherokee Village, AR 72525

Bodyciser
Bodyciser International Corp.
511 River Drive
Elmwood Park, NJ 07407
1-800-321-3664/201-791-9601

The Bodyciser is an aquatic exercise platform consisting of three unique floats. Unique hinge panels allow free-flowing movements. The floats accommodate any body weight and come in three sizes: small (5' to 5'5" body height), medium (5'6" to 5'11" body height), and large (6' to 6'4" body height). They weigh less than 6 pounds, fold and snap for storage, and are carried with a shoulder strap for easy transportation.

Body Logic Training System
Body Logic
P.O. Box 16201
Austin, TX 78716
512-327-0050

The Body Logic Training System is a complete information management system for sports training that can easily automate strength training, running sessions, or aerobics. A database provides information on strength, jumping, cardiovascular system, and body fat. Both individual and group reports can easily be printed. The TWIG Training Generator allows the user within two minutes to define individualized training sessions, producing training routines by the day, week, month, or year. The TWIG design also provides easy workout management.

Buoyancy Cuffs
Hydro-Fit, Inc.
3730 Donald Street
Eugene, OR 97405
1-800-346-7295

These colorful, durable resistance cuffs can be worn in a variety of ways to provide optimal muscle tone improvement and cardiorespiratory conditioning. When worn around the ankle, the cuffs provide comfortable buoyancy, maximizing the natural resistance of water.

Buoy Trunks
Buoyant Company
8455 Wabash Ave.
Saint Louis, MO 63134
314-524-2210

Buoy Trunks are a flotation suit designed to float the wearer at shoulder height, with no restriction of movement. Flotation-grade foam is sewn into trunks. They are to be worn over a regular swimsuit. Men and women wear the same trunks. Children's sizes are also available.

Double T-Bar
Kona Fitness, Inc.
P.O. Box 5775
Asheville, NC 28813
1-800-237-0469/704-252-8268

Two partners work at the same time with this water-resistance exerciser for the upper body, which elevates excitement, interest, and motivation. Two three-foot PVC bars with stainless steel end caps attach to Aquatoners (handle and three paddles only). The two bars hold four Aquatoners. Partners alternate pushing and pulling to the left and right sides to exercise the entire upper body with each rep; sets are accomplished with one partner guiding one end and vice versa.

Fins #635, #640, or #638
Sprint/Rothhammer
    International, Inc.
P.O. Box 5579
Santa Maria, CA 93456
1-800-235-2156

The Fins are used to build leg strength either while swimming or in deep water, giving better thrust with the legs.

Fitness Equipment— Weight Equipment
Pyramid Fitness Industries
115 High Street
Sharpsville, PA 16150
(412) 962-3200

Pyramid Fitness Industries manufacturers a complete line of single-station "selectorized" machines, rehab equipment, multistation gyms, free-weight equipment, and the innovative Selex line of free weights.

Foam Belts, Discs, Barbells

J & B Foam Fabricators, Inc.
P.O. Box 144
Ludington, MI 49431
1-800-621-3626/616-843-2448

J & B Foam products are to be used in water exercise instructional classes and rehabilitation programs.

– Foam Belts, Discs, Barbells

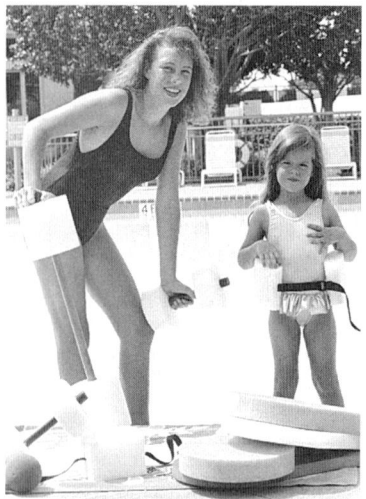

Hand Buoys

Hydro-Fit, Inc.
3730 Donald Street
Eugene, OR 97405
1-800-346-7295

Sturdy hand-held foam and plastic buoys provide a superior upper-body workout. Lightweight and sleek, the buoys are designed so that users can execute a wide range of exercises in a safe, hydrodynamically efficient manner.

Hand Paddles #750

Sprint/Rothhammer
  International, Inc.
P.O. Box 5579
Santa Maria, CA 93456
1-800-235-2156

These plastic paddles with straps are used to create more resistance for the arms while exercising.

Heart Rate Monitors and Biofeedback Devices

Biosig Instruments, Inc.
5471 Royalmount Avenue
Montreal, Quebec H4P 1J3
  Canada
514-733-3362/514-733-9554
U.S. Office
176 Rugar Street
Plattsburg, NY 12901
or
P.O. Box 860
Champlain, NY 12919

Hot Shot Diving Board Basketball

E.A. Favorite and Associates
P.O. Box 23252
Richfield, MN 55423
612-861-7008

The Hot Shot is a basketball backboard and hoop that attaches to a diving board for a game of aquatic basketball.

Hydro-Fit

1487 Oak Drive
Eugene, OR 97404
1-800-346-7295

Hydro Helpers (Model 8660)

Danmar Products, Inc.
221 Jackson Industrial Drive
Ann Arbor, MI 48103
1-800-783-1998

Hydro Helpers increase arm and leg strength through resistance training, gait re-education, and joint rehabilitation exercise programs. They are comprised of three bright yellow, extremely buoyant marine foam sections that strap around the arm or leg and foot. Two sizes are available (small and large).

– Hydro-Tone System One

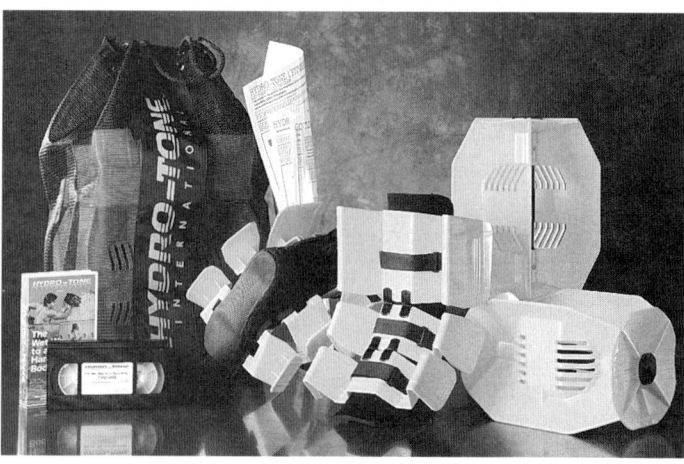

Hydro-Tone System One

Hydro-Tone International, Inc.
3535 N.W. 58th St., Suite #935
Oklahoma City, OK 73112
405-948-7754

or

Tom McPhillips
30727 Shiawassee, Suite 50
Farmington Hills, MI 48336

This three-dimensional system increases resistance, providing much greater muscle stimulation and calorie burning. It includes a pair of hand-held Hydro-Bells, a pair of foot-worn Hydro-Boots, an equipment travel bag, and a complete instructional package, including a video.

Kickboard

Speedo Activewear
11111 Santa Monica Blvd.
Los Angeles, CA 90025
213-473-0032

The Kickboard, a rectangular piece of styrofoam-based flotation material, allows the user to isolate the kick and strengthen leg muscles.

Kickboards #690, #605, #680, #606, or #695

Sprint/Rothhammer
   International, Inc.
P.O. Box 5579
Santa Maria, CA 93456
1-800-235-2156

Made of durable, high-density EVA foam, this Kickboard can be usedwith leg kick exercises or when hand held, it provides resistance as the participant moves through the water. Various sizes are available for different resistances and buoyancies.

Kickboards and Rescue Tubes

Creative Foam Corporation
300 N. Alloy Drive
Fenton, MI 48430
1-800-446-4644/313-629-4149

A variety of sizes of kickboards are available for use as a swim aid.

Limber Ladder (Model 8670)

Danmar Products, Inc.
221 Jackson Industrial Drive
Ann Arbor, MI 48103
1-800-783-1998

The Limber Ladder is a series of plastic-flotation rungs strung 3 inches apart with strong polypropylene rope. It is used to increase shoulder/upper-back flexibility. Two ladders may be strung together to make a longer ladder to accommodate individuals with less upper-back/shoulder flexibility. Ladders are sold in pairs.

Mateflex, Versaflex

Mateflex Mele Corp.
1712 Erie Street
P.O. Box 538
Utica, NY 13503-0538
1-800-926-3539/315-733-4600

These flow-through, interlocking, raised-grid safety floor tiles provide instant water drainage of water and good footing in wet areas.

Mindy McCurdy Waterballs

Mindy McCurdy, Inc.
P.O. Box 507
Naples, FL 33939-0507
813-262-1981

Mindy McCurdy Waterballs are especially effective for strengthening and toning the upper and lower body. They provide increased resistance to movement through water, as well as buoyancy. A series of exercises, designed by McCurdy using water exercise physiology principles, are detailed in the accompanying instruction manual.

Move It or Lose It Gloves

Essert Associates, Inc.
551 Roosevelt Road, Suite 304
Glen Ellyn, IL 60137
708-858-6348

Lycra gloves provide gentle resistance during upper-body water exercise.

M. S. Plastics and Package Company, Inc.

400 Union Ave.
Haskell, NJ 07420
201-831-1802

This manufacturer makes plastic wet sacks (small bags or rolls for wet clothes) and a full line of mesh gym bags. Other products include saniseats for saunas.

Plastazote Playmats, Swim Bars, Kickboards

H$_2$O Enterprises, Inc.
2925 Panorama Drive
North Vancouver, British
   Columbia V7G 2A4
   Canada
604-929-7316

Mats are designed for a variety of uses in teaching recreation. The swim bars and kickboards are used in teaching, exercise, and therapy programs. Other products include aquatic teaching games, such as Think Blocks and Pin the Tail on the Whale, an instructor newsletter, and the Little Waves Video/Teaching Guide. H$_2$O is the Western Canadian distributor of Hydro-Fit.

The Pool Lift

Aquatic Access, Inc.
417 Dorsey Way
Louisville, KY 40223
1-800-325-LIFT/502-425-5817

These water-powered swimming pool lifts enable handicapped people to enter and exit the pool. Prices are under $2,000 for an assisted lift and $2,800 for a self-operated lift.

Pool Splash and Slam Basketball Unit

Dunn-Rite Products, Inc.
210 S. 16th Street
Elwood, IN 46036
1-800-798-9646

This regulation-size basketball unit can be adjusted for height and has a patented breakaway system for safety.

Pool Towels

McArthur Towels, Inc.
P.O. Box 448
Baraboo, WI 53913
1-800-356-9168/608-356-8922

McArthur produces all types of terry bath towels (from 20" x 40" to 45" x 72"), in white and colors.

Pull Buoy

Speedo Activewear
11111 Santa Monica Blvd.
Los Angeles, CA 90025
213-473-0032

The Pull Buoy is constructed of two styrofoam cylinders, attached through the center by cording. Its purpose is to secure the legs, preventing them from kicking, in order to strengthen arms while pulling.

The Rebound Board

Gerstung Manufacturers
6310 Blair Lane
Baltimore, MD 21209
301-337-7781

The Rebound Board offers both resiliency and spring action through a unique bowed design that is supported on tough foam blocks. It is constructed of laminated hardwood (birch and maple) veneer plywood for maximum strength and is triple-polyurethane coated to ensure durability and beauty. The slip-free foam landing surface will not absorb perspiration and can be easily wiped off. A handle on the underside allows the board to be easily carried.

RODCO Products Company, Inc.

P.O. Box 944
2565 16th Ave.
Columbus, NE 68601
1-800-323-2799/402-563-3596

RODCO provides instant, accurate, and complete digital temperature information.

Running Water (Model 8680)

Danmar Products, Inc.
221 Jackson Industrial Drive
Ann Arbor, MI 48103
1-800-783-1998

This deep-water running aid helps the participant maintain a vertical position during running or other aerobic water exercise. Two marine-flotation foam pads curve to fit the body and are positioned in front and back. A crotch strap helps keep the foam sections in place around the waist.

Sears Healthy Care Specialties

Available through local Sears retail stores.

Sof-Turf

SEAMCO Laboratories, Inc.
Gordon McKinnon;
Paul L. Payne
119 S. Oregon Ave.
Tampa, FL 33606
813-251-1881

Granulated virgin rubber chips and epoxy are mixed together to form a soft, durable, decorative decking, or seamless floor. It provides excellent coating around pools and exercise rooms and can be used indoors or out. Sof-Turf is available in solid or mixed colors and supports the use of strips and logos.

Sprint Band #765
Sprint/Rothhammer
    International, Inc.
P.O. Box 5579
Santa Maria, CA 93456
1-800-235-2156

These Latex bands are held by the hands and then stretched to tone a number of muscle groups, depending on the position chosen. They are available in three different resistance levels.

Stabilizer Bar (Model 8729)
Danmar Products, Inc.
221 Jackson Industrial Drive
Ann Arbor, MI 48103
1-800-783-1998

The multipurpose bar may be used in place of a kickboard for gait training and to increase shoulder strength/flexibility. It is made of six rings of buoyant marine foam attached to a four-inch flotation-plastic rod. Rings may be added or subtracted to match the proficiency level of the user.

Step/Bench Equipment
Aerobic Workbench
P.O. Box 2575
Largo, FL 34649
813-391-7419

For more information see Aerobic Workbench earlier in this equipment section.

Step/Bench Equipment
BenchAerobix, Inc.
1775 The Exchange, Suite 180
Atlanta, GA 30339
1-800-25-BENCH

— Step/Bench Equipment

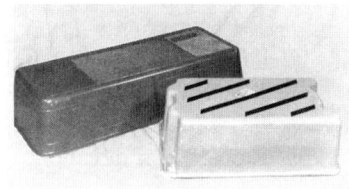

Step/Bench Equipment
CardioStep
1220 Freedom Road
Freedom, PA 15042
412-774-7720

Step/Bench Equipment
Peter H. Hand
The Aqua Step
280 Elizabeth Street
Suite A110
Atlanta, GA 30307
404-522-6202

SuitMate
Extractor Corporation
P.O. Box 99
South Elgin, IL 60177
708-742-3532 in Illinois
1-800-553-3353 outside
    Illinois

The SuitMate water extractor converts a dripping wet swimsuit into a dripless suit in five to ten seconds by extracting approximately 95% of the water.

Sweatwet
Basic Pool Products
5591 McAdam Road
Mississauga, Ontario L4Z
    1N4 Canada
416-890-0922

This pool exercise bar comes with various attachments that work different muscle groups in exercises and games, allowing the user to customize his workout routine. For example, the abdominal chair concentrates on the stomach area.

Swim Bug
Gerstung/Gym Thing
6308-10 Blair Hill Lane
Baltimore, MD 21209
301-337-7781

The SwimBug is a swim aid shaped like a lady bug. Made of soft but strong polyvinyl foam, it uses two straps to attach firmly to the body. Instructions are included.

— SuitMate

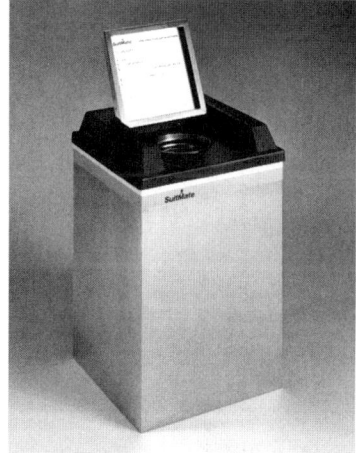

Swim Pak
Gerstung/Gym Thing
6308-10 Blair Hill Lane
Baltimore, MD 21209
301-337-7781

A soft but strong foam pad that is fitted below the chest with one or two straps that fasten in front, the Swim Pak serves as a swim aid.

T. H. & K. Aquatic Enterprises
30727 Shiawassee #50
Farmington Hills, MI 48024
313-476-8052

Aquatic exercise products.

Timing Devices
Accusplit, Inc.
2290A Ringwood Avenue
San Jose, CA 95131
408-432-8228

Timers are used for walking, jogging, auto racing, horse racing, and many other activities.

Training Paddle
Speedo Activewear
11111 Santa Monica Blvd.
Los Angeles, CA 90025
213-473-0032

These paddles are used on the hands and provide resistance when pulling to strengthen arms. A square plastic paddle secures to the hand with surgical tubing. Paddles come in small, medium, and large sizes.

Triangle Body Ball
SLM, Inc.
P.O. Box 1070
Gloversville, NY 12078
518-725-8101

This soft, round, weighted ball floats, providing resistance for muscle toning. It is available in two-, three-, and four-pound weights.

Underwater Treadmill
Life Tec, Inc.
1710 S. Wolf Road
Wheeling, IL 60090
1-800-822-5911/708-459-7500

The treadmill uses various water depths to change the weight-bearing capabilities of the user. It provides both cardiovascular and strengthening benefits.

Watercizer
AquaCizer, Inc.
Route 5, Lake Canton
Canton, IL 61520
(309) 647-1444

The Watercizer is made of closed-cell foam and fabric webbing. It weighs two pounds. It can support individuals weighing 200-plus pounds. One size adjusts to fit all.

Water Exercise Dumbbells #725
Sprint/Rothhammer
  International, Inc.
P.O. Box 5579
Santa Maria, CA 93456
1-800-235-2156

Each dumbbell is a plastic bar with durable high-density EVA foam floats. It is moved through the water using various positions and speeds, which provides resistance to develop arm strength. It also can be used to provide buoyancy while twisting the waist and legs.

Water Gloves #780
Sprint/Rothhammer
  International, Inc.
P.O. Box 5579
Santa Maria, CA 93456
1-800-235-2156

The gloves create webbed hands, increasing resistance and toning arms as they move through the water. The Lycra back covering allows for comfortable fit, and the neoprene palm assures firm pulling power.

Water Hoops
Water Hoops, Inc.
5235 E. Montecito
Scottsdale, AZ 85251
602-947-5503

Water Hoops can be used solely for entertainment and also for low- to no-impact aerobic exercise.

Water Wheel (Model 8640)
Danmar Products, Inc.
221 Jackson Industrial Drive
Ann Arbor, MI 48103
1-800-783-1998

The Wheel is a yellow and blue disc, 20 inches in circumference, made of flotation plastic. It has adjustable "windows" to allow modifications in resistance force, accommodating beginning through advanced training programs. Trunk, arm/shoulder, and back strength and flexibility are developed through progressive resistance

Equipment

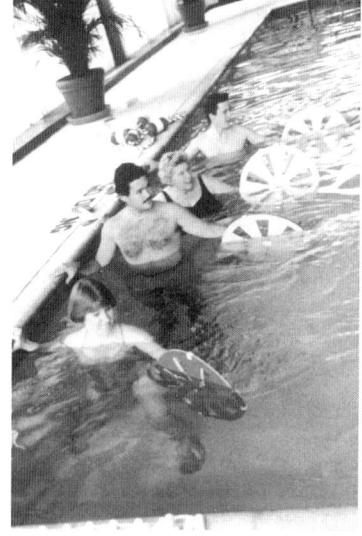

— Water Wheel (Model 8640)

training. The Wheel may be ordered individually or in pairs.

Water Wings #625
Sprint/Rothhammer International, Inc.
P.O. Box 5579
Santa Maria, CA 93456
1-800-235-2156

These inflatable buoys are hand held and moved through the water to tone muscles.

Wave Webs
Hydro-Fit, Inc.
3730 Donald Street
Eugene, OR 97405
1-800-346-7295

These specially designed webbed gloves enhance natural water resistance for safe and effective upper-body conditioning through a variety of means. They are lightweight and form fitting, made of a soft, durable nylon and Lycra blend. They come in three sizes and four colors.

Wrist and Ankle Weights #951, #952, #953, #933, or #935
Sprint/Rothhammer International, Inc.
P.O. Box 5579
Santa Maria, CA 93456
1-800-235-2156

Terrycloth O-ring wrist weights are available in weights of one, two, or three pounds per pair. Ankle weights made of neoprene strap on with Velcro and come in three- or five-pound weights per pair. They provide greater resistance while working out on land or in water. All weights are completely waterproof.

World Wide Aquatics
3814 Business Center Way
Cincinnati, OH 45246
1-800-543-4459

FILTERS, CHEMICALS, AND AIR PRODUCTS

Aquasol SPC Controller
Aquasol Controllers, Inc.
5600 Harvey Wilson Drive
Houston, TX 77220-5334
1-800-444-0675

Aquasol Controllers automatically sense the changing chemical needs of the water and then feed in the right chemical in the right amount. They automatically maintain continuous sanitation and chemical balance using ORP technology.

DH Series Industrial Dehumidifier
Dumont Refrigeration Corp.
Main Street
P.O. Box 149
Monmouth, ME 04259
207-933-4811

This dehumidifier operates on a refrigeration principle. It removes humidity from air space, decreasing the problems caused by humidity and condensation.

Dry-O-Tron
Dectrom, Inc.
P.O. Box 2076
South Burlington, VT 05407-9988
802-862-8342

This mechanical dehumidifier and closed-loop energy recycler dehumidifies the pool area while heating the pool water.

The Filter Saver
WING Enterprises, Inc.
P.O. Box 3100
Springville, UT 84663-3100
801-375-4455

The Filter Saver is a container made of PVC tubing for soaking cartridge filters. It eliminates the mess normally associated with soaking and can be reused. With the use of the optional T-BAR, the user's hands need not touch the cleaning solution. The Filter Saver saves time, money, and effort.

HydroTech Systems Ltd./ The Whitten Products Division
One Aquatic Center
P.O. Box 648
Cohoes, NY 12047
518-783-0038

HydroTech offers perimeter pool recirculation and filtration systems and associated competitive aquatic equipment.

Hydrozone
American Water Purification, Inc.
723 E. Skinner
Wichita, KS 67211
1-800-824-3821

Hydrozone is an ozone-generating system designed to reduce chemical costs by 40% to 60%. It greatly enhances water quality by virtually eliminating burning eyes, chlorine odor, and bleaching of hair, skin, and clothing.

Hypocell Water Purification System
Nature Pool Canada, Inc.
2133 Royal Windsor Drive, Unit 25
Mississauga, Ontario L5J 1K5 Canada
416-823-8557

The Hypocell System produces sparkling clear water by manufacturing its own hypochlorous acid to sanitize pools and spas. It eliminates the use of chlorine or bromine, further automating the pool, saving on maintenance and labor, and significantly reducing the environmental impact of pool chemicals. Hypocell is accepted by health authorities for commercial and public pool use.

Pool Water Chemistry Controller
Kruger and Eckels, Inc.
1406 E. Wilshire Avenue
Santa Ana, CA 92705
714-547-5165

An electronic controller allows the pool operator to set pH and ppm sanitizer levels and then activates chemical feeders only as needed to keep chemistry precisely controlled. Meter readouts constantly display pool water chemistry, and safety alarms warn of incorrect conditions. The controller comes in a nonmetallic, corrosion-proof, lockable cabinet with a front door viewing window.

Proteam Products
John Girvan Company, Inc.
11730 Phillips Highway
Jacksonville, FL 32256
1-800-356-6460

Proteam Supreme is created to reduce pool operating costs and maintenance work by denying algae their ability to reproduce. Without carbon dioxide to reproduce, Proteam Supreme enhances the pool sanitizer and acts as a buffer, neutralizing both strong acids and alkalies.

Water Analyzers and Controllers
Nature Pool Canada, Inc.
2133 Royal Windsor Drive, Unit 25
Mississauga, Ontario L5J 1K5 Canada
416-823-8557

Products available include the 2000D Analogue Controller and Water Analyzer with high or low alarm for pH and ORP (chlorine and bromine). A liquid crystal meter displays pH and ORP levels.

York Chemical Corporation
3309 E. Carpenter Freeway
Irving, TX 75062
214-438-6744

York offers a comprehensive line of chemical products for pool and spa water care: chlorine and bromine sanitizers, algaecides, pH control, water balancers, maintenance products, and winterizing chemicals.

Zephyr Dehumidifying Pool Water Heater
Dumont Refrigeration Corp.
Main Street
P.O. Box 149
Monmouth, ME 04259
207-933-4811

A refrigeration-based dehumidifier, the Zephyr captures energy in the warm humid pool air and recycles it through a heat exchanger to heat pool water and provide warm, dry air to the indoor pool enclosure. Use prevents condensation damage and keeps the pool area dry and comfortable.

HEALTH PRODUCTS

Alena Energy Drink/ Alena Energy Bar
Enreco
1926 S. 9th Street
Manitowoc, WI 54220
414-682-8796

Fortified Flax
Omega-Life, Inc.
15355 Woodbridge Road
Brookfield, WI 53005
1-800-328-3529/414-786-2070

This ground, premium-quality flax seed is fortified and stabilized with vitamins and minerals. It is loaded with Omega-3 (linolenic acid) and fiber. It also aids the body in metabolizing Omega-3 quickly and efficiently. It is used for extra energy and weight reduction.

Omega-Bar
15355 Woodbridge Road
Brookfield, WI 53005
1-800-328-3529/414-786-2070

A fruit and fortified flax energy bar, designed for use during athletic events or when on the go. It tastes great and is full of fiber and vegetable Omega-3.

Power Pack Energy Drink
15355 Woodbridge Road
Brookfield, WI 53005
1-800-328-3529/414-786-2070

Made with fortified flax, the Power Pack Energy Drink also contains oat bran, barley, lecithin, beta-carotene, and Omega-3 (vegetable, not fish oil). It provides lasting energy and power and is designed for use during an athletic event or as a between-meals snack.

Water Filtration Devices (Drinking Water) and Environmental Air Purifiers
Physicians Water Systems
630 Vernon Avenue, Suite F
Glencoe, IL 60022
708-835-4700

The water system removes contaminants that cause bad odor and taste from municipal water. The air system removes dust, pollens, and molds from the air, allowing easier breathing.

MUSIC SOURCES

Aerobic Beat
7985 Santa Monica Blvd. #109
Los Angeles, CA 90046
213-659-2503

"Aerobic Beat 1–4" contains uptempo, high-energy music for advanced workouts. The "Senior Workout" and "Step One" contain midtempo music for beginning/intermediate workouts.

Aerobics Power Mix Audiotape, Vol. 5
East Coast Music Productions, Inc.
P.O. Box 3812
Gaithersburg, MD 20878
1-800-777-BEAT/301-428-7963

The tape features 90 minutes of music (current releases and contemporary versions of past decades' hits) in either low-impact (130–145 beats per minute) or high impact (135–155 beats per minute). Floor work and cooldown segments are on side B.

Aerobics Tapes and Records, Inc.
P.O. Box 56
Cardiff, CA 92007
619-943-1649

This company sells motivating, safe exercise music designed and formatted specifically for workouts. Music is available on tapes and records. Custom music also is produced for aerobics.

Aqua Power
Strom-Berg Productions
253 Rhodes Court
San Jose, CA 95126
408-295-3898

The first in a new line of music for aqua professionals. This 60-minute tape is perfect for low-impact aerobic workouts and any strength training section of your aqua program. The instrumentals are uplifting with a strong steady beat that will carry in an indoor or outdoor pool setting.

David Shelton Productions
P.O. Box 310
Mendon, UT 84325
1-800-272-3411/801-753-2300

These tapes offer continuous 60- to 90-minute recordings of custom music for exercise, and many theme tapes are available. Most tapes are available in high- and low-impact versions.

Ease Down
Strom-Berg Productions
253 Rhodes Court
San Jose, CA 95126
408-295-3898

This relaxing music—with piano, string and flute instrumentation—is designed for cool-down, stretching, and aquatics programs. Side A contains synthesized instrumentals, and side B has piano solos.

Fitness Finders, Inc.
133 Teft Road
P.O. Box 160
Spring Arbor, MI 49283
517-750-1500

Each tape provides two 30-minute sessions for warm-up, muscle-toning, peak workout, and cooldown sections. The music is upbeat, and there are no vocals.

Infant Harmonies
Strom-Berg Productions
253 Rhodes Court
San Jose, CA 95126
408-295-3898

These special recordings relax infants, encourage the bonding process between mother and child, and also soothe the infant to sleep. Instrumentals are available for both infant and mother, including beautiful, original compositions, as well as remakes of two classics: "Simple Gifts" and "Over the Rainbow."

In-Lytes Productions
614 Sherburn Lane
Louisville, KY 40207
1-800-243-PUMP/
502-894-8008

Muscle Mixes
623 N. Hyer Avenue
Orlando, FL 32803
1-800-52-MIXES/
407-872-7576

Music-in-Sync, Volume I, Audio Cassettes
Medical and Sports Music Institute of America, Inc.
767 Willamette Street, Suite 104
Eugene, OR 97401
503-344-5323

AQUAMUSIC aquatic exercise and rehabilitation music audiotapes were medically tested in a three-year study. Inspirational music was composed to conform to the exact pace requirements needed by physicians, hydrotherapists, and water exercise enthusiasts.

New Cardio Jazz/Funk Video and Sound Track
Strom-Berg Productions
253 Rhodes Court
San Jose, CA 95126
408-295-3898

This hot, original music from Strom-Berg is good for low-impact exercise and perfect for aquatic programs.

Wet Steps
Strom-Berg Productions
253 Rhodes Court
San Jose, CA 95126
408-295-3898

Wet Steps is the first step tape developed for aqua bench aerobics. This 60-minute full format class tape is composed and mixed under the guidance of Ruth Sova of the Aquatic Exercise Association. It provides the correct beats per minute for an effective aqua step workout. The instrumentals make an exciting water workout.

ORGANIZATIONS

American Alliance for Health, Physical Education, Recreation and Dance: Aquatic Council (AAHPERD)
1900 Association Drive
Reston, VA 22091
703-476-3400

American National Red Cross
John Malatak
17th and D Streets N.W.
Washington, DC 20006
202-639-3686

Organizations

Aquatic Exercise Association
Ruth Sova, PRESIDENT
P.O. Box 497
Port Washington, WI 53074
414-284-3416

Aquatic Injury Safety Foundation
Ron Gilbert
1555 Penobscot Building
Detroit, MI 48226
1-800-342-0330/313-963-1600

Chlorine Institute
2001 L Street N.W., Suite 506
Washington, DC 20036

Council for National Cooperation in Aquatics (CNCA)
901 W. New York Street
Indianapolis, IN 46223
317-638-4238

Fitness/Wellness Program
Gwen Robbins, Director
Ball State University
School of Physical Education
Muncie, IN 47306

IDEA: The Association for Fitness Professionals
Kathie Davis, Executive Director
6190 Cornerstone Court East, Suite 204
San Diego, CA 92121-3773
1-800-999-IDEA/
619-535-8979

INFOFIT
Leisure Management and Education
Katherine MacKeigan
10814 75th Avenue
Edmonton, Alberta T6E 1K2
Canada

International Academy of Aquatic Art
Fran Sweeney/Jill White
2360 Hedge Row
Northfield, IL 60043
813-922-7528

International Swimming Hall of Fame
1 Hall of Fame Drive
Ft. Lauderdale, FL 33316
305-462-6536

IRSA: The Association of Quality Clubs
253 Summer Street, Suite 400
Boston, MA 02210
1-800-228-4772

Lifeguard Training USA
Bill Kirchhoff
12502 Niego Lane
San Diego, CA 92128
619-673-8576

National Advisory Committee on Aquatics for Young Children
Stephen Langendorder
Motor Development Lab
Kent State University
Kent, OH 44242
216-672-2117

National Advisory Committee on Lifeguarding
Stan Anderson
800 Cloverdale Avenue
Victoria, British Columbia
V8X 2S8 Canada
604-598-8685/604-386-7528

National Advisory Committee on SCUBA
Robert Smith
1213 Seventeenth Street
Key West, FL 33040
305-296-9081

National Recreation and Park Association: Aquatic Section (NRPA)
Walter Johnson
Director Great Lakes Region NRPA
650 W. Higgins Road
Hoffman Estates, IL 60195
1-800-626-6772/312-843-7529

National Spa and Pool Institute (NSPI)
Chuck Whitmer, President
2111 Eisenhower Avenue
Alexandria, VA 22314
703-838-0083

President's Council on Physical Fitness and Sports
Suite 303, Donahoe Building
6th and D Streets N.W.
Washington, DC 20201
202-272-3430

POOL PRODUCTS

Aqua Plunge Spas
Box 677
Muscatine, IA 52761-0677
1-800-553-9664/319-263-6642

Aqua Plunge sells 3 shell designs, 15 different sizes of swim spas, and 11 different sizes of commercial spas.

AquaCiser System
Ferno Ille
70 Well Way
Willmington, OH 45177
1-800-541-8360/
513-382-1461

This underwater treadmill system was created originally to rehabilitate racehorses. It is now used as a therapy system either as a treadmill or as a therapeutic pool by using the resting seat. It combines the benefits of treadmill exercise with the healing effect of hydrotherapy.

Aquarius Rehabilitation Tank
631 U.S. Highway One, Suite 300
North Palm Beach, FL 33408
407-585-0754

The self-contained free-standing, stainless steel rehabilitation tank is manufactured by Aquarius Health and Fitness Products, Inc. It is ideal for nursing homes, training camps, institutions and doctors' offices. It is available in 42-inch, 63-inch and 84-inch heights. Its cost is billable to insurance companies, workers' compensation and Medicare. It is designed for those with sports injuries, lower back pain, obesity, and arthritis; and it can be used for cardiovascular conditioning, muscle toning and general body strengthening. The tank includes protocol for lower back pain, weakness on the lubopelvic girdle, abdominal and lumbar paraspinals, and loading of pathological structures by gravity.

AquaSwim'n'Spa
Pool Technology Ltd.
P.O. Box 3707
Brownsville, TX 78523
512-831-2715

AquaSwim'n'Spas are available in 14', 16', and 19' models with special individual features; all are 7'6" wide. Also available is a 14' exercise pool without the spa, with steps going into the pool, no benches, and swimjets at end. All units may be installed inground, partially inground, or aboveground.

ATRIA (Supersky)
Skylight and Enclosure Systems
P.O. Box 800074
Bethany, OK 73008
405-232-1956

The use of aluminum frames, triple-walled poly-carbonate glazing, sliding glass doors, and opening roof systems allows year-round use of the Atria.

BaduJet
Speck Pumps—Pool Products, Inc.
7775 Bayberry Road
Jacksonville, FL 32256
904-739-2626

The Speck BaduJet creates an adjustable flow of water in any swimming pool, making it possible to swim a long distance without turning at pool walls. The user can exercise with the full force of the BaduJet, swim at a leisurely pace, or relax with a pulsating massage. This air-supported, reinforced vinyl airdome enclosure is custom made; maximum size is 15,000 square feet.

Clycan Alpha Ltd.
625 E. Third Street
Lexington, KY 40505
606-259-3779

This air-supported fabric enclosure allows year-round use of pool facilities. The structure generally can be erected or taken down in one day.

EZ Steps Drop-In Stairs
Quaker Plastic Corporation
103 Manor Street
Mountville, PA 17554

The unit includes two stainless steel handrails and hardware. Side panel grillwork allows water circulation behind the unit. Special edging along the bottom and sides guards against pool bottom damage. A built-in ballast prevents the stairs from floating.

Kiefer Sports Group
1750 Harding Road
Northfield, IL 60093
708-446-8866

Kiefer offers aquatic products, specialty flooring, and pool construction.

Proteam Products
John Girvan Company, Inc.
11730 Phillips Highway
Jacksonville, FL 32258
904-260-4505

Proteam Supreme is a long-lasting algae suppressant that produces 35% to 60% sanitizer savings, a reduction in filter maintenance, and less eye and skin irritation.

Sau Sea Swimming Pool Products, Inc.
Vincentown, NJ 08088
609-859-8500

Sau Sea manufactures swimming pool paint and repair products for masonry (concrete and plaster) swimming pools.

SwimEx Aquatic Exercise Machine
SwimEx Systems, Inc.
P.O. Box 328
Warren, RI 02885
401-245-7946

The SwimEx compact lap pool provides a smooth, even current that allows the user to swim in place or perform nonimpact aerobic exercises. With over 30 different water speeds up to 4.5 mph, the SwimEx meets all abilities. Its unique paddlewheel propulsion system creates a natural, smooth flow of water—no high pressure swimjets.

Swim Gym
Swim Gym, Inc.
2175 Agate Court
Simi Valley, CA 93065
213-457-9242

A high-volume pumping system provides the current for swimming in place, jogging, aerobics, and other activities.

Swim-N-Place
Leisure Workshop
P.O. Box 1783
North Brunswick, NJ 08902
(201) 828-9568

Swim-N-Place enables the user to swim against an adjustable flow of water in any type swimming pool. Hydrotherapy jets lend themselves to the therapeutic experience bathers seek, and it is especially appropriate for special populations.

Total Spa and Bath
4445 S.W. 35th Terrace #100
Gainesville, FL 32608
1-800-647-7727 outside Florida/904-372-3508

Total Spa and Bath offers the finest spas, saunas, whirlpools, steamers, and related components in the industry.

PUBLICATIONS
Books

AKWA Bookstore
Aquatic Exercise Association
P.O. Box 497
Port Washington, WI 53074
(414) 284-3416

AKWA Bookstore offers to the public current books and videos on aquatic fitness. A listing of books and videos is available for purchase from AEA on the subjects of aquatic fitness and aquatic therapy.

American Heart Association
Contact your local affiliate
A free brochure, called "Risko," provides information to help individuals compute their current chances of ever getting heart disease, as well as suggestions for reducing the odds. "Risko" scores are based on four of the most important modifiable heart disease risk factors: weight, blood pressure, blood cholesterol level, and use of tobacco. Call the local AHA office to receive a brochure.

Aqua Dynamics Handbook
F.I.R.M. Fitness Instructor's Resource Materials
Karen Westfall, President
1352 W. Southwind Street
St. George, UT 84770
801-628-3160

The Aqua Dynamics program is a combination of aquatic toning, strengthening, and cardiovascular conditioning. The book includes sections on warm-up, upper-body strengthening and toning, lower-body toning, locomotive aerobics, and deep-water aerobics (with flotation devices). Each movement is thoroughly explained and illustrated. The "helpful hint" sections describe safety, form, and proper technique.

AQUATICS: The Complete Reference Guide for Aquatic Fitness Professionals
Ruth Sova, Author
Aquatic Exercise Association
P.O. Box 497
Port Washington, WI 53074
414-284-3416

This book is an encyclopedia for aquatic fitness professionals. It is the only book currently available covering both the complete spectrum of the aquatic fitness industry and peripheral disciplines affecting it. *AQUATICS* covers all the information needed by the aquatic professional to begin a safe, effective, successful aquatic program. It includes a safety inspection checklist, sample emergency action plans, accident and incident reports, health history, medical clearance, informed consent, and class policy forms. A sample marketing plan, information on legal issues and guidelines regarding selection of equipment and music are included. The price is $45.

Aqua-X, Make Waves
Aqua-X/A-X Enterprises
Pauline B. Foord
P.O. Box 842
San Marcos, CA 92079-0842
619-743-5760

This manual of exercises describes 130 exercises and includes numerous pictures, showing what movements to perform and how to perform them. It also gives program formats and information on using music for exercising. It is indexed by exercise level, body part benefited, and exercise title. This is a practical and easy-to-use guide for the instructor and participant. The cover is water resistant and strong enough to stand alone at poolside.

At Home Water Workout with Wendy
WW Enterprises of Wisconsin, Ltd.
P.O. Box 371
DePere, WI 54115
414-336-2142

An audiocassette and instruction booklet guide the user through approximately 50 minutes of water exercise. Popular background music sets the perfect pace for a total body workout.

Choreographed Routines
WW Enterprises of Wisconsin, Ltd.
P.O. Box 371
DePere, WI 54115
414-336-2142

Choose from more than 150 routines to make a session package that's ready to use. Routines include a counted (beats) page, "cheat sheets," and a detailed cue sheet.

Chlorine Institute
2001 L Street Northwest, Suite 506
Washington, DC 20036

The full-color booklet "Chlor-Alkali Chemicals and the Chlorine Institute" includes information on the physical properties of chlorine, health and environmental effects associated with it, and what to do if exposed to it. Another booklet, the pocket-style "Chlorine and Your Health," gives comprehensive information on acute and chronic health effects from chlorine exposure and tips on first aid, how to avoid exposure at home, and how to get help during a chlorine emergency.

How to Deep Water Jog
WW Enterprises of Wisconsin, Ltd.
P.O. Box 371
DePere, WI 54115
414-336-2142

This instruction manual gives suggestions for making deep-water jogging fun and effective, such as descriptions of class format, the variety of ways to jog, and games.

IDEA Resource Library: Aqua Exercise
IDEA: The Association for Fitness Professionals
6190 Cornerstone Court E., Suite 204
San Diego, CA 92121-3773
1-800-999-4332/619-535-8979

This collection of articles from *IDEA Today* magazine and conference presentations offers guidelines for developing, teaching, and marketing safe, effective aqua programs. It includes a list of aqua resources, including books, tapes, and products.

Instructor Teaching Kit
Aquamotion
P.O. Box 31208
Santa Barbara, CA 93130
805-682-9493

This 150-page manual covers how to set up a business, including information on advertising, fitness screening, and music selection. It details over 30 movements proven to work in water, which are demonstrated on a VHS video.

Instructor Training Manual
Aerobics for Health
Welsh Church Road
Erieville, NY 13061
315-662-7416

A well-organized instructor training manual, this book was designed to make learning the scientific aspects of fitness easy to understand and the practical aspects of teaching easy to implement.

Jumping Into Water Exercise: A Student Manual
WW Enterprises of Wisconsin, Ltd.
P.O. Box 371
DePere, WI 54115
414-336-2142

This easy-to-follow guide for the water exercise student contains general information about the components of water exercise, heartrates, modifying workouts to meet individual needs, and more.

"Just Jugging" 101 Exercises
Judy's Splash Aerobics
1738 Briarwood Drive
Lansing, MI 48917
517-321-2669

Just Jugging describes water exercises using plastic jugs for support or resistance. Easy-to-follow illustration is provided in booklet form.

Moves You Can Use
WW Enterprises of Wisconsin, Ltd.
P.O. Box 371
DePere, WI 54115
414-336-2142

This manual lists a variety of moves that may be incorporated into the water exercise program. The moves are categorized for each component of the class (warm-up, aerobic, etc.) for easy reference.

Shape-Up with Splash
Judy's Splash Aerobics
1738 Briarwood Drive
Lansing, MI 48917
517-321-2669

This how-to-water-exercise book is well illustrated and easy to follow. It outlines exercises done at the wall and with jugs. It has been printed on stiff paper to stand up at pool edge.

The Water Power Workout Book
Huey's Athletic Network
3014 Arizona Avenue
Santa Monica, CA 90404
213-829-5622

This guide provides eight different water exercise or water rehabilitation programs appropriate for all fitness levels. Over 100 photos of champion athletes are included.

Young at Heart Older Adult Exercise Manual
Young Enterprises, Inc.
107 N. Main
Lansing, KS 66043
913-727-2263

This 120-page manual educates fitness professionals on how to adapt programs to meet the needs of older adults.

Catalogs

The Aerobic Connection
Box 4612
Carlsbad, CA 92008

The Connection sells fitness equipment and audiopromotional items.

Aqua Accessories
15 Atwood Street
Wakefield, MA 01880
617-246-2508

This company provides high-quality therapeutic and aquatic exercise programs, products, and apparel for children and adults.

The Finals
21 Minisink Avenue
Port Jervis, NY 12771
1-800-431-9111

The Finals offers an extensive line of performance swimwear and related products and accessories.

Fitness, Inc.
P.O. Box 786
Mandeville, LA 70470
1-800-777-9255

Products include T-shirts, bumper stickers, newsletters, aerobi-test, music tapes, fit-test, video, books, power vest, and power bench.

Fitness Wear
Instructor's Choice—
  Oakbrook Sales Corp.
1750 Merrick Avenue
Merrick, NY 11566
516-546-5800

This catalog is an "off-price" source for brandname fitness wear, as well as Instructor's Choice basic fitness. Bathing suits are available in season.

Fitness Wholesale
3064 W. Edgerton
Silver Lake, OH 44224
1-800-537-5512

Products include tank tops, Dynabands, exercise mats, fitness charts, aquatic products, hand weights, videos, tubing, audiotapes, educational books and materials, music, aquatic equipment, products for fitness professionals, maps, charts, bands, weights, and more.

Gulbenkian Swim, Inc.
70 Memorial Plaza
Pleasantville, NY 10570
914-747-3240

Gulbenkian sells Lycra swimsuits designed for the women over 25. They are reasonably priced, functional, and fashionable.

Gymtile
Pawling Corporation
157 Charles Colman Blvd.
Pawling, PA 12564
814-855-1005

This catalog is a source of cut-resistant, interlocking rubber flooring.

Kast-A-Way Swimwear, Inc.
9356 Cinti-Columbus Road
Cincinnati, OH 45241
1-800-543-2763

This 42-page catalog includes swimwear, training devices, awards, and books, for anyone involved in aquatic sports.

Pro-Fit
12012 156th Avenue S.E.
Renton, WA 98055-6317
(206) 255-3817

This catalog includes fitness and nutrition teaching supplies.

Recreation Supply Company, Inc.
P.O. Box 2757
Bismarck, ND 58502
701-222-4860

This catalog lists common pool equipment and supplies. The company stocks hundreds of parts for all types of pool equipment, and it also supplies complete pool systems for new pools or for major renovations.

Recreonics Corporation
7696 Zionsville Road
Indianapolis, IN 46268
1-800-792-3489 in Indiana/
1-800-428-3254/317-872-4400

Recreonics offers over 5,000 pool products for handicapped access, safety, decks, new construction, and renovation systems.

Road Runner Sports
6310 Nancy Ridge Road,
  Suite 101
San Diego, CA 92121
1-800-551-5558

Products include Reef Runners, clothes, and AquaJogger.

Sport Club
1-800-345-3610

Sport Club offers fitness apparel and some equipment.

SportWide
P.O. Box 16134
San Luis Obispo, CA 93406
1-800-631-9684

SportWide represents three apparel manufactures—Arina, Hind, and Speedo—and carries all their suits, goggles, caps, and accessories. They also represent other equipment vendors, offering a full line of pool equipment.

Sprint/Rothhammer International, Inc.
P.O. Box 5579
Santa Maria, CA 93456
1-800-235-2156/
1-800-445-8456 in California

This source offers 42 new water-related products. Sprint/Rothhammer is the #1 leading supplier for aquatic equipment. The have over 180 items for activities ranging from aerobics to water polo. They are always looking for new and exciting equipment for water. Call for a free catalog.

Swim Time
United Industries, Inc.
1913 Ohio
P.O. Box 338
Wichita, KS 67201-9829
1-800-835-3272/316-267-4341

This supplier sells swimming pool equipment.

TYR Sport
15661 Container Lane
Huntington Beach, CA 92649
714-897-0799

TRY offers competitive and active swimwear and related swimming accessories.

Uniflex, Inc.
Workout/Active Wear
B1217 Port Plaza Mall
Green Bay, WI 54301
414-432-6629

Uniflex sells workout wear for aerobics, ballet, gymnastics, weightlifting, swimming, and running, along with a line of casual wear.

Vital Signs
Country Technology, Inc.
P.O. Box 87
Gays Mills, WI 54631
608-735-4718

This is a complete source for quality fitness testing and conditioning equipment featuring an expanded selection of aquatic fitness products. New items include an underwater heartrate monitor; Aqua Jazz, a no-impact aerobic exercise system; hydrotherapy weights, the Rehab Wet Vest; the Swim Flex Trainer tethered swimming belt; and the Aquasense pool water quality meter.

ZIFFCO
333B W. Aloutra Blvd.
Gardena, CA 90248
213-532-3452

ZIFFCO sells pool products.

Magazines and Newsletters

AKWA Letter
Aquatic Exercise Association
P.O. Box 497
Port Washington, WI 53074
414-284-3416

Aquatics Magazine
6255 Barfield Road
Atlanta, GA 30328
404-256-9800

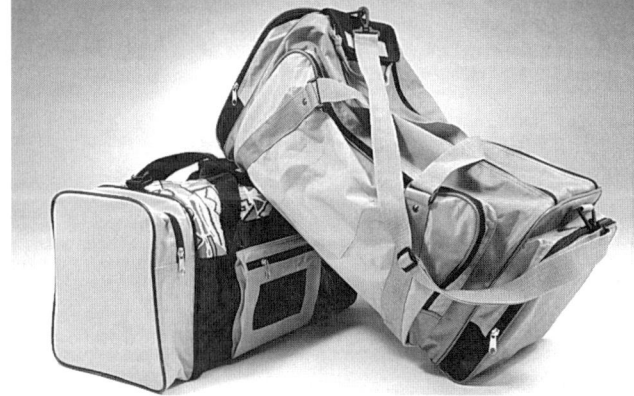
— Sport bags from Sprint/Rothhammer

Fitness Management
3923 W. 6th Street
Los Angeles, CA 90020
213-385-3926/619-481-4155

IDEA Today
IDEA: The Association of Fitness Professionals
6190 Cornerstone Court East, Suite 204
San Diego, CA 92121
619-535-8227

Journal of Physical Education, Recreation and Dance
AAHPERD
1900 Association Drive
Reston, VA 22091
703-476-3400

National Aquatics Journal
CNCA
901 W. New York Street
Indianapolis, IN 46223

Parks and Recreation
National Recreation and Park Association
3101 Park Center Drive
Alexandria, VA 22302
1-800-626-6772

SHOES

Aqua Sock
NIKE
One Bowerman Drive
Beaverton, OR 97005-6453
503-644-9000

The Sock has a four-way stretch Spandex mesh upper with interior toe reinforcement, a closed-cell EVA midsole, and a minilug outsole for excellent cushioning and traction.

Aqua Sock Too
NIKE
One Bowerman Drive
Beaverton, OR 97005-6453
503-644-9000

This Sock has a stretch Spandex mesh upper with interior toe reinforcement, a molded heel counter, an adjustable Velcro closure on the foot strap, a molded natural rubber cupsole, a minilug outsole pattern, and EVA midsole cushioning.

Aqua Walkers #906
Sprint/Rothhammer International, Inc.
P.O. Box 5579
Santa Maria, CA 93456
1-800-235-2156

Aqua Walkers have a molded rubber, nonslip sole and a nylon mesh upper. Velcro straps provide a secure fit. The shoe is available in six different sizes, in assorted neon and basic color combinations.

NIKE, Inc.
Attn: Dept RLH
One Bowerman Drive
Beaverton, OR 97005-6453
1-800-535-NIKE

Puddle Puppies #908
Sprint/Rothhammer International, Inc.
P.O. Box 5579
Santa Maria, CA 93456
1-800-235-2156

This shoe has a molded, nonslip rubber sole and a soft, comfortable neoprene upper. It is available in five sizes, in assorted neon and basic color combinations.

Reebok Professional Instructor Alliance
1-800-435-7022/
1-800-445-1165 in Massachusetts

Reef Warrior and Reef Runner
Omega Corporation
130 Condor Street
East Boston, MA 02128
617-569-3400

Constructed with neoprene/mesh materials, Reef Runners and Reef Warriors both offer superior slip resistance and are lightweight and quick drying. They are perfect for any activity in or near the water.

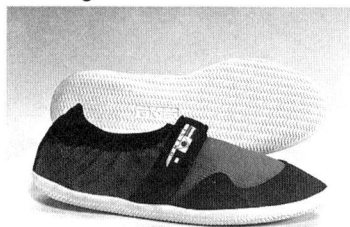
— Omega Reef Runner

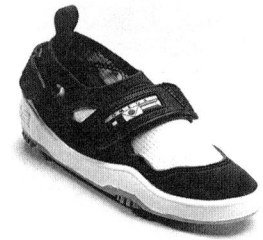
— Omega Reef Warrior

— Surfwalker

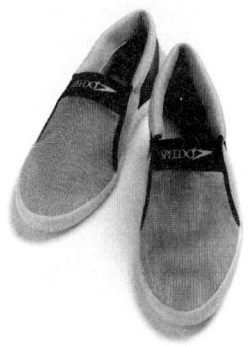

Surfwalker
Speedo Activewear
11111 Santa Monica Blvd.
Los Angeles, CA 90025
213-473-0032

The Surfwalker shoe is a slip-on with a rubber sole and neoprenelike upper. It is designed for kicking, water aerobics, and other exercise programs both in and out of the water.

SIGNS AND CHARTS

Aerobic Intensity Charts
Young Enterprises, Inc.
107 North Main
Lansing, KS 66043
913-727-2263

These teaching tools are intended for fitness professionals to determine students' heart-rates and perceived exertion rates. Eleven different, 11" x 24" charts are available, on aluminum and posterboard—some four-color, some black and white.

Andrus Aquatics Exercise Chart
Andrus Fitness, Inc.
351 Scott Drive
Silver Spring, MD 20904
301-384-8138

The Andrus is a laminated chart with pictures that guide an individual through a safe, energizing aquatic workout.

Custom Signs
Alison Osinski
3833 Lamont Street, 4C
San Diego, CA 92109
619-270-3459

Custom-made signs are available in your choice of materials and sizes, along with reusable stencils. All signs are available in English, Spanish, or bilingual formats.

Just Jugging Poster
Judy's Splash Aerobics
1738 Briarwood Drive
Lansing, MI 48917
517-321-2669

This heavy, laminated, waterproof poster displays approximately 40 jugging exercises.

SKIN AND HAIR CARE PRODUCTS

A.C.T. Swimmers-Shampoo, Conditioner, and Body Lotion
Dena Corporation
850 Nicholas Blvd.
Elk Grove Village, IL 60007
708-593-3041

Body Drench
Bill Heyne
P.O. Box 37
Highway 53
Alexandria, TN 37012
1-800-722-BODY

Malibu 2000 Products
MALIBU 2000
24955 Pacific Coast Highway
Malibu, CA 90265
213-456-7557

Malibu shampoos are formulated with gentle, effective cleansing agents for frequent shampooing. Combined with moisturizing nutrients and proteins, these shampoos provide soft manageability, with volume and shine. Conditioners are formulated with natural antioxidants to provide residual protection from hard water minerals and chemicals while rinsing the hair. Design spray shapes the hair during and after styling.

Soothing Touch
Sunshine Products Group
1919 S. Burnside Avenue
Los Angeles, CA 90035
213-939-6400

These products enhance a speedy recovery after workouts. Natural analgesics combined with pure, essential oils heal bruises and sore muscles.

UltraSwim Shampoo, Conditioner, and Soap
Chattem Consumer Products
1715 W. 38th Street
Chattanooga, TN 37409
1-800-366-6833

UltraSwim Shampoo removes chlorine through a unique approach. It converts chlorine in the hair and skin into a water-soluble chloride, similar to table salt, which is easily washed away.

TRAINING AND WORKSHOPS

Aqua Extravaganza
Aquatic Exercise Association
P.O. Box 497
Port Washington, WI 53074
414-284-3416

This workshop covers choreography of safe, effective water exercise routines, music selection, special-populations programming, money matters, and marketing. Participants receive a "water moves" glossary and a program package with written routines and a music cassette.

Aqua Power—The New Wave in Fitness
Sandra K. Nicht/The Re-Construction Project
P.O. Box 18259
Baltimore, MD 21227-8259
301-536-0419

This seminar for the aerobic and aquatic professional and novice instructor gives an overview of the basic components and safety considerations of leading a water exercise class.

Aquatic Fitness Instructor Certification
Aquatic Exercise Association
P.O. Box 497
Port Washington, WI 53074
414-284-3416

This program prepares water exercise instructors to design and teach safe, effective classes. Topics covered include exercise physiology, anatomy, kinesiology, injury prevention, leadership techniques, emergency training, health screening, legal issues, and weight control. Written and practical exams are given.

Bench Aquatix: The No-Sweat Workout
Sandra K. Nicht/The Re-Construction Project
P.O. Box 18259
Baltimore, MD 21227-8259
301-536-0419

Bench Aquatix adapts the movements of bench-step training to the aquatic environment. The seminar and workshop provide the aerobic and aquatic professional with the basic information needed to create and lead a safe, progressively challenging, and enjoyable alternative to traditional aquatic and land-group exercise classes.

The Choreographic Challenge
Sandra K. Nicht/The Re-Construction Project
P.O. Box 18259
Baltimore, MD 21227-8259
301-536-0419

By learning the basics of music and song structure, instructors can create blueprints for creative and progressively challenging choreography.

Maternity Fitness Perinatal Instructor Manual/Seminar and Certification
Maternity Fitness, Inc.
130 Cecilia Court
Waukesha, WI 53188
414-524-8777

Maternity Fitness, Inc., has developed the perinatal exercise certification to provide experienced instructors with the basic knowledge needed to offer a complete and safe prenatal/postnatal class in an educational and supportive environment. Topics include basic prenatal exercise physiology, anatomy, and kinesiology, as well as specific discussions on using the ACOG guidelines as an industry standard, which includes: health screening and risk-factor identification; teaching and monitoring the signs and symptoms of exercise intolerance; rational program development; controversial aspects of exercise and pregnancy; common orthopedic problems during pregnancy; and nutrition and legal responsibilities. Each participant receives an instructor's manual ahead of time for advanced preparation. At the conclusion of the seminar, practical and written exams are given. Upon successful completion of each seminar, certification is awarded. AEA, IDEA, AFAA, or ACSM certification is prerequisite for these seminars.

Mini-Training Workshops
WW Enterprises of
   Wisconsin, Ltd.
P.O. Box 371
De Pere, WI 54115
414-336-2142

Workshops are given dealing with the basics of water exercise and how to teach aquatics classes. Workshops can be custom made to fit the needs of instructors in a given program.

Supermarket Tours
Supermarket Savvy
P.O. Box 7069
Reston, VA 22091
703-620-4410

Learn how to raise additional revenue for a club by selling supermarket tours by conducting 2-1/2 hour, aisle-by-aisle tours, explaining the nutritional value of supermarket foods. Leni Reed's Supermarket Savvy Tour Training Kit includes a 100-page manual and two audiocassette tapes.

VIDEO- AND AUDIOCASSETTES

AKWA Bookstore
Aquatic Exercise Association
P.O. Box 497
Port Washington, WI 53074
414-284-3416

A listing of books and videos is available for purchase from the Aquatic Exercise Association on the subjects of aquatic fitness and aquatic therapy.

Aqua Abdominals
Aquatic Exercise Association
P.O. Box 497
Port Washington, WI 53074
414-284-3416

Can you work abdominals in the pool? You bet you can . . . and it's fun. This video workshop includes foolproof methods, positions, and safety hints, along with abdominal functions, and aquatic principles that affect the abdominals. Correct and incorrect body positioning is shown.

Aquabics!
Niehoff Associates
2416 Heathercrest
Arlington, TX 76017
817-467-5496

This VHS video includes over 60 exercises for a great aerobic workout, as well as a section of relaxation and visualization routines. It comes with a pool-proof laminated exercise card.

Aquacize
Mindy McCurdy, Inc.
P.O. Box 507
Naples, FL 33939-0507
813-262-1981

This state-of-the-art, underwater, VHS video demonstrates an action-packed, uniquely choreographed aquatic exercise workout. The package includes an instructional audiocassette tape with music and cues.

Aqua Dynamics Video
F.I.R.M. Fitness Instructor's
   Resource Materials
1352 W. Southwind
St. George, UT 84770
801-628-3160

The Aqua Dynamics Video offers a combination of aquatic toning, strengthening, and cardiovascular conditioning. The 40-minute video includes a 10-minute informative section explaining the benefits of aquatic strength training and exploring the principles and application of the nine principles of increasing water's resistance. Participants are taught how to increase the water's resistance to provide the ultimate aquatic workout.

Dawn Brown—Aquasize
Parade Video (P.P.I. Ent.
   Group)
88 St. Francis Street
Newark, NJ 07105
201-344-4214
or
Dawn Brown
503 S. Second Avenue
Absecon Highlands, NJ 08201
609-652-2545

This 30-minute video demonstrates 65 basic calisthenic and aerobic exercises done in a pool. Both surface and underwater filming are used for clarity. The video comes with a laminated card listing all exercises for use poolside. Also available is the EXER-CARD, a laminated sheet showing 16 water exercises. It hangs from a cord and is designed to wear around the neck while exercising in the pool.

Easy Listening Piano Instrumental
Billie C. Lange
P.O. Box 822
Umatilla, FL 32784
1-800-888-3866 in Florida/
904-483-0606
1-800-772-5928 in Texas

This 30-minute tape includes ten selections of good piano music.

Rehabilitation Through Aquatics
Ruth L. Elvedt
17 Jewett Lane
South Hadley, MA 01075
413-532-4760

Phase I (25 minutes) is an introduction to the program. Phase II (11 minutes) demonstrates specific therapeutic exercises for treatment of various disabilities, promoting relaxation, circulation, reduction of swelling and pain. Exercises are geared to individual needs of both swimmers and nonswimmers. Emphasis is placed on self-motivation and disciplined participation.

Ruth Sova's Aqua Challenge Program
Aquatic Exercise Association
P.O. Box 497
Port Washington, WI 53074
414-284-3416

This complete package for the water exercise instructor offers guidance for starting or improving an aqua dance program. It includes glossaries, suggested music, routines, and helpful hints on nutrition, muscle development, and program safety. The package includes a manual, a VHS or Beta video cassette, and audio cassettes, with and without cues.

Slim and Trim with Billie In and Out of Pool
Billie C. Lange
37 Cayman Circle
P.O. Box 822
Umatilla, FL 32784
904-483-0606

The "in-pool" color videotape consists of eight different segments for working all parts of the body designed to delete inches, reduce stress, build endurance, and increase flexibility. This is an excellent starting program for new classes. A 10-week measuring sheet is included.

Step Up Aquatics
Aquatic Exercise Association
P. O. Box 497
Port Washington, WI 53074
414-284-3416

Learn the fundamentals, class information and choreography in this bench stepping aquatics video workshop. It includes a sample class and gives you a chance to view several step variations.

Swimnastics Instructional Video
Swimnastics by Nancy Benson
P.O. Box 1258
Oak Brook, IL 60522-1258
708-393-4224

The Swimnastics water exercise video provides 30 minutes of instruction. The VHS tape comes with a water exercise booklet for poolside reference. Proper exercise techniques are taught for beginner, intermediate, and advanced workouts.

Water Walk and Jog Package
Aquatic Exercise Association
P.O. Box 497
Port Washington, WI 53074
414-284-3416

This complete instructional workout program includes a two-hour video (half lecture, half workout), lecture outline, sample moves and variations, and a 60-minute audio cassette with music and verbal cues.

GLOSSARY

A

Abduction—Movement away from the midline of the body, out of anatomical position; to move similar parts apart; the reverse movement from adduction (see **Adduction**).

Acceleration—An increase in speed or velocity; for a given object, acceleration depends on its mass and the applied force.

ACSM—American College of Sports Medicine.

Active rest—A time of low impact or low intensity that helps the body restore itself before moving to the next, more exertive mesocycle; occurs within periodization (see **Periodization**); also known as the transition phase.

Adaptation—An improvement in fitness that results when the body adjusts to overload conditions; also called training.

Adduction—Movement toward the midline of the body, into anatomical position; to move similar parts together; the return movement from abduction (see **Abduction**).

Aerobic—Technically, that which is living or active in the presence of oxygen; generally used to describe a type of exercise that produces cardiorespiratory benefits; also the most active portion of a typical workout.

Agility—The ability to change movement rapidly, accurately, and gracefully.

Agonist—A muscle that contracts with the simultaneous lengthening action of the antagonist with which it is paired (see Antagonist).

Amplitude—The difference between a totally contracted muscle and a totally extended muscle.

Angina pectoris—A feeling of pressure in the heart or center of the chest caused by deficient oxygenation of the heart muscles; often mistaken for heart attack.

Antagonist—A muscle that is lengthened with the simultaneous contraction of the agonist muscle with which it is paired (see **Agonist**).

Anterior—Positioned before or toward the front of the body.

Apical pulse—The pulse felt at the chest, most strongly after heavy exercise.

Appendicular skeleton—The bones in the arms and legs.

Aquatic aerobics—A type of aerobic program done in the water (see also **Aerobic**).

Aquatic therapy—Rehabilitation through water movement for populations including injured athletes, the chronically diseased, the disabled, or the handicapped.

Archimedes principle—The physical principle that states that when a body is immersed in fluid, it experiences an upward thrust equal to the weight of the fluid displaced; also called buoyancy.

Arthritis—An inflammation of the joints (see also **Osteoarthritis; Rheumatoid arthritis**).

Articulation—See **Joint.**

Atherosclerosis—The abnormal thickening and hardening of the walls of the arteries.

Athletic rehabilitation—A form of therapy used with adults who are injured but otherwise conditioned and healthy.

Atrophy—The wasting away of muscle strength and size from lack of use; progressive decline.

Autogenic training—A form of relaxation in which the body is trained to produce sensations of heaviness and warmth.

Axial skeleton—The bones in the head and trunk.

B

Balance—The stability produced by an equal distribution of weight on either side of an axis; maintaining equilibrium while stationary or moving.

Ballistic—A fast, jerky, bouncing type of movement (such as stretching) that can easily cause injury.

Bench workout—See **Step workout.**

Beta blocker—A medication taken to control hypertension by lowering the heartrate.

Body composition—Overall body makeup in terms of relative proportions of lean body mass and fat.

Buoyancy—The ability to float or rise in water.

C

Calisthenics—Athletic exercises that use the body's weight and gravity as resistance.

Calorie—A unit of energy, namely, that needed to raise the temperature of 1 gram of water by 1 degree Celsius. (A kilocalorie is the amount of energy needed to raise the temperature of 1 kilogram of water 1 degree Celsius.)

Carcinogenic—The quality of being cancer causing.

Cardiac cycle—The time period from one heartbeat to the next.

Cardiorespiratory endurance—The ability of the heart to supply oxygen from the respiratory system to the rest of the body during sustained exercise; one of five components of physical fitness.

Cardiorespiratory system—The body system comprised of the heart, lungs, and blood vessels (which includes the veins, arteries, and capillaries); its purpose is to carry oxygenated blood to the muscles and return deoxygenated blood to the heart; also called the *cardiovascular system.*

Carotid artery—One of two arteries found on the neck to either side of the throat.

Carotid pulse—The pulse felt at the carotid artery in the neck.

Cervical vertebrae—The bones of the spine found in the neck.

Cholesterol—Technically, steroid alcohol found in cells and body fluids and important in many physiological processes; more commonly, a fatty substance found in the blood and correlated with atherosclerosis (see Atherosclerosis).

Chondromalacia patella—A disorder in which the cartilage of the undersurface of the patella (kneecap) is softened or irritated; most often found in women.

Circuit training—An aerobic workout combining strength training and aerobic conditioning in a variety of activities, usually completed as a series in a certain order and/or on a course.

Circumduction—Movement in a circular pattern.

Concentric contraction—The phase of contraction in which the muscle shortens; also called the positive phase (see also Eccentric contraction).

Coordination—The integration of separate motor activities in the smooth, efficient execution of an activity.

Coronary heart disease (CHD)—A major form of cardiovascular disease; the result of atherosclerosis (see *Atherosclerosis*).

D

Deep-water exercise—Any type of water exercise program done in water depth greater than the height of the participant.

Depression—Squeezing the scapula together, causing the shoulders to lower and adduct; done by the shoulder girdle depression muscles.

Diastasis recti—A condition in prenatal women characterized by separation of the abdominal muscles through the middle of the long rectus abdominus.

Dive reflex—A primitive reflex that prompts lowering of the heartrate and blood pressure when the face is submerged in water; associated with a nerve found in the nasal area.

Dorsal—Positioned behind or toward the back of the body; also the top of the foot.

Dorsiflex—Flexion of the toes up toward the shin.

Duration—The length of an individual workout; ACSM guidelines suggest a continuous aerobic portion of 20 to 60 minutes.

E

Eccentric contraction—The phase of contraction in which the muscle lengthens; also called the negative phase (see also Concentric contraction).

Edema—An accumulation of fluid; swelling.

Elasticity—The quality of being able to stretch or expand and then resume former shape; a property of muscles.

Elevation—Lifting the scapula, causing the shoulders to lower and abduct; done by the shoulder girdle elevation muscles.

Endorphin—A powerful hormone that may be related to pain, emotions, the immune system, exercise, and the reproductive system; thought to be responsible for the so-called "runner's high," the feeling of euphoria experienced during exertive exercise.

Ergometer—An instrument used to measure the amount of energy used or being worked on.

Eversion—Turning the foot so the bottom faces outward.

Extensibility—The ability of the muscle to extend.

Extension—The straightening or unbending of a joint, increasing the angle between bones; the return movement from flexion (see **Flexion**).

Extensor—A muscle that extends a joint, generally working with gravity; usually, the weaker of the muscle pair.

F

Flexibility—The ability of the muscles to flex and extend the joints, providing movement through a normal range of motion; one of five components of physical fitness.

Flexion—The bending or flexing of a joint, decreasing the angle between bones; the opposite of extension (see **Extension**).

Flexor—A muscle that bends or flexes a joint, generally working against gravity; usually, the stronger of the muscle pair.

Footstrike—The foot hitting a surface.

Frequency—The number of times a workout is repeated, usually in terms of hours per week.

G

Gastrocnemius—The calf muscle.

Glycogen—The chief carbohydrate stored in the muscles and liver; the body's main source of energy.

Glycogen depletion—Depletion of the body's primary source of energy, causing graduated and overall fatigue; it can be avoided by following the principle of progressive overload (see **Progressive overload**).

H

Heat cramp—A muscle spasm caused by loss of body fluids during physical exertion in intense heat.

Heat exhaustion—Weakness and sometimes collapse caused by loss of body fluids during physical exertion in intense heat.

Heatstroke—A life-threatening condition in which the body's cooling mechanisms have ceased to function; body temperature continues to rise with no thermoregulatory system functioning to stop it.

High-density lipoprotein (HDL)—A cholesterol-carrying protein molecule that deposits fat in the liver, where it is eliminated from the body; HDL level is increased by exercise.

Hydrostatic pressure—The pressure exerted by any fluid on any body at rest.

Hyperextension—Moving a joint past anatomical position.

Hyperthermia—A condition in which the body temperature is too high, resulting in an overall loss of energy; likely to occur when exercising in warm water or an area with very little circulation.

Hyperventilation—A very rapid rate and/or depth of breathing, which results in the loss of too much carbon dioxide from the blood; faintness may result.

Hypokinetic—The quality of insufficient movement.

Hypokinetic disease—A condition caused or aggravated by inactivity.

Hypothermia—A condition in which the body temperature is too low, resulting in disorientation, uncoordination, and inactivity; a life-threatening condition.

I

Iliopsoas—The muscle that flexes the hip; also called a *hip flexor*.

Immersion—Putting a limb or the body into the water.

Inferior—Positioned below another area of the body.

Inflammation—A condition characterized by localized redness, pain, heat, or swelling; may result from injury, infection, or irritation to a given area of the body.

Insomnia—The inability to sleep.

Intensity—The degree of challenge a workout poses for the cardiorespiratory system.

Interval training—An exertive exercise program, combining high-intensity segments with moderate- or low-intensity segments.

J

Joint—A place where two bones are joined, usually (although not exclusively) to allow motion; also called an articulation.

K

Karvonen formula—A mathematical formula used to determine target heartrate.

Kinetic—Characterized by motion and the forces and energy associated with it.

Kyphosis—Excessive curvature of the upper portion of the thoracic spine.

L

Lactic acid—A product of anaerobic glycosis that results when the oxygen supplied to the muscle is insufficient; it causes a burning sensation that usually comes on suddenly and is focused on one muscle group; can be avoided by varying the nature of the workout, especially by shortening duration and intensity.

Lateral—Positioned away from the midline of the body, toward the outside.

Lateral flexion (of the spine)—Bending the torso toward the outside; generally used to describe sidebends.

Lordosis—Excessive curvature of the lumbar area of the spine (see **Lumbar area**).

Low-density lipoprotein (LDL)—A cholesterol-carrying protein molecule that builds up plaque formations that tend to collect on arterial walls, leading to atherosclerosis (see **Atherosclerosis**).

Lumbar area—The five vertebrae of the lower back, just above the sacrum and just below the thoracic vertebrae.

M

Maximal heartrate—The greatest number of times per minute the heart is capable of beating.

Maximum working heartrate—The upper end of the working heartrate range (see **Working heartrate range**); the maximum number of times the heart should beat per minute during exercise for cardiorespiratory training to take place.

Medial—Positioned toward the midline of the object or body.

Medication—A prescription drug.

Metabolic rate—The level at which physical and chemical demands are processed in the body, providing energy for life support; regular exercise enhances metabolic rate.

Minimum working heartrate—The lower end of the working heartrate range (see **Working heartrate range**); the minimum number of times the heart should beat per minute during exercise for cardiorespiratory training to take place.

Mode—The type of exercise selected for a cardiorespiratory workout; the optimal mode is based on large-muscle activity, maintained continuously and rhythmic in nature.

Muscle balance—The condition achieved when the muscles in a muscle pair have equal strength and flexibility.

Muscle cramp—An acute involuntary contraction (i.e., muscle spasm) caused by fluid loss from physical exertion in warm weather or as a result of lactic acid buildup (see **Lactic acid**).

Muscular endurance—The ability of a muscle to repeat a contraction with a moderate workload over a sustained period of time; one of five components of physical fitness.

Muscular strength—The ability of a muscle to exert great force in a single effort, usually achieved by lifting weights; one of five components of physical fitness.

Musculoskeletal fatigue—Fatigue brought on by the overuse of any muscle; characterized by pain in a bone, joint, or muscle.

O

Obesity—The condition of having an excessive level of body fat (approximately 25% for men and 33% for women), usually in combination with being overweight; frequently results in significant health impairment.

Optimum working heartrate—The middle portion of the working heartrate range (see Working heartrate range); the ideal number of times the heart should beat per minute during exercise for cardiorespiratory training to take place; varies with fitness goal.

Osteoarthritis—A disease in which the cartilage of the bones and joints wears away or simply degenerates; symptoms include pain, decreased range of motion, and muscular atrophy; the most common type of arthritis; often associated with aging (see also Rheumatoid arthritis).

Osteoporosis—A condition characterized by loss of bone mineral due to calcium deficiency; a potentially crippling condition that often afflicts older women.

Overload principle—See **Progressive overload.**

Overtraining—An excessive level of exercise frequency, duration, or intensity, causing fatigue and/or injury.

Overuse injury—A physical problem caused by putting too much stress on one area of the body over a long period of time.

Oxygen consumption—The rate at which oxygen is used to produce energy for cellular work; also called *oxygen uptake*; used to measure exercise intensity or energy expenditure (the more efficient the consumption, the greater the level of fitness).

P

Patella—The kneecap.

Pelvic tilt—A physical position in which the abdominal muscles are pulled in and the buttocks are tucked under.

Perceived exertion—An individual's ability to judge the intensity at which he is exercising.

Peripheral circulation—The small, subsidiary blood vessels and the ability to use and expand them when the main, large vessels are nonfunctional.

Physiological—Characteristic of or appropriate to a body's normal functioning.

Plantar—Positioned along the bottom surface, such as the sole of the foot.

Plantarflex—Flexion in which the toes are pointed toward the floor (as in ballet).

Plyometric—A type of exercise characterized by a series of jumping, bounding, and hopping moves; doing so preloads and forces the stretching of the muscle immediately prior to concentric action.

Positive affirmation—A statement of a current goal or purpose regarding an individual or situation.

Posterior—Positioned toward the back (dorsal) side of the body.

Poststretch—The flexibility segment of the workout that occurs after the aerobic portion; helps the muscles relax and return to their normal resting state.

Power—In fitness terms, transferring energy into force at a fast rate; a combination of strength and speed in one explosive action.

Prestretch—The flexibility segment of the workout that occurs after the thermal warm-up but before activities requiring high intensity and full range of motion.

Progressive overload—A philosophy of exercise that purports that the body (or one of its systems) will adapt to meet an increase in the demand made on it, resulting in improved physical fitness; in terms of physical conditioning, the level of demand should be controlled and increase gradually; also called *progressive resistance.*

Pronation—Turning the palms down or the soles of the feet out to the sides.

Prone—Positioned lying face down.

Proprioception—The reception of stimuli generated from within one's body.

Psychosomatic—Resulting from the interrelationship between psychological and physical (somatic) factors; namely, illness that is brought on by mental conflict.

R

Radial pulse—The pulse felt at the base of the thumb on the wrist.

Reaction time—The amount of time that elapses between stimulation and response to that stimulation.

Recovery heartrate—The number of times the heart beats per minute when monitored 5 to 10 minutes after vigorous exercise; an indication of how quickly the cardiorespiratory system is able to return to its pre-exercise condition, which is a reflection of fitness.

Relaxin—A hormone that softens the joint structure and causes increased flexibility in pregnant women.

Repetitions—The number of times a particular movement is repeated during a set (see **Set**); also called *reps*.

Resistance—The load, force, or weight applied against the muscle.

Respiration rate—The number of breaths taken per minute.

Resting heartrate—The number of times the heart beats per minute when the body is at rest; the average is 72; a low resting heartrate usually indicates fitness.

Reversibility—The principle that fitness benefits cannot be stored by the body but must be maintained through regular exercise; training levels begin to decline after several days of inactivity.

Rheumatoid arthritis—An autoimmune disease that causes inflammation in the tissues surrounding the joint.

Rotation—Turning on an axis; spinal rotation is twisting to the right and then to the left.

Rotator—A type of muscle that serves to rotate a part of the body.

S

Set—A number of movement repetitions performed in sequence (see **Repetitions**); a rest period is allowed between sets to allow the muscles to recover.

Shallow-water jogging—Jogging in waist- to chest-deep water at a fast enough pace to cause the necessary overload for cardiorespiratory benefits.

Skeletal system—The body's framework of bones and how they function in supporting tissues and protecting organs.

Skeleton—The assembly of bones.

Specificity—The principle that states that only that part of the body being exercised according to progressive overload will adapt and improve (see also **Progressive overload**).

Speed—The act or state of moving quickly.

Step workout—A type of exercise program based upon a stepping movement on and off a bench; also called a *bench workout* or *step aerobics*; the original step workout was the Harvard Step Test for fitness testing.

Sport-specific workout—A type of aerobic program designed to train athletes in a specific sport, such as bicycling or tennis; emphasis is on developing the muscle strength, flexibility, and skills specific to the given sport.

Static stretch—A type of stretch in which the extended position is held without bouncing to increase muscle flexibility.

Stretch reflex—A type of reflex that causes the muscle fibers to contract when a stretch is begun; may result in muscle tears if ballistic stretching is used, which is why static stretching is recommended (see **Ballistic; Static stretching**).

Submaximal—Employing about 60% of the maximum ability of the heart or a muscle group; working out at this level increases cardiovascular endurance and/or muscular strength.

Superior—Positioned above another part of the body.

Supination—Turning the palms upward or rolling the soles of the feet in, toward each other.

Synovial fluid—The transparent, viscous, and lubricating fluid secreted by the membranes of articulations, bursa, and tendon sheaths; enhances movement.

T

Talk test—A method of testing workout intensity; namely, an individual should work out at an intensity that enables him or her to talk while exercising.

Target zone—The range on a scale of heartrate—delineated by the minimum and maximum working heartrates—that represents the appropriate intensity for safe and effective exercise; also called the *working heartrate range, target heartrate range,* or *training zone* (see **Maximum working heartrate; Minimum working heartrate**).

Temporal pulse—The pulse felt at the temple.

Tendon—A fibrous band that connects muscle to bone.

Thermal warm-up—The initial segment of the workout in which the muscles are gradually stimulated; this increases the muscles' demand for oxygen and releases synovial fluid into the joints.

Thermoregulatory system—The body system that regulates the core temperature.

Thorax—The cavity between the neck and abdomen that contains the heart and lungs.

Tibia—The inner, thicker of the two bones between the knee and ankle (i.e., the shin).

Toning—The segment of the workout that develops muscular endurance.

Torque—A type of force or combination of forces that produces twisting or rotation.

Transverse abduction/adduction—Abduction and adduction done across the body; also called *horizontal abduction/adduction*. (*Transverse abduction* is when the leg is straight, the hip is flexed, and one leg moves laterally toward the outside of the body; *transverse adduction* is when the leg is straight, the hip is flexed, and one leg moves laterally to the inside, across the other.)

Triglyceride—The format in which fat is stored, consisting of three free fatty acids and glycerol.

Turbulent—The disruptive movement through water produced when an object encounters extreme resistance because it is not streamlined; resistance is proportional to velocity squared.

V

VO_2 max—The level of maximal oxygen consumption.

Valsalva maneuver—A technique used involving forced exhalation with the breath held (against a closed glottis); causes increased pressure in the thoracic cavity and major increases in both systolic and diastolic blood pressure. (This is like taking a deep breath and holding it while trying to exhale with great force. Weight lifters often do this, against good medical advice.)

Variability—The principle that adaptation or fitness improvements are enhanced by varying the intensity, length, or type of workout.

Vasodilation—The dilation of blood vessels.

Ventral—The front surface of the body.

Vital capacity—The measurement of lung capacity; depressed by hydrostatic pressure.

W

Water walking—Striding in waist- to chest-deep water at a pace fast enough to create the necessary overload for cardiorespiratory benefits.

Working heartrate range—The range on a scale of heartrate—delineated by the minimum and maximum working heartrates—that represents the appropriate intensity for safe and effective exercise; also called the *target zone, target heartrate range,* or *training zone* (see **Maximum working heartrate; Minimum working heartrate**).

Z

Zero-to-peak—A mathematical formula for determining heartrate range; also called the maximal heartrate formula.

REFERENCES

AEA Heart Rate Study. (1987, September). *The AKWA Letter, 2* (3), p. 7.

Aerobic and Fitness Association of America. (1982). *Aerobics: Theory and Practice.* Atlanta: Author.

Aldridge, M. (1990, May). Step. *Fitness Management,* pp. 32-38.

American Cancer Society. (1988). *Facts on Skin Cancer.*

American College of Sports Medicine. (1990a, July). ACSM Guidelines for Fitness Updated. *Running & Fitnews, 8,* 1.

American College of Sports Medicine. (1990b). *ACSM Position Stand: The Recommended Quantity and Quality of Exercise for Developing and Maintaining Cardiorespiratory and Muscular Fitness in Healthy Adults.* Indianapolis: Author.

American College of Sports Medicine. (1982). *Guidelines for Graded Exercise Testing and Exercise Prescription.* Indianapolis: Author.

American Heart Association. (1989). *1989 Heart Facts.* Dallas: Author.

Artal, R., Friedman, M. J., & McNitt-Gray, J. (1990, September). Orthopedic Problems in Pregnancy. *The Physician and Sportsmedicine, 18* (9), 93-100.

Beasley, R. L. (1989, January). Aquatic Exercise. *Sports Medicine Digest,* pp. 1-3.

Borg, G. A. V. (1982). Pyschophysical Bases of Physical Exertion. *Medicine and Science in Sport and Exercise, 14,* 377-387.

Brehm, B. A. (1990, August). Why Exercise Should Be A Lifelong Priority. *Fitness Management,* p. 20.

Brehm, B. A. (1990, May). Making an Impact on Bone Density. *Fitness Management,* p. 14.

Chase, S. (1977). *Moving to Win—The Physics of Sports.*

Chossek V., Delzeit, L., Lindle, J., Sova, R., & Windhorst, M. (1990). *Aquatic Concepts.* Port Washington, WI: Aquatic Exercise Association.

Chossek, V. (1988, January). AKWA Network: In my Opinion. *The AKWA Letter, 1* (5), 4.

Chrisman, D. C. (1983). *Body Recall* (2nd ed.). Berea, KY: Berea College Press.

Cirullo, J. (1989, May). Part I: Attaining and Maintaining a Healthy Back Through Wise Water Work. *The AKWA Letter, 3* (1), 1.

Cirullo, J. (1989, July). Part II: Attaining and Maintaining a Healthy Back Through Wise Water Work. *The AKWA Letter, 3* (2), 5-6.

Cisar, C. J., & Kravitz, L. (1989, January). Interval Training. *IDEA Today,* pp. 13-17.

Close, S. (1990). Equipment and Props for Exercise. *Reebok Instructor News, 3* (4), 7.

Conrad, C. C. (1979, February). Why Your Organization Should Consider Starting a Physical Fitness Program. *TRAINING, The Magazine of Human Resources Development,* pp. 30-31.

Consistent Training. (1989, Fall). *The Pursuit of Excellence, 4* (3), 1-2.

Cooper, K. (1982). *The Aerobics Program for Total Well-Being.* New York: Bantam Books.

Couzens, G. S. (1989, March). Plunging into Therapy. *Newsday,* p. 11.

DeCluitt, M. M. (1988, July). Water Exercise for Older Bodies. *The AKWA Letter, 2* (2), 10.

Dougan, T. (1989, July). Silver Splash: A Water Workout for Seniors. *The AKWA Letter, 3* (2), 12–13.

Essert, M. B. (1989, May). Water Walking. *The AKWA Letter, 3* (1), 3.

Evans, B., Cureton, K., & Purvis, J. (1978). Metabolic and Circulatory Responses to Walking and Jogging in Water. *Research Quarterly, 49* (4), 442–449.

Every Body in the Pool. (1989, September). *The Pursuit of Excellence, 4* (4), 1–2.

Exercising in Hot Weather. (1989, July). *The AKWA Letter, 3*, (2), 1.

Flatten, K., Wilhite, B., & Reyes-Watson, E. (1988). *Exercise Activities for the Elderly.* New York: Springer.

Francis, L., & Francis, P. (1990). Step Training. *Reebok Instructor News, 3* (5), 12.

Growing Up Fit. (1989, November/December). *IDEA Today,* p. 7.

Herman, E. (1989, December 11). Saving Your Skin. *Pool and Spa News,* pp. 46–47.

Horstmeyer, B. (1989a, March). Aquatics for Expectant Mothers. *The AKWA Letter, 2* (6), 1.

Horstmeyer, B. (1989b). *Perinatal Certification Instructor's Manual.* Milwaukee, WI: Maternity Fitness.

Huttner, B. (1988, November). Aquatic Exercise Equipment: Flugels. *The AKWA Letter, 2* (4), 3.

Increase in Bone Density? (1988, March). *Fitness Management,* 6.

Institute for Aerobics Research. (1981). Management of Exercise and Fitness Programs. Dallas: The Aerobics Center.

Johnson, B. L. et al. (1977). Comparison of Oxygen Uptake and Heart Rate During Exercises on Land and in Water. *Physical Therapy, 57* (3), 273–278.

Kendall, F. P., Kendall, F., & Wadsworth, P. (1971). Muscle Testing & Function. Baltimore: Williams and Wilkins.

Koszuta, L. (1988, September). Splash On By. *Walking Magazine,* pp. 65, 66, 68, 70.

Lindle, J. (1989). Water Exercise Research. *The AKWA Letter, 3* (4), 11, 13.

Luttgens, M., & Wells, L. (1982). *Kinesiology—Scientific Basis of Human Motion* (7th ed.). Philidelphia: W. B. Saunders.

McArdle, W., Katch, F., & Katch, V. (1986). *Exercise Physiology, Energy, Nutrition, and Human Performance.* Philadelphia: Lea and Febiger.

McWaters, G. (1988). *How the Older Become Younger and the Impaired Become Repaired.* Birmingham, AL.

Mitchell, T. (1989, May). The Use of Props in Water Exercise for Muscle Conditioning. *The AKWA Letter, 3* (1), 6.

Monroe, E. (1988, July). The Sun and Your Skin. *The AKWA Letter, 2,* (2), 7–9.

Murphy, J. (1985, July). Shopwalk. *Sports Illustrated,* p. 12.

Nelson, A. T. (1989, April). Workshop on Aquatic Circuit Training. International Aquatic Fitness Conference, Chicago, IL.

Nelson, A. T. (1989, April). Workshop on Deep Water Fitness. International Aquatic Fitness Conference, Chicago, IL.

Osinski, A. (1990, February). The Complete Aquatic Guide. *Parks & Recreation,* pp. 36–43.

Osinski, A. (1989, Spring). Water Running. *National Aquatics Journal,* pp. 3-6.

Osinski, A. (1988, September). Water Myths. *The AKWA Letter, 2* (3), 1.

Pitts, E. H. (1990c, July). Getting Strong After Age 90. *Fitness Management,* p. 12.

Pollock, M. L. et al. (1982). Comparison of Methods for Determining Exercise Training Intensity for Cardiac Patients and Healthy Adults. *Advanced Cardiology, 31,* 129–133.

Pollock, M. L., Wilmore, J. H., & Fox, S. M. (1984). *Exercise in Health and Disease.* Philadelphia: W. B. Saunders.

Research Abstracts. (1990). *Reebok Instructor News, 3* (4), 4.

Research Project. (1988, May). *The AKWA Letter, 2* (1), 6.

Rikli, R., & McManis, B. (1990, September). Effects of Exercise on Bone Mineral Content in Postmenopausal Women. *Research Quarterly for Exercise and Sport, 61* (3), 243–249.

Riposo, D. (1990). *Fitness Concepts.* Port Washington, WI: Aquatic Exercise Association.

Riposo, D. (1985). *America's Certification Trainers Manual*. Port Washington, WI: The Fitness Firm.

Robbins, G. et al. (1989). *The Wellness Way of Life*. Dubuque, IA: Wm. C. Brown.

See, J. (1990, January). Aqua Power Aerobics. *The AKWA Letter, 3* (5), 1.

Seibert, G. R. (1990, July). Here Come the Kids, Are You Ready? *Fitness Management*, p. 22.

Shortley, G., & Williams, D. (1965). *Elements of Physics*. Englewood Cliffs, NJ: Prentice Hall.

Sova, R. (1990a, May). Heartrates in Aquatic Exercise. *IDEA Today*, p. 9.

Sova, R. (1989a, July). Body Alignment: How to Maintain It. *The AKWA Letter, 3* (2), 10.

Sova, R. (1989b, July). Exercising in Hot Weather. *The AKWA Letter, 3* (2), p. 6.

Special Considerations for Special Seniors. (1990). *Reebok Instructor News, 3* (4), 8.

Spitzer, T. A. et al. (1989). *A Comparison of Selected Training Responses to Water Aerobics and Low-Impact Aerobics*. Prepared by Boise State University; Idaho Sports Medicine Institute; and Indiana State University.

Spodnik, J. O., & Cogan, D. P. (1989). *The 35-Plus Good Health Guide for Women*. New York: Harper and Row.

Strovas, J. (1990, September). 90-year-olds Increase Strength Dramatically. *The Physician and Sportsmedicine, 18* (9), 26.

U.S. Department of Agriculture and Department of Health and Human Services (1979). *Nutrition and Your Health, Dietary Guidelines for Americans*. Washington, DC: Authors.

U.S. Department of Health and Human Services (1984). *What You Need to Know About Cancer of the Skin*. Washington, DC: National Cancer Institute.

VanCamp, G., & Boyer, B. (1989, May). Exercise Guidelines for the Elderly. *The Physician and Sportsmedicine, 17* (5), 14-16.

Vickery, S. R., Cureton, K. J., & Langstaff, J. L. (1983, March). Heart Rate and Energy Expenditure During Aqua Dynamics. *The Physician and Sportsmedicine, 11* (3), 67-72.

Walters, J. (1990, April). Handout from Children's Creative Movement Workshop. International Aquatic Fitness Conference, Chicago, IL.

Warm Up: It Pays Dividends. (1987, July). *The AKWA Letter, 1* (2), 1.

Water Exercise: A Better Fat Burner. (1988, January). *The AKWA Letter, 1* (5), 5.

Weider, J. (1990, October). Quality Time. *Shape*, p. 7.

Welch, D. (1989, July). Water Dancing. *Health*, pp. 46-51.

Wigglesworth, J. K. et al. (1990, September). Aquatic Exercise Research: The Effect of Water Exercise on Various Parameters of Physical Fitness. *The AKWA Letter, 4* (3), 3.

Windhorst, M., & Chossek, V. (1988). *Aquatic Exercise Association Manual*. Port Washington, WI: Aquatic Exercise Association.

Young, T. (1990). *Older Adult Exercise Manual* (4th ed.). Lansing, KS: Young Enterprises.

INDEX

Adaptation, 6
Aquawear, 84–85
Arthritis, 69–70
Back pain, 70–71
    prevention of, 155–156
Buoyancy, 1–2, 48
    equipment, 73–74
Body composition
    definition of, 5
Caloric consumption, 47, 53–54
Cardiorespiratory endurance
    definition of, 3
    warm-up, 9–10
    workout guidelines, 10–12
Certification, 37
    standards for, 154
Children, 71–72
Circuit training
    sample workout for, 148–149
    workout guidelines, 33–34
Contraindicated exercises, 154–156
Coronary heart disease, 4
Depth, 63
Equipment guidelines, 75–76
Extensors, 47, 136–137
Flexibility
    definition of, 4
    sample workout, 147
    workout guidelines, 22–24
Flexors, 47, 136–137
Fitness
    major components of, 3
    minor components of, 5
    definition of, 2
Format
    cardiorespiratory class, 8
Heartrate
    aquatic, 54–55
    definitions of, 50–52
    formulas, 52–53
Hypokinetic disease, 2
Injuries, 157–161
Intensity, 11
    comparing land and water, 57
    heartrates, 50–58
    increasing, 59–60
    measuring, 50
    methods to check, 58–59
Interval training
    workout guidelines, 30–31
Knee pain, 71
    prevention of, 155
Muscular endurance, 11–12
    definition of, 4
    sample workout, 146–147
    workout guidelines, 18–19
Muscular strength, 12–13
    definition of, 4
    sample workout, 142–143
    workout guidelines, 20–22
Muscle
    balance, 47, 87, 136
    groups of, 137–141
Music, 85–86, 156
Nutrition, 40–42
Obesity, 68–69
Older adults, 66–68
    and heat, 159
Overload, 5
    progressive, 5–6
Prenatal, 69
Plyometrics
    workout guidelines, 35–36
Relaxation, 36–37
Resistance, 46
    equipment, 74
Reversibility, 6
Shoes, 83–84, 156–157
Specificity, 6
Sports conditioning
    sample workout, 149–150
    workout guidelines, 26–28
Step aerobics
    sample workout, 150–151
    workout guidelines, 28–30
Temperature, 63
    arthritis, 70
Variability, 6–7
Weight control, 42–45
Warm-up, 8–10
Water aerobics, 17–18
    sample workouts, 145–146
Water jogging, 14–17
Water walking, 12–14
    sample workout, 143–145

NOTES

NOTES